EXERCISES IN SONOGRAPHY

Introduction to Normal Structure and Function

EXERCISES IN SONOGRAPHY

Introduction to Normal Structure and Function

REVA ARNEZ CURRY, PhD, RT(R), RDMS, FSDMS
Dean of Student Services
Salem Community College
Carney's Point, New Jersey

BETTY BATES TEMPKIN, BA, RT(R), RDMS
Ultrasound Consultant
Formerly, Clinical Director
Diagnostic Medical Sonography Program
Hillsborough Community College
Tampa, Florida

SECOND EDITION

with 1160 *illustrations*

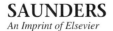

SAUNDERS
An Imprint of Elsevier

SAUNDERS
An Imprint of Elsevier

11830 Westline Industrial Drive
St. Louis, Missouri 63146

Exercises in Sonography: Introduction to
Normal Structure and Function
Copyright © 2004, Elsevier. All rights reserved.

Previous edition copyrighted 1995

ISBN-13: 978-0-7216-9781-9
ISBN-10: 0-7216-9781-X

Publisher: Andrew Allen
Acquisitions Editor: Jeanne Wilke
Senior Developmental Editor: Linda Woodard
Publishing Services Manager: Pat Joiner
Project Manager: David Stein
Design Manager: Gail Morey Hudson

Printed in the United States of America

Last digit is the print number: 9 8 7 6 5 4

Contributors

PEGGY MALZI BIZJAK, BBA, RDMS, RT(R)(M)
Imaging Chief/Manager
Department of Radiology, Ultrasound Division
University of Virginia Health System
Charlottesville, Virginia
The Female Pelvis, First Trimester Obstetrics, Second and Third Trimester Obstetrics, High-Risk Obstetric Sonography

REVA ARNEZ CURRY, PhD, RT(R), RDMS, FSDMS
Dean of Student Services
Salem Community College
Carney's Point, New Jersey
The Pancreas, The Urinary System, The Neonatal Brain, Three-Dimensional Ultrasound

MARILYN DICKERSON, MEd, MPH, RDMS
Vascular Technologist
Department of Radiology
Crawford Long Hospital of Emory Hospital
Atlanta, Georgia
The Liver, The Gastrointestinal System

KATHRYN A. GILL, MS, RT, RDMS
Program Director
Institute of Ultrasound Diagnostics
Daphne, Alabama
Introduction to Ultrasound of Human Disease

CANDYCE JAMES, BS, RDMS
Sonographer
The Imaging Center of Aiken
Aiken, Georgia
The Abdominal Aorta, The Inferior Vena Cava, The Portal Venous System, The Biliary System, The Pancreas, The Urinary System, The Spleen

MICHAEL J. KAMMERMEIER, BSRT, RDMS, RVT
Clinical Specialist
GE Ultrasound, Inc.
Milwaukee, Wisconsin
The Male Pelvis, Three-Dimensional Ultrasound

ALEXANDER LANE, PhD
Coordinator of Anatomy and Physiology
Triton College
River Grove, Illinois
Anatomy Layering and Sectional Anatomy

WAYNE C. LEONHARDT, BA, RT, RDMS, RVT, APS
Lead Sonographer,
Technical Director and Continuing Education Coordinator
Alta Bates Summit Medical Center
Summit Campus Ultrasound Section
Oakland, California
Clinical Instructor, Foothill College School of Ultrasound
Los Altos, California
The Thyroid and Parathyroid Glands

VIVIE MILLER, BA, BS, RDMS, RDCS
Clinical Specialist
Hephizabah, Georgia
The Abdominal Aorta, The Inferior Vena Cava, The Portal Venous System, The Biliary System, The Pancreas, The Urinary System, The Spleen, Pediatric Echocardiography

MARSHA M. NEUMYER, BS, RVT
Director, Vascular Diagnostic Educational Services
A Division of Inside/Outside, L.L.C.
Harrisburg, Pennsylvania
Abdominal Vasculature, Vascular Technology

M. NATHAN PINKNEY, BS, RDMS
Medical Physicist, Sonicor, Inc.
West Point, Pennsylvania
Physics, Instrumentation

J. CHARLES POPE III, PAC, RDCS, RVS
Assistant Clinical Professor
Director, Echocardiography Laboratory
Cardiovascular Associates of Augusta
Augusta, Georgia
Adult Echocardiography

LISA STROHL, BS, RT(R), RDMS, RVT
Marketing Manager
Jefferson City Imaging
Philadelphia, Pennsylvania
Breast Sonography

BETTY BATES TEMPKIN, BA, RT(R), RDMS
Ultrasound Consultant, Formerly, Clinical Director
Diagnostic Medical Sonography Program
Hillsborough Community College
Tampa, Florida
Body Systems, Anatomy Layering and Sectional Anatomy, The Pancreas, The Urinary System, The Female Pelvis, First Trimester Obstetrics, Second and Third Trimester Obstetrics, High-Risk Obstetric Sonography, The Neonatal Brain, Introduction to Ultrasound of Human Disease, Interventional and Intraoperative Ultrasound

Contents

Instructions for Students

The purpose of this manual is to assist you in studying concepts presented in the textbook SONOGRAPHY: NORMAL STRUCTURE AND FUNCTION. The following are suggestions that may help you.

1. Pay attention to the key words and objectives. The key words are highlighted in the text to guide you on what is important. Keep the objectives in mind as you read the chapter.

2. Notice how most chapters are divided into main sections, including Location, Anatomy, Physiology, Sonographic Appearance, and Reference Charts. You may want to divide your reading by sections. For example, one evening you may read the Location and Gross Anatomy sections. The next evening, you might read the Physiology and Sonographic Appearance sections. We suggest you finish reading or studying an entire section before ending your study time. That way, you can pick up with a new concept the next time you study.

3. The Student Manual contains review questions designed to test you at a basic level on your ability to retain information you've just read. How well you answer these questions is an indicator of your comprehension. (The answers are located in the back of the manual so you can test and grade yourself.) The next step will be for you to get very comfortable with the material. Read other textbooks in the library and increase your knowledge on what we've presented.

4. This manual contains unlabeled images and illustrations from every chapter in the textbook to test your comfort level with sonograms and identifying anatomy. Make sure you understand the images that have been presented for you. Can you identify structures without labels? Do you know how to describe them? If you're still confused about the images presented here, go back and reread the section in the textbook. We encourage you to color the structures on the illustrations to better differentiate the anatomy.

5. Make sure you understand which things in the text are important *to your instructor.* Think of these as guidelines. Write these guidelines down and refer to them as you study. This technique should help you prepare for major tests on the material.

Sonography is an exciting and challenging profession; we wish you the best in your career.

INTRODUCTION

Your First Scanning Experience

REVIEW QUESTIONS

1. The primary role of the sonographer is
   a. to provide the interpreting physician with a technical observation
   b. to provide the interpreting physician with a diagnosis
   c. to provide interpretable images for diagnosis by a physician
   d. to provide the patient with a technical observation

2. A reason(s) for using a scanning protocol is
   a. to learn how to take nice images
   b. standardization, quality, and use with comparable studies
   c. to accommodate physicians
   d. to give a good technical observation

3. The best patient position for imaging the abdominal aorta is
   a. supine
   b. decubitus
   c. determined by whichever position provides the optimal view
   d. determined by patient respiration

4. If a patient did not fast for at least 8 hours prior to an aorta sonogram you should
   a. still attempt the examination
   b. cancel the examination
   c. postpone the examination for 4 hours
   d. postpone the examination for 1 hour

5. For retroperitoneal structures like the aorta the transducer of choice is usually
   a. a higher number megahertz transducer
   b. a lower number megahertz transducer
   c. a curved linear array
   d. a phased array

6. What is *not* done during a survey?
   a. adjust technique
   b. rule out any normal variants or abnormalities
   c. examine the areas of interest
   d. document findings

7. What is the first recommended view to be performed when scanning the abdominal aorta?
   a. transverse survey from a posterior approach in the transverse plane
   b. longitudinal survey from an anterior approach in the coronal plane
   c. longitudinal survey from a right lateral approach in the coronal plane
   d. longitudinal survey from an anterior approach in the sagittal plane

8. When initiating the first scanning approach of the aorta, where should the sonographer begin?

    a. with the transducer perpendicular, to the far right of midline of the body, under the costal margin

    b. with the transducer parallel and at the midline of the body, at the symphysis pubis

    c. with the transducer perpendicular and at the midline of the body, just inferior to the xyphoid process

    d. with the transducer perpendicular and at the midline of the body, at the suprasternal notch

9. The transverse survey of the aorta consists of

    a. a posterior approach in the transverse plane

    b. an anterior approach in the longitudinal plane

    c. a posterior approach in the longitudinal plane

    d. an anterior approach in the transverse plane

10. Images taken during the examination should contain the following:

    a. patient's name

    b. patient's identification number

    c. date

    d. scanning site

    e. sonographer's initials

    f. all of the above

CHAPTER 1

Physics

REVIEW QUESTIONS

1. What is the primary difference between x-rays and ultrasound energy?

   a. x-rays are ionizing and sound is electromagnetic

   b. sound is mechanical

   c. sound can travel through a vacuum

   d. ultrasound is electromagnetic

2. Which of the following frequencies is not typically used for medical diagnostic ultrasound?

   a. 100 kHz

   b. 2.25 MHz

   c. 3.5 MHz

   d. 5.0 MHz

3. What determines the velocity of sound in a material?

   a. stiffness and density

   b. stiffness and frequency

   c. density and intensity

   d. density and frequency

4. What is the velocity of sound in human soft tissue?

   a. 1540 mm/sec

   b. 1.54 mm/sec

   c. 1540 m/μsec

   d. 1540 m/sec

5. What is a typical pulse repetition frequency in a diagnostic ultrasound system?

   a. 1 MHz

   b. 100 Hz

   c. 1000 Hz

   d. 1000 kHz

6. What does a backing material provide when used in a pulse-echo ultrasound transducer?

   a. improved lateral resolution

   b. damping

   c. focusing

   d. impedance matching

7. If the transducer frequency is doubled,

   a. the period is doubled

   b. the period is halved

   c. the period is the same

   d. none of the above

8. The wavelength is halved if

   a. the frequency is halved

   b. the frequency is doubled

   c. the velocity is doubled

   d. none of the above

9. What is the approximate reflection percentage from a fat-bone interface?

   a. 1%

   b. 25%

   c. 50%

   d. 100%

10. The angle of reflection at an interface is determined by

    a. the angle of incidence

    b. the angle of transmission

    c. the frequency of the transducer

    d. the velocity

11. A change in velocity as sound passes through an interface can cause
    a. refraction
    b. sidelobes
    c. enhancement
    d. none of the above

12. What affects the axial resolution?
    a. spatial pulse length
    b. wavelength
    c. damping
    d. all of the above

13. What affects the lateral resolution?
    a. spatial pulse length
    b. damping
    c. focusing
    d. all of the above

14. What is the effect of higher frequencies on attenuation and penetration?
    a. less attenuation, less penetration
    b. more attenuation, less penetration
    c. more attenuation, more penetration
    d. less attenuation, more penetration

15. What are the three categories of bioeffects?
    a. heat, thermal, other
    b. heat, thermal, cavitation
    c. heat, cavitation, other
    d. none of the above

16. Frequencies used for medical diagnostic ultrasound normally range from
    a. 20 Hz to 20,000 Hz
    b. 20 kHz to 20 MHz
    c. 2 MHz to 15 MHz
    d. 20 MHz to 40 MHz

17. The velocity of sound is greatest through
    a. bone
    b. fat
    c. water
    d. air

18. The value of 1% is related to a fat-muscle interface. This parameter is the
    a. reflection coefficient
    b. attenuation coefficient
    c. refraction coefficient
    d. transmission coefficient

19. Ultrasound includes only those frequencies greater than
    a. 20 Hz
    b. 20 kHz
    c. 100 kHz
    d. 1 MHz

20. Intensity can be measured in
    a. mW/cm
    b. W/m
    c. mW
    d. W/m^2

21. What does not cause attenuation?
    a. enhancement
    b. absorption
    c. scattering
    d. reflection

22. If the velocities of the two materials that form an interface are not equal, and if the angle of incidence is not zero,
    a. the reflected angle will not be the same as the incident angle
    b. refraction may occur
    c. the transmitted angle will always equal the incident angle
    d. the quality factor will increase

23. Red blood cells
    a. are specular reflectors
    b. do not cause Rayleigh scattering
    c. are nonspecular reflectors
    d. do not reflect diagnostic ultrasound frequencies

24. The velocity of sound through a material is not affected by
    a. stiffness
    b. density

c. frequency

d. elasticity

25. A perpendicular angle of incidence is
    a. normal incidence
    b. oblique incidence
    c. critical incidence
    d. an incident angle of 90 degrees

26. The velocity of sound through bone is in the range of
    a. 300 to 1650 m/sec
    b. 4000 to 5000 m/sec
    c. 6000 to 8000 m/sec
    d. 8000 to 10,000 m/sec

27. A nonspecular reflector will produce
    a. transient cavitation
    b. stable cavitation
    c. 100% reflection coefficient
    d. backscatter

28. What is one difference between audible and inaudible sound?
    a. audible sound is greater than 20 kHz
    b. inaudible sound waves are never longitudinal
    c. audible sound is used for therapeutic applications
    d. inaudible sound has a higher frequency

29. If the frequency is doubled,
    a. the period will not change
    b. the period will be doubled
    c. the wavelength will be halved
    d. the wavelength will be doubled

30. Extraneous energy components that are not in the primary direction of the ultrasound beam
    a. will not affect the lateral resolution
    b. will affect the axial resolution
    c. are called sidelobes
    d. can be eliminated by increasing the PRF

31. Which of the following does not affect axial (longitudinal) resolution?
    a. focusing
    b. frequency

c. spatial pulse length

d. damping

32. Lateral resolution is affected by all of the following except
    a. frequency
    b. beam width
    c. focusing
    d. bandwidth

33. A decrease in the thickness of the piezoelectric element will result in
    a. a decrease in the quality factor
    b. an increase in the frequency of the transducer
    c. an increase in the velocity of sound
    d. a greater pulse duration

34. Lateral resolution is determined by
    a. the angle of refraction
    b. damping
    c. spatial pulse length
    d. beam width

35. The duty factor in a pulse-echo system
    a. is greater than the duty factor in a continuous wave Doppler system
    b. is normally less than 1%
    c. is typically 50%
    d. is normally 100%

36. An ultrasound wave leaves the transducer, travels through tissue, and returns 10 microseconds later. What is the distance to the reflector?
    a. 1.54 mm
    b. 15.4 mm
    c. 7.7 mm
    d. 1540 m

37. Bioeffects have not been confirmed for SPTA intensities below
    a. 100 mW/m
    b. 100 W/cm^2
    c. 100 mW/cm^2
    d. 10,000 mW/cm^2

CHAPTER 2

Instrumentation

1. Which of the following does not produce a sector image?
   a. annular array
   b. phased linear array
   c. flat sequenced array
   d. convex array

2. Increasing the dynamic range in a pulse-echo ultrasound system does not
   a. ensure a wider range of displayed gray levels
   b. decrease the amount of compression of the received signal
   c. decrease the attenuation of sound in tissue
   d. increase the ratio of the largest signal to the smallest signal that the system can handle

3. The component that generates ultrasound energy is the
   a. transducer
   b. receiver
   c. pulsar
   d. cathode ray tube

4. If the pulse repetition frequency is increased, the real-time frame will have
   a. a higher frame rate
   b. a lower frame rate
   c. more acoustic lines
   d. fewer acoustic lines

5. Read-magnification is performed by
   a. controlling the A to D converter
   b. enlarging each pixel
   c. placing a large magnifying glass over the television screen
   d. varying the depth setting

6. What is the size of a typical image memory matrix?
   a. 10×10
   b. 10×256
   c. 256×256
   d. 512×512

7. How many horizontal scan lines are contained in a television frame?
   a. 525
   b. $262\frac{1}{2}$
   c. 60
   d. 30

8. The maximum number of displayed gray shades in an 8-bit system is
   a. 8
   b. 256
   c. 64
   d. 512

9. The output of the scan converter is fed to the
   a. transducer
   b. receiver

c. television monitor

d. spectrum analyzer

10. What is the scan converter function that determines the assignment of echoes to predetermined gray scale levels?

a. postprocessing

b. preprocessing

c. bit mapping

d. D to A conversion

11. Which of the following performs digital storage of echo-signal information?

a. scan converter

b. television monitor

c. receiver

d. A to D converter

12. An advantage of continuous wave Doppler over pulsed Doppler is

a. a lower Nyquist limit

b. a lower PRF

c. a wider range of shift frequencies

d. spectral analysis is not required

13. Aliasing will be present if the Doppler shift exceeds

a. the PRF

b. twice the PRF

c. one half the Nyquist limit

d. the Nyquist limit

14. When using pulse Doppler, a low PRF

a. detects wider range of shift frequencies than continuous wave Doppler

b. will not result in aliasing if the Doppler shift is higher than the PRF

c. may result in aliasing when high velocity flow is present

d. will not result in aliasing if the Doppler shift is equal to the PRF

15. If the fundamental frequency is 3.5 MHz, a harmonic frequency is

a. 3.0 MHz

b. 7.0 MHz

c. 7.5 MHz

d. none of the above

16. An ultrasound scanner that uses a single probe to display a real-time image along with spectral information is

a. a duplex system

b. nonexistent

c. not susceptible to aliasing

d. used only with continuous wave Doppler

17. A Doppler system measures

a. frequency shift and calculates blood velocity

b. frequency shift and calculates sound velocity

c. frequency shift and calculates attenuation

d. blood velocity and calculates frequency shift

18. Which one of the following does not use frequency shift information to detect blood flow?

a. continuous wave Doppler

b. power Doppler

c. pulsed wave Doppler

d. color flow Doppler

19. Angle correction is used to obtain accurate frequency shift values for

a. Doppler angles less than 10 degrees

b. Doppler angles greater than 45 degrees

c. color flow Doppler

d. none of the above

20. Which transducer produces a sector image?

a. flat sequenced array

b. continuous wave Doppler probe

c. flat linear array

d. curved linear array

21. What is the shape of the image produced by a phased array transducer?

a. sector (pie-shaped)

b. linear (rectangular)

c. linear (pie-shaped)

d. linear (trapezoidal)

22. What is the shape of the image produced by a flat sequenced array?

  a. sector (pie-shaped)

  b. linear (rectangular)

  c. linear (trapezoidal)

  d. linear (pie-shaped)

23. What is the shape of the image produced by a vector array?

  a. sector (rectangular)

  b. sector (pie-shaped)

  c. sector (trapezoidal)

  d. linear (rectangular)

24. Electronic focusing is possible with

  a. single-element transducers

  b. transducer arrays

  c. two-element continuous wave Doppler probes

  d. none of the above

25. Which of the following does not produce a sector image?

  a. annular array

  b. phased linear

  c. flat sequenced linear array

  d. convex array

26. The transmitter, acoustic power, or energy output control

  a. affects the amplification of received echoes

  b. varies the frequency of the transducer

  c. affects the amount of energy entering a patient

  d. varies the dynamic range

27. If the real-time frame rate is increased, the result will be

  a. increased line density

  b. decreased line density

  c. a smoother image

  d. none of the above

28. With phased array transducers, the transmitted sound beam is steered by

  a. mechanically rotating three or more piezoelectric elements

  b. increasing the PRF with each applied shock pulse

  c. varying the delay of pulses to the transducer's elements

  d. varying the frequency applied to the transducer's elements

29. The number of television fields per second is

  a. 10

  b. 30

  c. 60

  d. $262\frac{1}{2}$

30. A digital picture is a

  a. bit

  b. voxel

  c. pixel

  d. none of the above

31. Which of the following is a "hard copy?"

  a. floppy disk recording

  b. multiimage film

  c. video tape recording

  d. optical disk recording

32. What is the scan converter function that determines the emphasis given to the various gray scale levels?

  a. log compression

  b. A to D conversion

  c. preprocessing

  d. postprocessing

33. A Doppler angle of 90 degrees results in

  a. no Doppler shift

  b. maximum Doppler shift

  c. a shift to a higher frequency

  d. a shift to a lower frequency

35. The difference between red and blue hues in a color flow Doppler image represents a difference in

  a. reflection coefficient

  b. reflector amplitude

  c. flow intensity

  d. flow direction

35. A high PRF, when using pulsed Doppler

  a. increases the possibility of aliasing

  b. increases the chances for depth ambiguity

c. eliminates the refraction artifact

d. decreases the chance of depth ambiguity

36. Which one of the following factors does not affect the frequency of the Doppler shift?

a. angle with which the probe is pointed at a vessel

b. velocity of blood in a vessel

c. the transmitted frequency

d. size of the Doppler probe

37. Continuous wave Doppler systems

a. are capable of detecting higher velocities than are gated Doppler systems

b. detect all movement in the path of the Doppler beam

c. both of the above

d. none of the above

CHAPTER 3

Body Systems

REVIEW QUESTIONS

1. All of the following are tasks performed by bones except
   a. protection
   b. support
   c. blood cell formation
   d. hormone release

2. Voluntary muscles include all of the following except
   a. biceps
   b. cardiac
   c. triceps
   d. quadriceps

3. All of the following act as storage areas except
   a. spleen
   b. liver
   c. bone
   d. brain

4. Which of the following organs has two sets of capillary beds?
   a. liver
   b. kidneys
   c. pancreas
   d. spleen

5. Which organ allows free mixing of oxygenated and deoxygenated blood within sinusoids?
   a. liver
   b. kidneys
   c. pancreas
   d. spleen

6. Which organ is dependent on subatmospheric pressures to perform properly?
   a. liver
   b. skin
   c. kidneys
   d. lungs

7. Which glands release a watery substance that assists in temperature control?
   a. ovaries
   b. testicles
   c. pancreas
   d. sweat glands
   e. sebaceous glands

8. Which of the following does not excrete urea?
   a. lungs
   b. kidneys
   c. skin

9. The ovum is released on approximately the _____ day of the menstrual cycle.
   a. 5th
   b. 10th
   c. 14th
   d. 21st

10. Which region of the brain is responsible for detecting changes in blood chemistry (receptors)?
    a. pituitary
    b. hypothalamus
    c. vermis
    d. cortical mantle

11. Which system requires a pump to circulate fluids?
    a. arterial flow
    b. venous flow
    c. lymphatic flow

12. The structures within the gastrointestinal tract that allow for expansion and contraction of the digestive wall, similar to an accordion, are
    a. villi
    b. rugae
    c. tunica media

13. Which cavity contains the brain?
    a. abdominopelvic
    b. thoracic
    c. spinal
    d. cranial

14. Venous and lymphatic flow is primarily accomplished via
    a. subatmospheric pressure
    b. cardiac systolic contractions
    c. muscle contraction
    d. gravity

15. Which system is primarily responsible for removing excess fluids and preventing edema?
    a. lymphatic
    b. circulatory
    c. digestive
    d. endocrine

16. The pleural sac is associated with the
    a. heart
    b. lungs
    c. kidneys
    d. spleen

17. Fertilization usually occurs in the
    a. uterus
    b. ovary
    c. fallopian tube
    d. cervix

18. Which hormone causes a decrease in blood sugar levels?
    a. epinephrine
    b. norepinephrine
    c. glucagon
    d. insulin

19. Which organ is not part of the excretory system?
    a. skin
    b. kidney
    c. adrenal gland
    d. lung

20. The peritoneal cavity is
    a. the cavity whose boundaries are the pubic bone inferiorly and the diaphragm superiorly
    b. the anterior area of the abdominopelvic cavity within the peritoneal lining
    c. separated from the abdominal cavity by the diaphragm
    d. the posterior area of the abdominopelvic cavity, located posterior to the peritoneal lining

21. The dorsal cavity is composed of the
    a. peritoneal and spinal cavities
    b. spinal and ventral cavities
    c. spinal and cranial cavities
    d. cranial and peritoneal cavities

22. Which body cavity is the posterior area of the abdominopelvic cavity, located posterior to the peritoneal lining?
    a. peritoneal cavity
    b. ventral cavity
    c. thoracic cavity
    d. retroperitoneal cavity

23. Which body cavity is the enclosed area that basically corresponds to the rib cage and is separated from the abdominal cavity by its inferior boundary, the diaphragm?
    a. peritoneal cavity
    b. ventral cavity
    c. thoracic cavity
    d. retroperitoneal cavity

24. The ventral cavity is composed of the
   a. cranial, abdominopelvic, peritoneal, and thoracic cavities
   b. abdominopelvic, peritoneal, thoracic, and retroperitoneal cavities
   c. abdominopelvic, peritoneal, thoracic, and spinal cavities
   d. cranial, abdominopelvic, peritoneal, and spinal cavities

25. Interdependent body systems
   a. cannot exist without the aid of each other
   b. do not interrelate
   c. do not exist
   d. are normally exclusive

26. Which comprises the endocrine glands?
   a. pituitary gland, thyroid gland, parathyroid glands, ovaries, testes, kidneys, pancreas
   b. pituitary gland, thyroid gland, parathyroid glands, adrenal glands, ovaries, testes, pancreas
   c. pituitary gland, thyroid gland, parathyroid glands, ovaries, testes, kidneys, pancreas, spleen
   d. pituitary gland, adrenal glands, ovaries, testes, pancreas

27. Which hormone can be detected via blood or urine to detect a pregnancy?
   a. FSH (follicle stimulating hormone)
   b. GH (growth hormone)
   c. ACTH (adrenocorticotropin)
   d. BhCG (human chorionic gonadotropin)

28. Which is the "master" endocrine gland?
   a. pineal gland
   b. brain
   c. pancreas
   d. pituitary gland

29. Which body system does nothing directly to contribute to the survival of the human body?
   a. central nervous system
   b. endocrine system
   c. reproductive system
   d. digestive system

Identify the structures indicated in the following illustrations. These figures duplicate those found in *Sonography: Introduction to Normal Structure and Function.* Refer to the textbook if you need help.

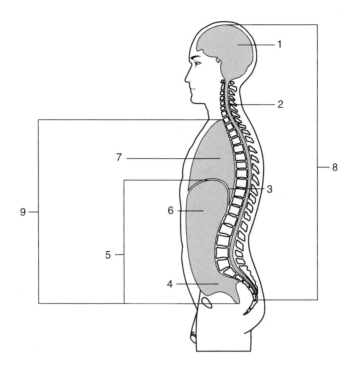

1 _____   6 _____

2 _____   7 _____

3 _____   8 _____

4 _____   9 _____

5 _____

Figure 3-1 Body cavities.

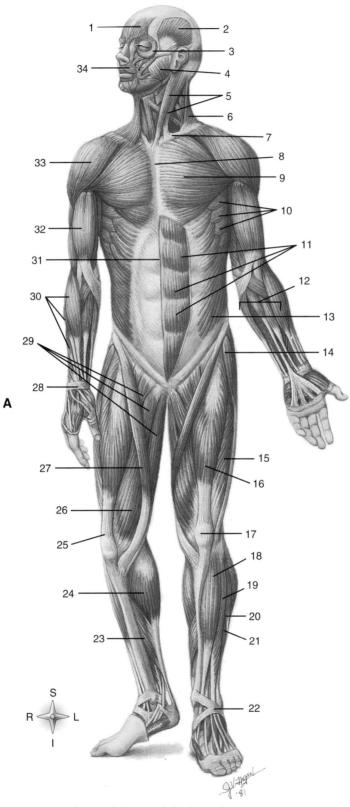

Figure 3-2 A, Skeletal muscles, anterior view.

1 _____

2 _____

3 _____

4 _____

5 _____

6 _____

7 _____

8 _____

9 _____

10 _____

11 _____

12 _____

13 _____

14 _____

15 _____

16 _____

17 _____

18 _____

19 _____

20 _____

21 _____

22 _____

23 _____

24 _____

25 _____

26 _____

27 _____

28 _____

29 _____

30 _____

31 _____

32 _____

33 _____

34 _____

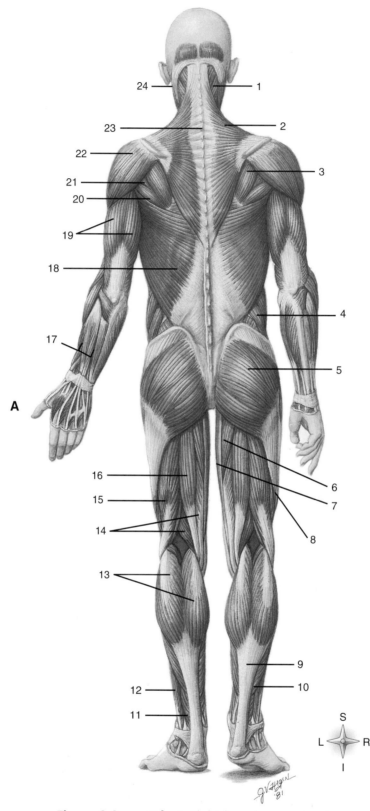

Figure 3-2, cont'd A, Skeletal muscles, posterior view.

1 _____

2 _____

3 _____

4 _____

5 _____

6 _____

7 _____

8 _____

9 _____

10 _____

11 _____

12 _____

13 _____

14 _____

15 _____

16 _____

17 _____

18 _____

19 _____

20 _____

21 _____

22 _____

23 _____

24 _____

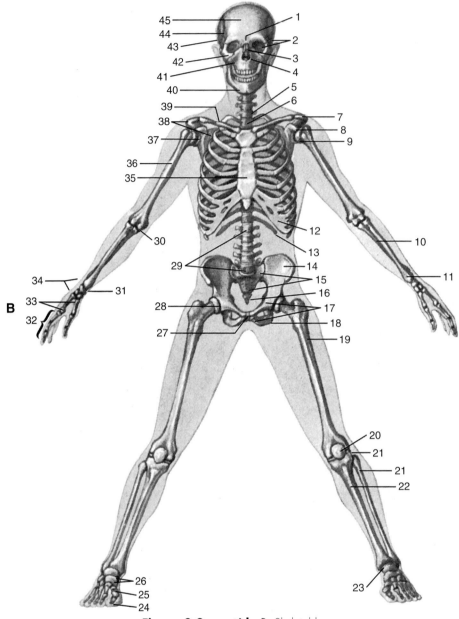

B

Figure 3-2, cont'd B, Skeletal bones.

1 _____

2 _____

3 _____

4 _____

5 _____

6 _____

7 _____

8 _____

9 _____

10 _____

11 _____

12 _____

13 _____

14 _____

15 _____

16 _____

17 _____

18 _____

19 _____

20 _____

21 _____

22 _____

23 _____

24 _____

25 _____

26 _____

27 _____

28 _____

29 _____

30 _____

31 _____

32 _____

33 _____

34 _____

35 _____

36 _____

37 _____

38 _____

39 _____

40 _____

41 _____

42 _____

43 _____

44 _____

45 _____

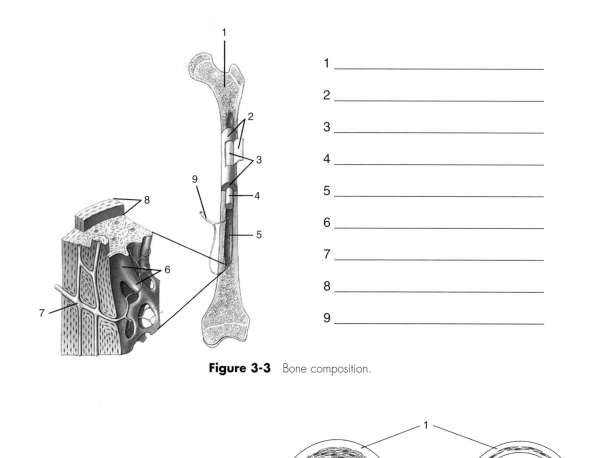

1 _____

2 _____

3 _____

4 _____

5 _____

6 _____

7 _____

8 _____

9 _____

Figure 3-3 Bone composition.

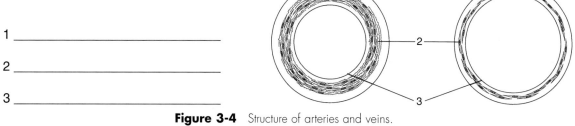

1 _____

2 _____

3 _____

Figure 3-4 Structure of arteries and veins.

1 _____

2 _____

3 _____

4 _____

5 _____

6 _____

7 _____

8 _____

9 _____

10 _____

11 _____

12 _____

13 _____

14 _____

15 _____

16 _____

17 _____

18 _____

19 _____

20 _____

21 _____

22 _____

23 _____

24 _____

25 _____

26 _____

27 _____

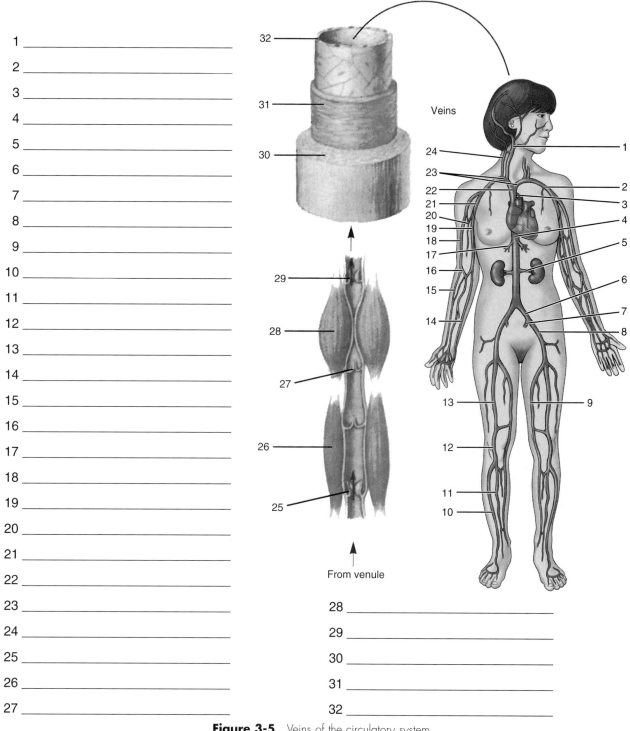

From venule

28 _____

29 _____

30 _____

31 _____

32 _____

Figure 3-5 Veins of the circulatory system.

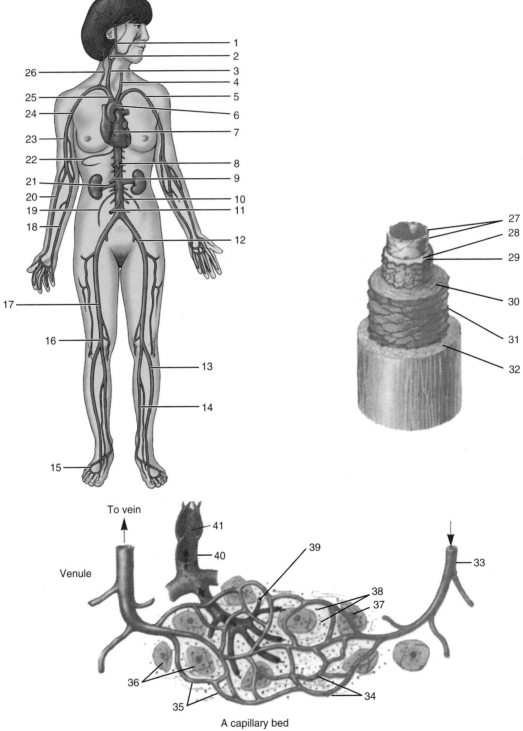

1
2
3
4
5
6
7
8
9
10
11
12
13
14
15
16
17
18
19
20
21
22
23
24
25
26

27
28
29
30
31
32

To vein

Venule

41
40
39
38
37
36
35
34
33

A capillary bed

Figure 3-6 Arteries of the circulatory system.

1 _____

2 _____

3 _____

4 _____

5 _____

6 _____

7 _____

8 _____

9 _____

10 _____

11 _____

12 _____

13 _____

14 _____

15 _____

16 _____

17 _____

18 _____

19 _____

20 _____

21 _____

22 _____

23 _____

24 _____

25 _____

26 _____

27 _____

28 _____

29 _____

30 _____

31 _____

32 _____

33 _____

34 _____

35 _____

36 _____

37 _____

38 _____

39 _____

40 _____

41 _____

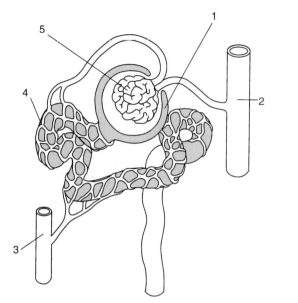
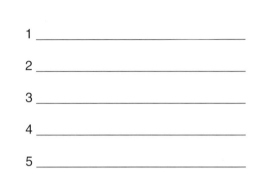
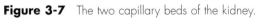

1 _____

2 _____

3 _____

4 _____

5 _____

Figure 3-7 The two capillary beds of the kidney.

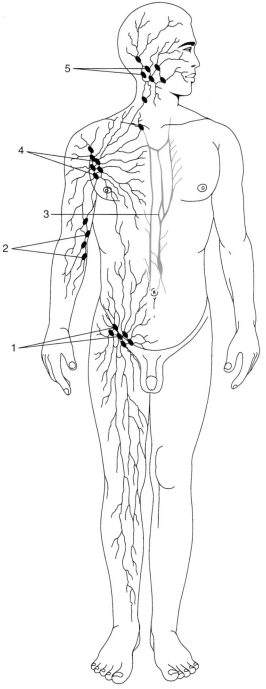

Figure 3-8 The lymphatic system.

1 _____

2 _____

3 _____

4 _____

5 _____

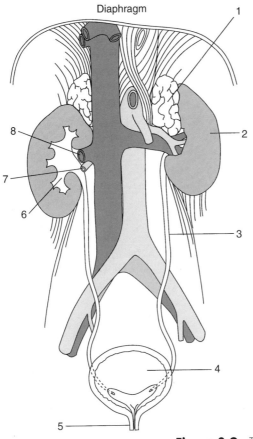

Diaphragm

1 _____

2 _____

3 _____

4 _____

5 _____

6 _____

7 _____

8 _____

Figure 3-9 The urinary system.

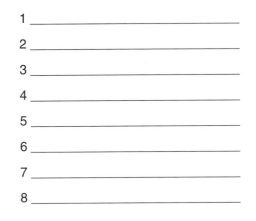

1 _____

2 _____

3 _____

4 _____

5 _____

6 _____

7 _____

8 _____

9 _____

10 _____

11 _____

12 _____

Figure 3-10 A nephron and surrounding capillaries.

1 _____

2 _____

3 _____

4 _____

5 _____

6 _____

7 _____

8 _____

9 _____

10 _____

11 _____

12 _____

13 _____

14 _____

15 _____

16 _____

17 _____

18 _____

19 _____

20 _____

21 _____

22 _____

23 _____

24 _____

25 _____

26 _____

27 _____

28 _____

29 _____

30 _____

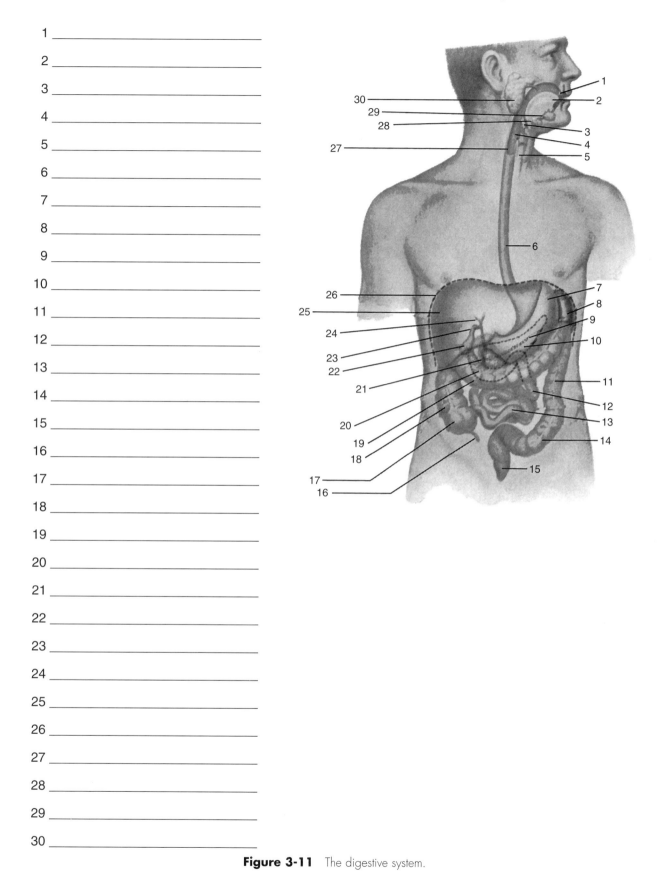

Figure 3-11 The digestive system.

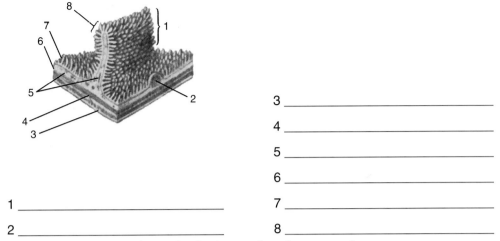

3 _____

4 _____

5 _____

6 _____

1 _____   7 _____

2 _____   8 _____

Figure 3-12 Section of small intestine wall.

1 _____

2 _____

3 _____

4 _____

5 _____

6 _____

7 _____

8 _____

9 _____

10 _____

11 _____

12 _____

13 _____

14 _____

15 _____

16 _____

17 _____

18 _____

19 _____

20 _____

21 _____

22 _____

23 _____

24 _____

25 _____

26 _____

27 _____

28 _____

29 _____

30 _____

31 _____

32 _____

33 _____

34 _____

35 _____

36 _____

37 _____

38 _____

39 _____

40 _____

41 _____

42 _____

43 _____

44 _____

45 _____

46 _____

47 _____

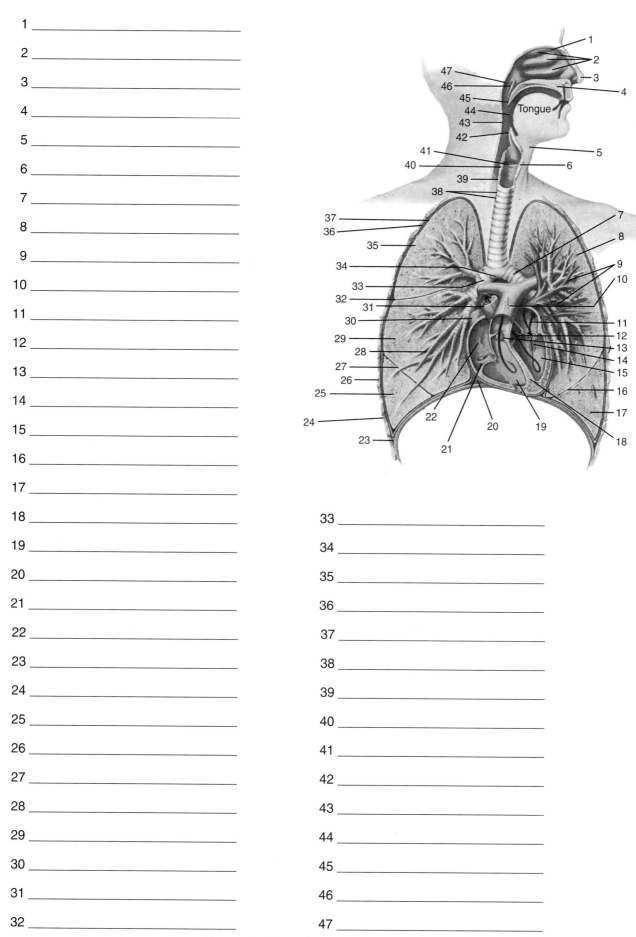

Figure 3-13 A, The respiratory system and heart.

1 _____

2 _____

3 _____

4 _____

5 _____

6 _____

7 _____

8 _____

9 _____

10 _____

11 _____

12 _____

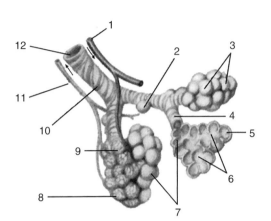

Figure 3-13, cont'd B, Primary respiratory lobule.

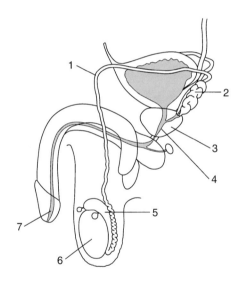

1 _____

2 _____

3 _____

4 _____

5 _____

6 _____

7 _____

Figure 3-14 Male reproductive system.

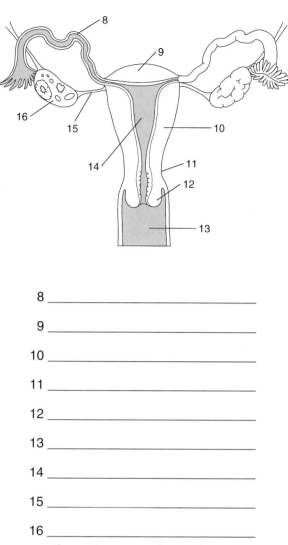

8 _____

9 _____

10 _____

11 _____

12 _____

13 _____

14 _____

15 _____

16 _____

Figure 3-15 Female reproductive system.

1 _____

2 _____

3 _____

4 _____

5 _____

6 _____

7 _____

8 _____

9 _____

10 _____

11 _____

12 _____

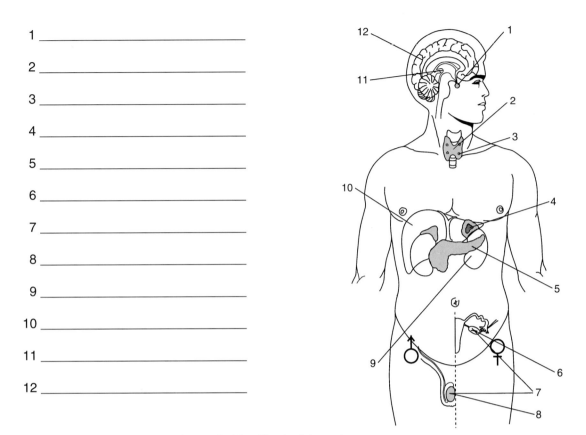

Figure 3-16 Glands of the endocrine system.

1 _____

2 _____

3 _____

4 _____

5 _____

6 _____

7 _____

8 _____

9 _____

10 _____

11 _____

12 _____

13 _____

14 _____

15 _____

16 _____

17 _____

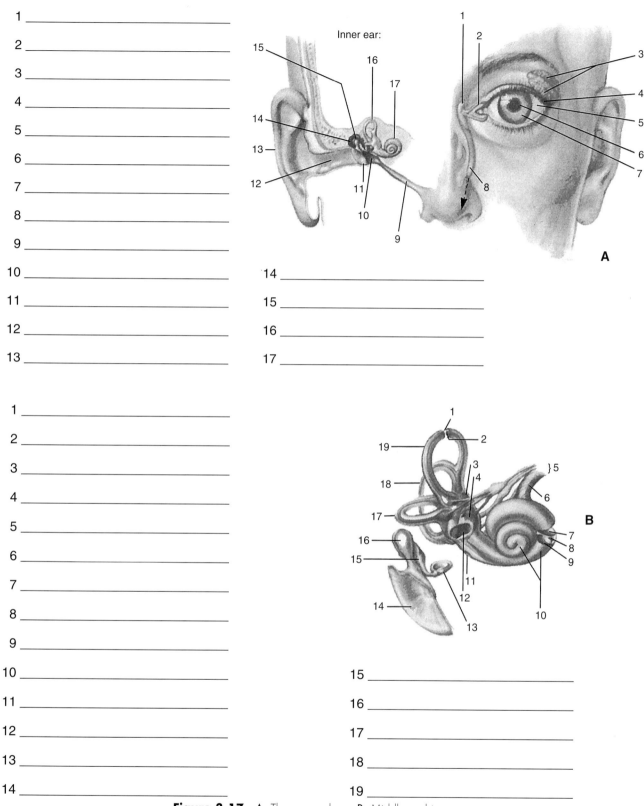

1 _____

2 _____

3 _____

4 _____

5 _____

6 _____

7 _____

8 _____

9 _____

10 _____

11 _____

12 _____

13 _____

14 _____

15 _____

16 _____

17 _____

18 _____

19 _____

Figure 3-17 A, The eye and ear. B, Middle and inner ear.

1 _____

2 _____

3 _____

4 _____

5 _____

6 _____

7 _____

8 _____

9 _____

10 _____

11 _____

12 _____

13 _____

14 _____

15 _____

16 _____

17 _____

18 _____

19 _____

20 _____

21 _____

22 _____

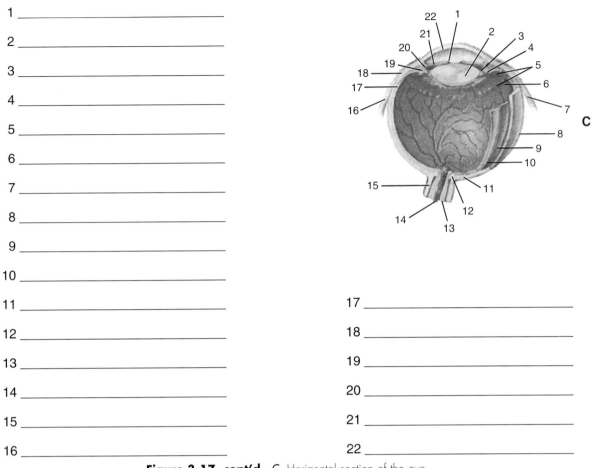

Figure 3-17, cont'd C, Horizontal section of the eye.

CHAPTER 4

Anatomy Layering and Sectional Anatomy

REVIEW QUESTIONS

1. Which structure is not intraperitoneal?
   a. gallbladder
   b. pancreas
   c. liver
   d. spleen

2. Which structure is not retroperitoneal?
   a. gallbladder
   b. pancreas
   c. urinary bladder
   d. aorta

3. Which structure does not lie in a vertical position within the body?
   a. abdominal aorta
   b. superior mesenteric vein
   c. left renal vein
   d. superior mesenteric artery

4. Which structure does not lie transversely within the body?
   a. left renal vein
   b. left renal artery
   c. portal vein
   d. right renal vein

5. Which anatomic area is not seen on a sagittal section?
   a. posterior
   b. inferior
   c. anterior
   d. medial

6. Which anatomic area is not seen on a coronal section?
   a. medial
   b. lateral
   c. anterior
   d. superior

7. Which anatomic area is not seen on a transverse section?
   a. superior
   b. right lateral
   c. anterior
   d. medial

8. The scanning planes used in sonography are the same as anatomic body planes, but their interpretations depend on
   a. the size of the transducer
   b. the shape of the transducer and how it is held
   c. body habitus
   d. the location of the transducer and the sound wave approach

9. The single difference between structures seen on an ultrasound image section and a cadaver section is
   a. size
   b. sonographic appearance
   c. adjacent relationships
   d. shape

10. Which term is not used to describe sonographic appearance?

    a. isosonic

    b. annular array

    c. anechoic

    d. hypoechoic

11. Using the figure below: the pancreas is located _____ to the splenic artery.

    a. inferior

    b. anterior

    c. posterior

    d. superior

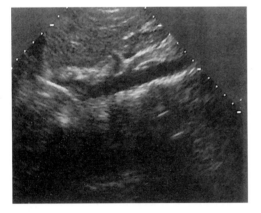

12. Using the figure below: the psoas muscle is located _____ to the aorta.

    a. superior

    b. lateral

    c. medial

    d. inferior

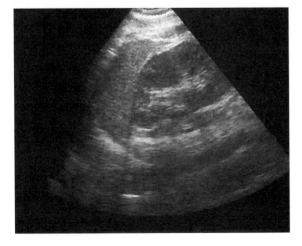

13. Using the figure below: the left renal vein is located _____ to the superior mesenteric artery.

    a. anterior

    b. posterior

    c. left lateral

    d. right lateral

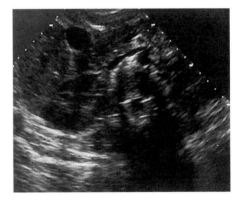

14. Using the same figure as in Question 13: the superior mesenteric vein is located _____ to the superior mesenteric artery.

    a. left lateral

    b. posterior

    c. right lateral

    d. anterior

15. Using the same figure as in Question 13: the superior mesenteric vein runs between the _____ and _____.

    a. splenic vein/inferior vena cava

    b. splenic vein/aorta

    c. pancreas neck/uncinate process

    d. pancreas head/inferior vena cava

16. Which group of structures is not retroperitoneal?

    a. kidneys, ureters, adrenal glands, inferior vena cava, aorta, abdominal lymph nodes, pancreas, urinary bladder, uterus, and prostate gland

    b. kidneys, adrenal glands, pancreas, inferior vena cava, aorta, spleen, ascending colon, descending colon

    c. inferior vena cava, aorta, adrenal glands, pancreas, urinary bladder, uterus, prostate gland, most of the duodenum, abdominal lymph nodes

    d. inferior vena cava, aorta, abdominal lymph nodes, ascending colon, descending colon, somatic nerves

17. Which group of structures is not intraperitoneal?
    a. liver (except bare area), gallbladder, spleen
    b. liver (except bare area), spleen, stomach
    c. ovaries, uterus, majority of the intestines
    d. spleen, gallbladder, stomach

18. The greater sac
    a. extends from the diaphragm to the pelvis and covers the width of the abdomen
    b. is the omental bursa
    c. is a double layer of peritoneum that extends from the stomach to adjacent abdominal organs
    d. is a diverticulum of the mesentery located posterior to the stomach

19. The lesser sac
    a. extends from the diaphragm to the pelvis and covers the width of the abdomen
    b. is a diverticulum of the greater sac located posterior to the stomach
    c. is a double layer of peritoneum that extends from the stomach to adjacent abdominal organs
    d. attaches to the anterior surface of the transverse colon

20. Intraperitoneal structures are connected to the cavity wall by the
    a. omentum
    b. greater sac
    c. lesser sac
    d. mesentery

21. Crura of the diaphragm are
    a. folds of peritoneum that insert into the diaphragm
    b. visceral tissue layers that insert into the diaphragm
    c. bands arising from the diaphragm that attach to the abdominal aorta and inferior vena cava
    d. muscular bands that arise from the lumbar vertebrae and insert into the diaphragm

22. The left and right renal arteries are _____ to the left and right renal veins
    a. inferior
    b. posterior
    c. anterior
    d. lateral

23. The quadratus lumborum muscle is a bilateral muscle tissue that is _____ to the psoas major muscle and _____ to the kidneys and adrenal glands.
    a. medial/posterior
    b. medial/lateral
    c. lateral/posterior
    d. lateral/anterior

24. Muscle echo texture is usually _____ the organ(s) they are adjacent to.
    a. more echogenic than
    b. isogenic to
    c. less echogenic than
    d. hyperechoic compared with

25. Which group of structures is not routinely imaged by sonography?
    a. normal lymph nodes, nerves, collapsed bowel
    b. normal lymph nodes, normal fallopian tubes, normal ureters
    c. normal fallopian tubes, ovarian follicles, normal ureters
    d. second-order vascular branches, gastroduodenal artery, appendix

Identify the structures indicated in the following illustrations. These figures duplicate those found in *Sonography: Introduction to Normal Structure and Function.* Refer to the textbook if you need help.

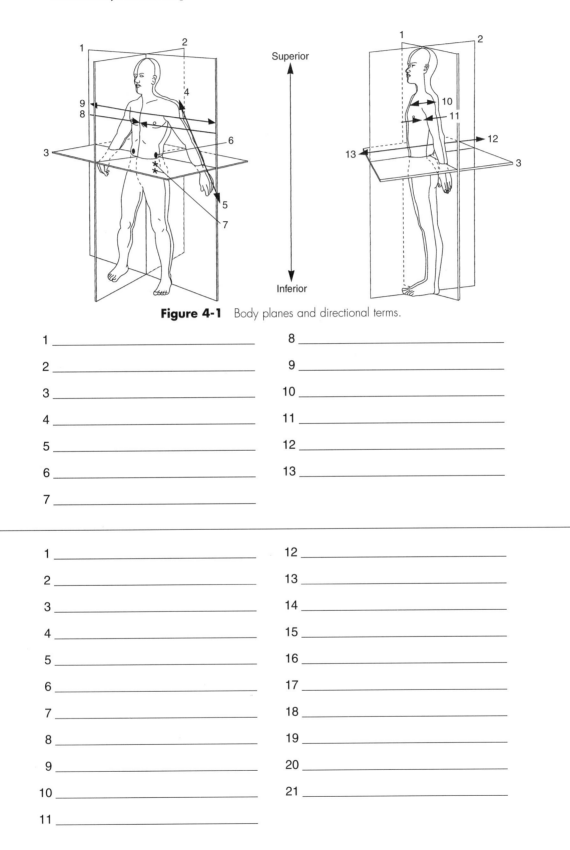

Figure 4-1 Body planes and directional terms.

1 _____   8 _____

2 _____   9 _____

3 _____   10 _____

4 _____   11 _____

5 _____   12 _____

6 _____   13 _____

7 _____

1 _____   12 _____

2 _____   13 _____

3 _____   14 _____

4 _____   15 _____

5 _____   16 _____

6 _____   17 _____

7 _____   18 _____

8 _____   19 _____

9 _____   20 _____

10 _____   21 _____

11 _____

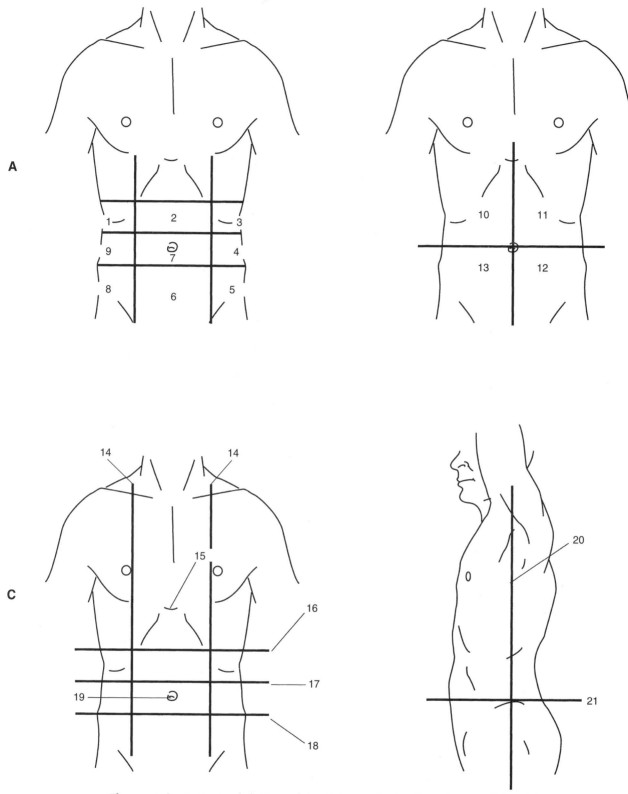

Figure 4-2 A, Regional divisions of the abdomen. B, Quadrant divisions of the abdomen. C, Surface landmarks of the abdominal wall.

A. POSTERIOR MUSCLES

Right   Left

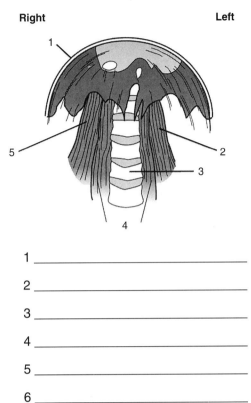

1 _____

2 _____

3 _____

4 _____

5 _____

1 _____

2 _____

3 _____

4 _____

5 _____

6 _____

7 _____

8 _____

9 _____

10 _____

B. KIDNEYS AND ADRENAL GLANDS

Right   Left

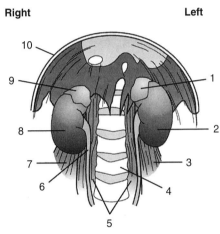

1 _____

2 _____

3 _____

4 _____

5 _____

6 _____

7 _____

8 _____

9 _____

10 _____

11 _____

12 _____

13 _____

C. VENA CAVA

Right   Left

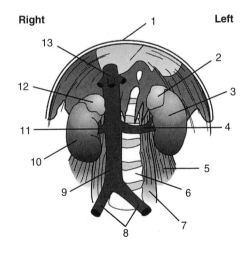

Figure 4-3 The layers of the abdomen.

1 _____
2 _____
3 _____
4 _____
5 _____
6 _____
7 _____
8 _____
9 _____
10 _____
11 _____
12 _____
13 _____
14 _____
15 _____
16 _____
17 _____

D. AORTA

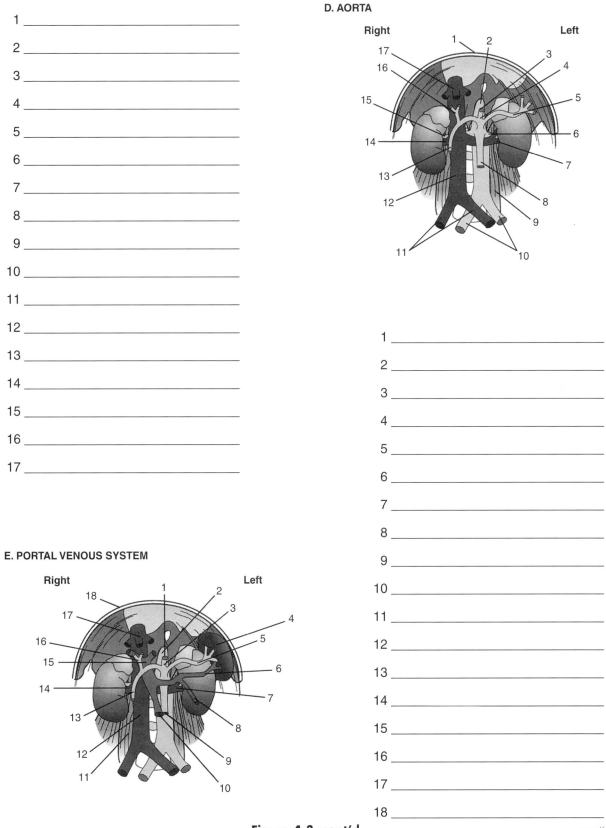

E. PORTAL VENOUS SYSTEM

1 _____
2 _____
3 _____
4 _____
5 _____
6 _____
7 _____
8 _____
9 _____
10 _____
11 _____
12 _____
13 _____
14 _____
15 _____
16 _____
17 _____
18 _____

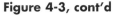

Figure 4-3, cont'd

continued

F. PANCREAS

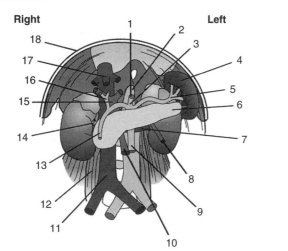

Right   Left

5 _____

6 _____

7 _____

8 _____

9 _____

10 _____

11 _____

12 _____

13 _____

14 _____

15 _____

16 _____

17 _____

18 _____

1 _____

2 _____

3 _____

4 _____

1 _____

2 _____

3 _____

4 _____

5 _____

6 _____

7 _____

8 _____

9 _____

10 _____

11 _____

12 _____

13 _____

14 _____

15 _____

G. GALLBLADDER AND BILIARY TRACT

Right   Left

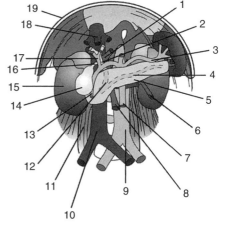

16 _____

17 _____

18 _____

19 _____

Figure 4-3, cont'd

H. GASTROINTESTINAL TRACT

Right   Left

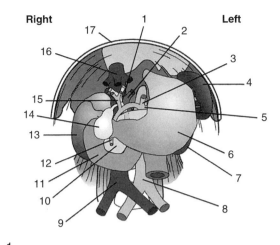

1 _____

2 _____

3 _____

4 _____

5 _____

6 _____

7 _____

8 _____

9 _____

10 _____

11 _____

12 _____

13 _____

14 _____

15 _____

16 _____

17 _____

1 _____

2 _____

3 _____

4 _____

5 _____

6 _____

7 _____

8 _____

9 _____

I. LIVER

Right   Left

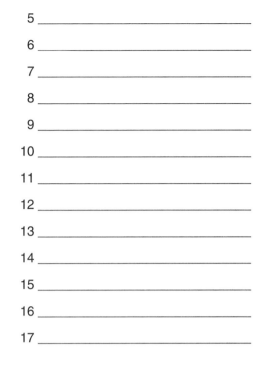

10 _____

11 _____

J. ANTERIOR MUSCLES

Right   Left

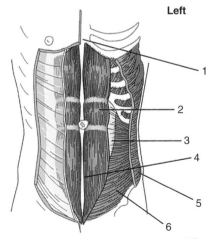

1 _____

2 _____

3 _____

4 _____

5 _____

6 _____

Figure 4-3, cont'd

A. POSTERIOR MUSCLES/TRUE PELVIS

Right   Left

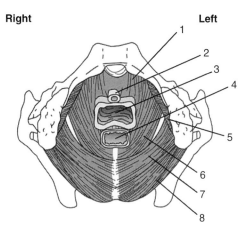

1 _____

2 _____

3 _____

4 _____

5 _____

6 _____

7 _____

8 _____

1 _____

2 _____

3 _____

4 _____

5 _____

B. POSTERIOR MUSCLES/FALSE PELVIS

Right   Left

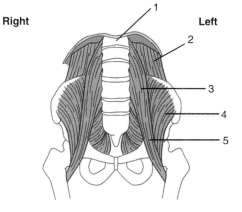

C. RECTUM/COLON

Right   Left

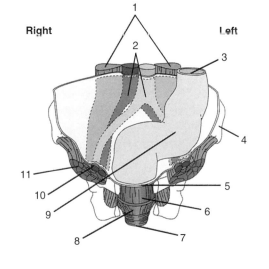

1 _____

2 _____

3 _____

4 _____

5 _____

6 _____

7 _____

8 _____

9 _____

10 _____

11 _____

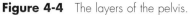

Figure 4-4 The layers of the pelvis.

1 _____

2 _____

3 _____

4 _____

5 _____

6 _____

7 _____

8 _____

9 _____

10 _____

D. UTERUS/BLADDER

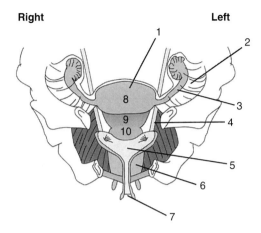

E. PROSTATE GLAND/BLADDER

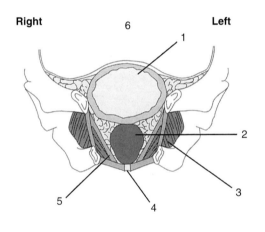

1 _____

2 _____

3 _____

4 _____

5 _____

6 _____

F. ANTERIOR MUSCLE

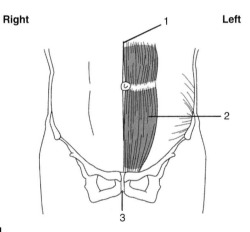

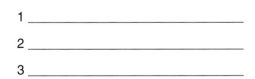

1 _____

2 _____

3 _____

Figure 4-4, cont'd

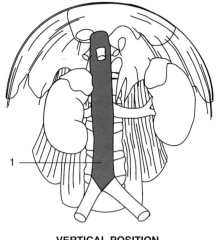

VERTICAL POSITION

1 _____

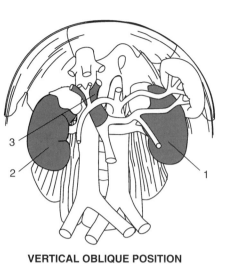

VERTICAL OBLIQUE POSITION

1 _____

2 _____

3 _____

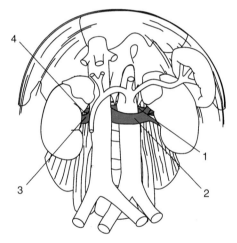

TRANSVERSE POSITION

1 _____

2 _____

3 _____

4 _____

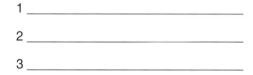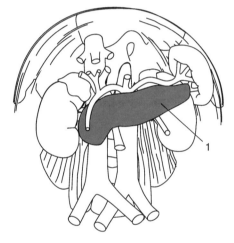

TRANSVERSE OBLIQUE POSITION

1 _____

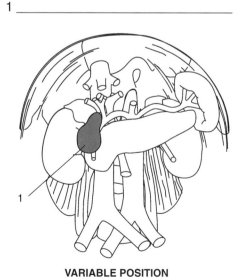

VARIABLE POSITION

1 _____

Figure 4-5

A. ANTERIOR APPROACH/SAGITTAL PLANE

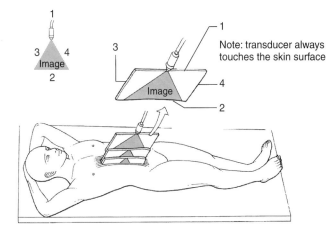

Note: transducer always touches the skin surface

1 _____

2 _____

3 _____

4 _____

B. PCSTERIOR APPROACH/SAGITTAL PLANE

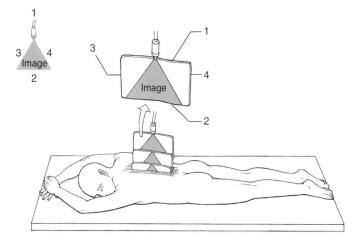

1 _____

2 _____

3 _____

4 _____

C. ANTERIOR APPROACH/TRANSVERSE PLANE

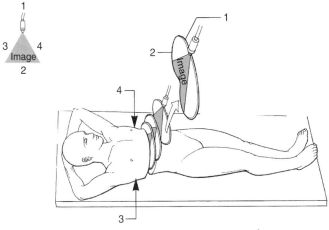

1 _____

2 _____

3 _____

4 _____

Figure 4-6

continued

D. POSTERIOR APPROACH/TRANSVERSE PLANE

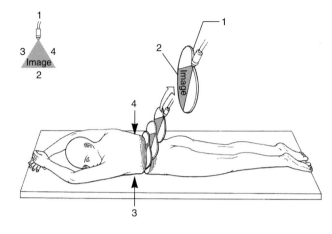

1 _____

2 _____

3 _____

4 _____

E. LATERAL APPROACH/TRANSVERSE PLANE

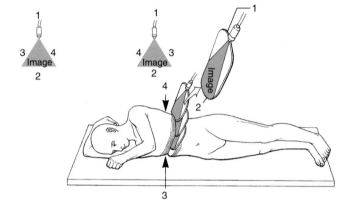

1 _____

2 _____

3 _____

4 _____

F. LATERAL APPROACH/CORONAL PLANE

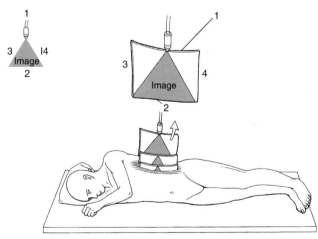

1 _____

2 _____

3 _____

4 _____

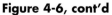

Figure 4-6, cont'd

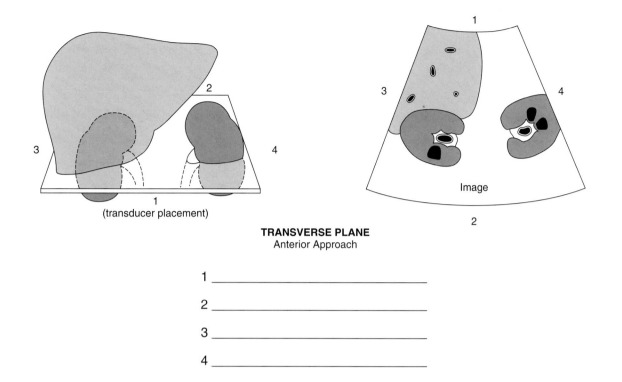

TRANSVERSE PLANE
Anterior Approach

1 _____

2 _____

3 _____

4 _____

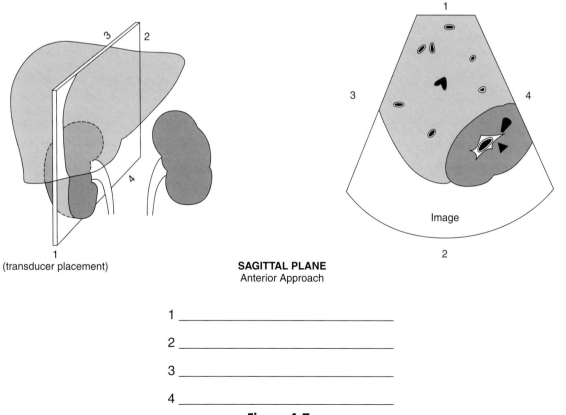

SAGITTAL PLANE
Anterior Approach

1 _____

2 _____

3 _____

4 _____

Figure 4-7

continued

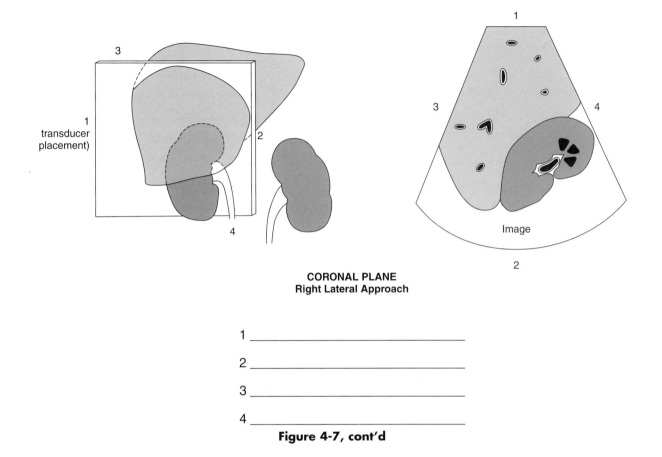

CORONAL PLANE
Right Lateral Approach

1 _____

2 _____

3 _____

4 _____

Figure 4-7, cont'd

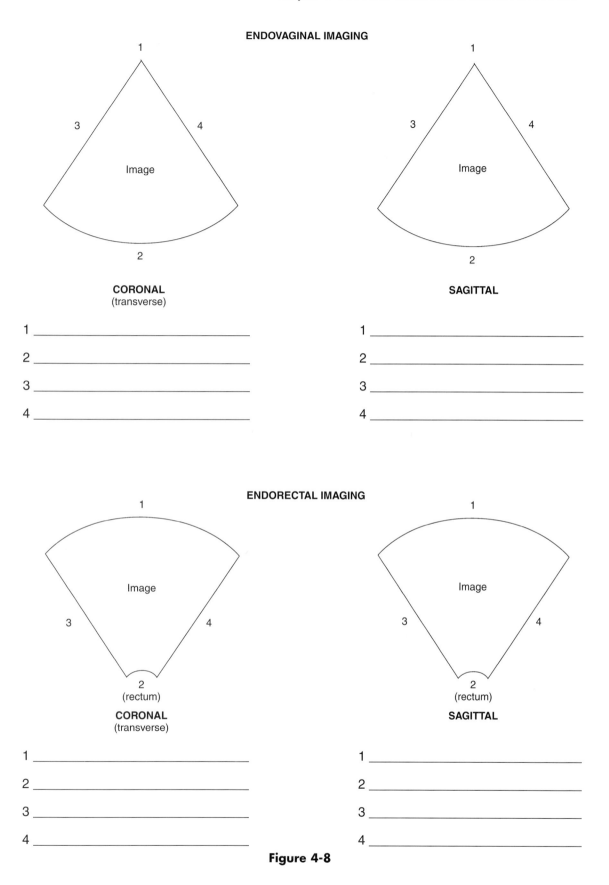

Figure 4-8

NEUROSONOGRAPHY IMAGING
(Brain Imaging)

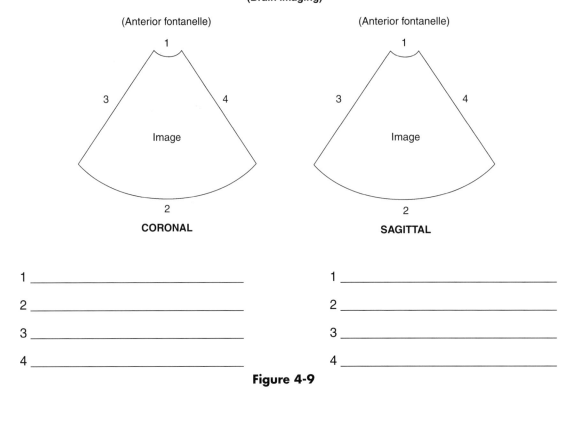

CORONAL

SAGITTAL

1 _____

2 _____

3 _____

4 _____

1 _____

2 _____

3 _____

4 _____

Figure 4-9

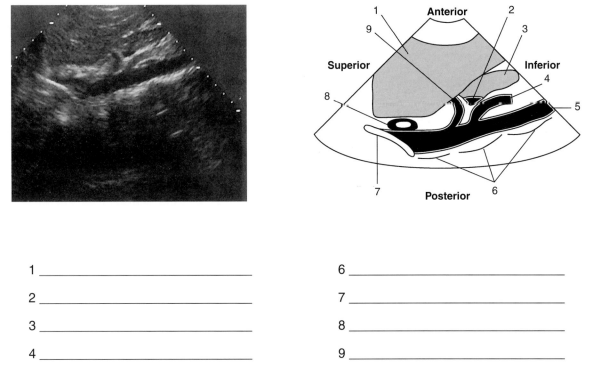

1 _____

2 _____

3 _____

4 _____

5 _____

6 _____

7 _____

8 _____

9 _____

Figure 4-10 In this sagittal section, the area of interest is the body of the pancreas.

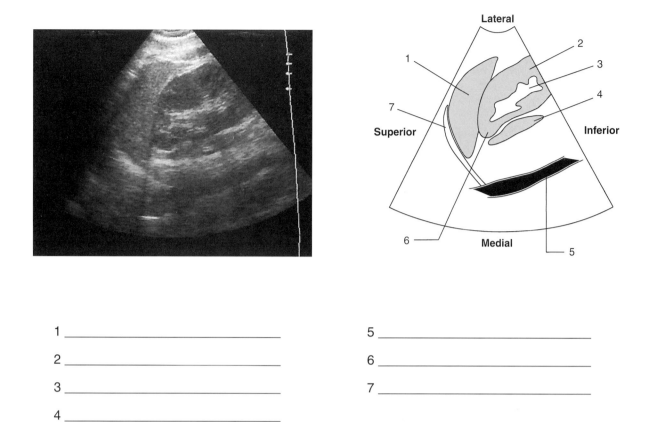

1 _____

2 _____

3 _____

4 _____

5 _____

6 _____

7 _____

Figure 4-11 In this coronal section, the area of interest is the superior pole of the left kidney.

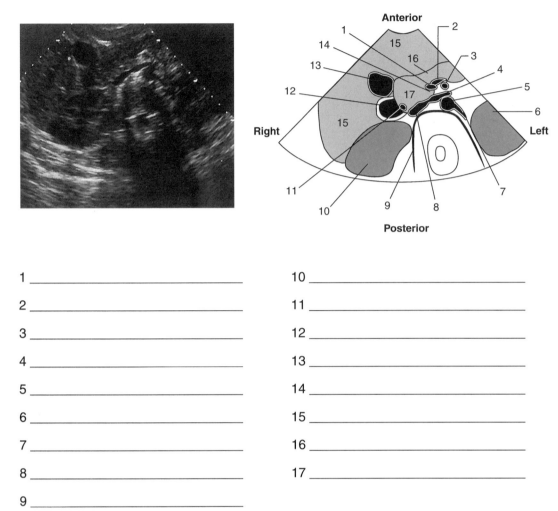

1 _____   10 _____

2 _____   11 _____

3 _____   12 _____

4 _____   13 _____

5 _____   14 _____

6 _____   15 _____

7 _____   16 _____

8 _____   17 _____

9 _____

Figure 4-12 In this transverse section, the area of interest is the head of the pancreas.

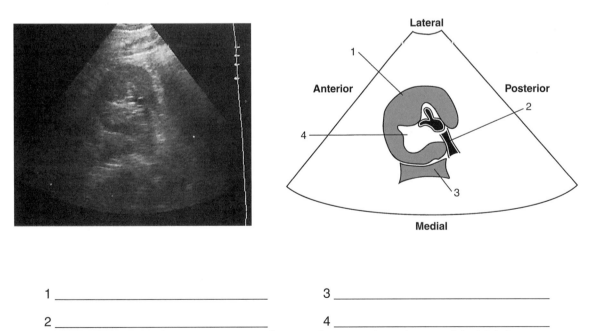

1 _____   3 _____

2 _____   4 _____

Figure 4-13 In this transverse section, the area of interest is the midportion of the left kidney.

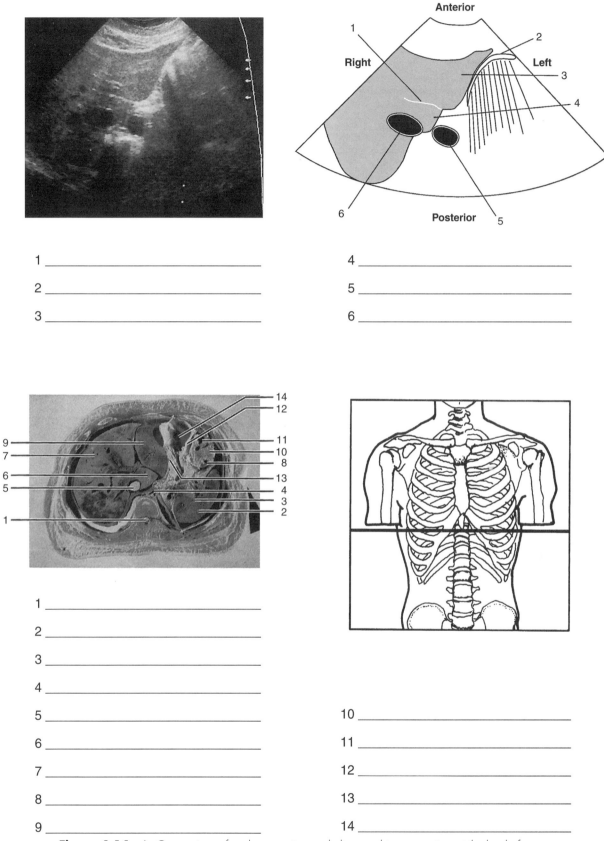

1 _____   4 _____

2 _____   5 _____

3 _____   6 _____

1 _____

2 _____

3 _____

4 _____

5 _____   10 _____

6 _____   11 _____

7 _____   12 _____

8 _____   13 _____

9 _____   14 _____

Figure 4-14   A, Comparison of cadaver section and ultrasound image section at the level of the tenth thoracic vertebrae.

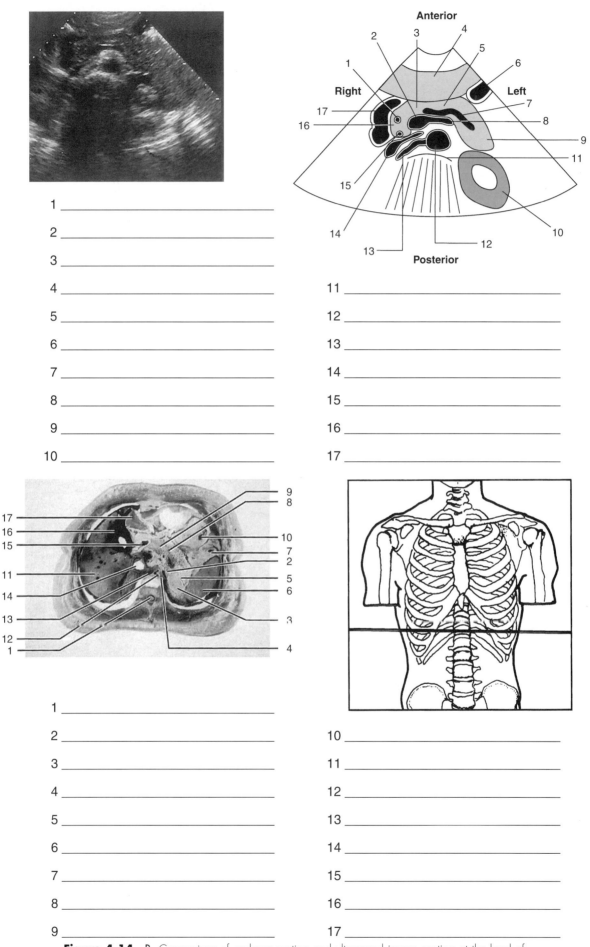

1 _____

2 _____

3 _____

4 _____   11 _____

5 _____   12 _____

6 _____   13 _____

7 _____   14 _____

8 _____   15 _____

9 _____   16 _____

10 _____   17 _____

1 _____

2 _____

3 _____

4 _____

5 _____   10 _____

6 _____   11 _____

7 _____   12 _____

8 _____   13 _____

9 _____   14 _____

                           15 _____

                           16 _____

                           17 _____

Figure 4-14 B, Comparison of cadaver section and ultrasound image section at the level of the twelfth thoracic vertebra.

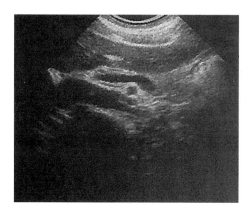

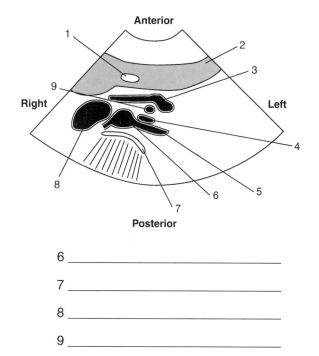

1 _____   6 _____

2 _____   7 _____

3 _____   8 _____

4 _____   9 _____

5 _____

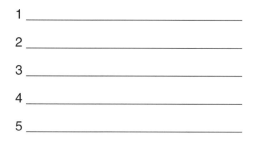

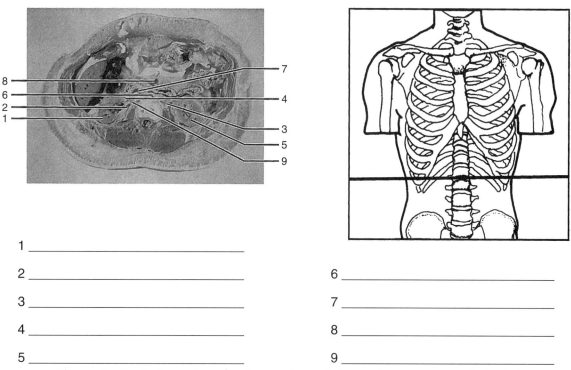

1 _____

2 _____   6 _____

3 _____   7 _____

4 _____   8 _____

5 _____   9 _____

Figure 4-14 C, Comparison of cadaver section and ultrasound image section at the level of the second lumbar vertebra.

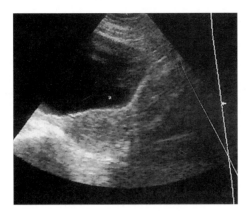

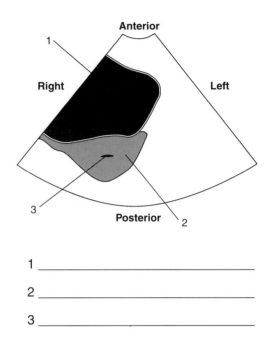

1 _____

2 _____

3 _____

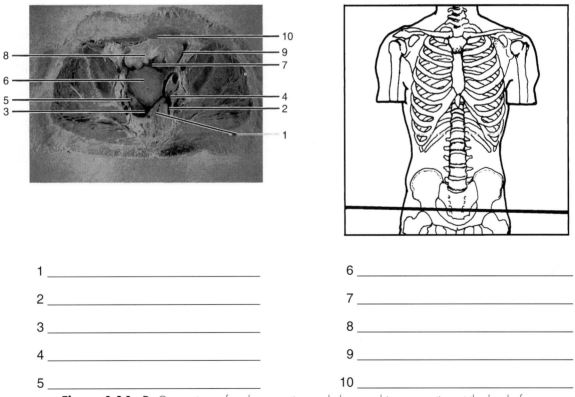

1 _____   6 _____

2 _____   7 _____

3 _____   8 _____

4 _____   9 _____

5 _____   10 _____

Figure 4-14   D, Comparison of cadaver section and ultrasound image section at the level of the fifth vertebra of the sacrum.

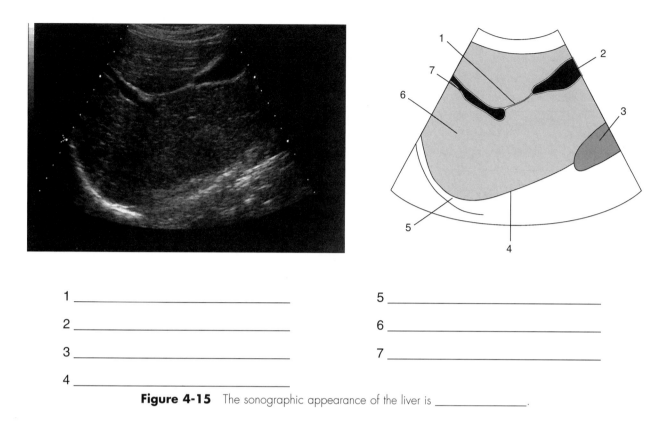

1 _____   5 _____

2 _____   6 _____

3 _____   7 _____

4 _____

Figure 4-15 The sonographic appearance of the liver is _____.

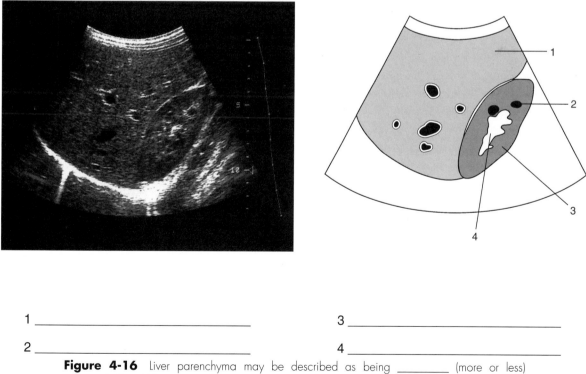

1 _____   3 _____

2 _____   4 _____

Figure 4-16 Liver parenchyma may be described as being _____ (more or less) echogenic than kidney parenchyma.

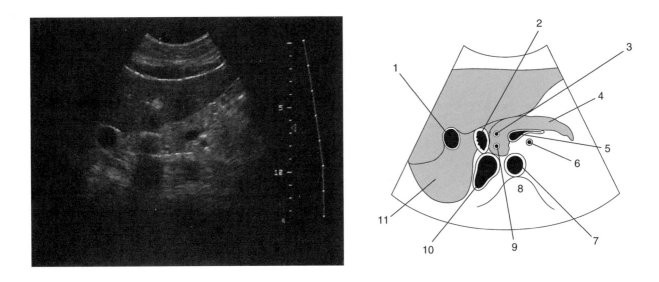

1 _____	7 _____
2 _____	8 _____
3 _____	9 _____
4 _____	10 _____
5 _____	11 _____
6 _____	

Figure 4-17 Liver parenchyma may be described as being _____ (more or less) echogenic than pancreatic parenchyma.

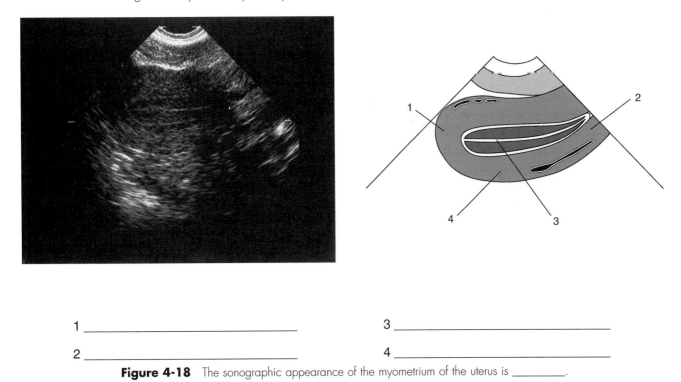

1 _____	3 _____
2 _____	4 _____

Figure 4-18 The sonographic appearance of the myometrium of the uterus is _____.

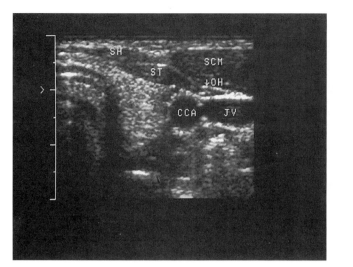

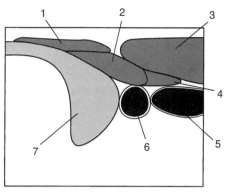

1 _____   5 _____

2 _____   6 _____

3 _____   7 _____

4 _____

Figure 4-19 The sonographic appearance of muscles is _____. Muscles are _____ (more or less) echogenic than the thyroid.

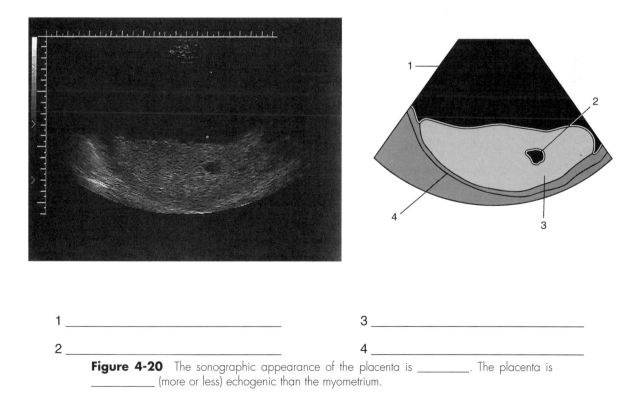

1 _____   3 _____

2 _____   4 _____

Figure 4-20 The sonographic appearance of the placenta is _____. The placenta is _____ (more or less) echogenic than the myometrium.

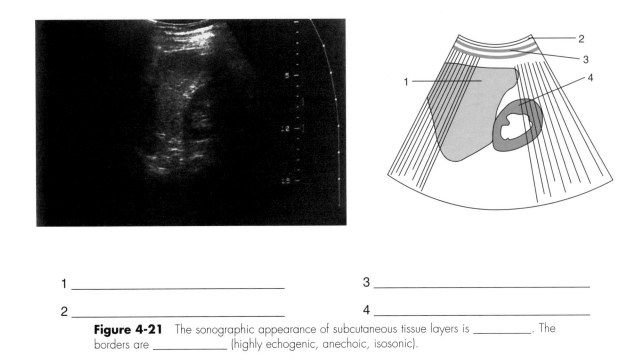

1 _____   3 _____

2 _____   4 _____

Figure 4-21 The sonographic appearance of subcutaneous tissue layers is _____. The borders are _____ (highly echogenic, anechoic, isosonic).

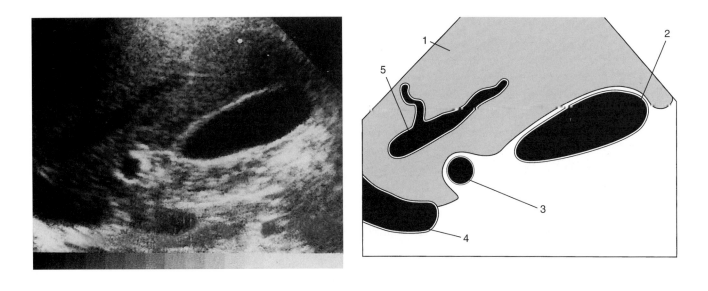

1 _____   4 _____

2 _____   5 _____

3 _____

Figure 4-22 A, The gallbladder is _____(highly echogenic, anechoic, isosonic).

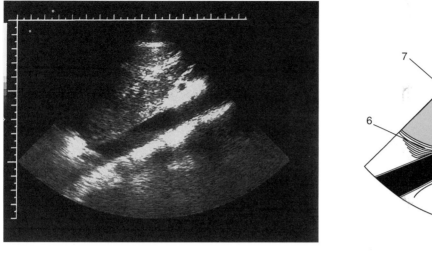
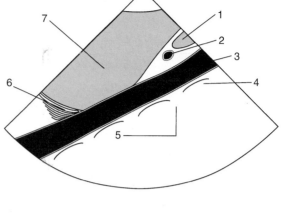

1 _____   5 _____

2 _____   6 _____

3 _____   7 _____

4 _____

Figure 4-22 B, The aorta and splenic artery are _____ (highly echogenic, anechoic, isosonic).

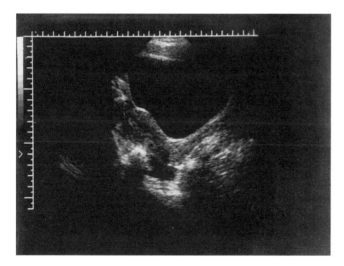
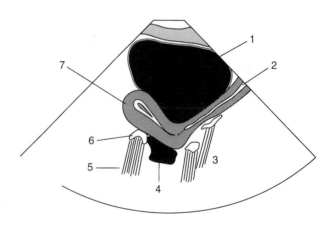

1 _____   5 _____

2 _____   6 _____

3 _____   7 _____

4 _____

Figure 4-22 C, The urinary bladder is _____ (highly echogenic, anechoic, isosonic).

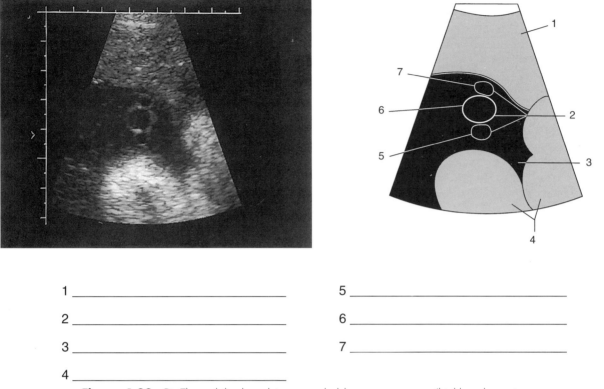

1 _____   5 _____

2 _____   6 _____

3 _____   7 _____

4 _____

Figure 4-22 D, The umbilical cord is surrounded by _____ (highly echogenic, anechoic, isosonic) amniotic fluid.

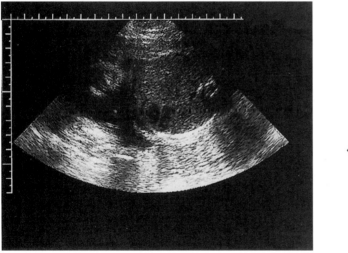
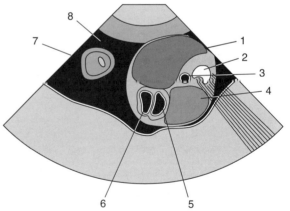

1 _____   5 _____

2 _____   6 _____

3 _____   7 _____

4 _____   8 _____

Figure 4-22 E, The ventricles of the fetal heart and fetal aorta are _____ (highly echogenic, anechoic, isosonic).

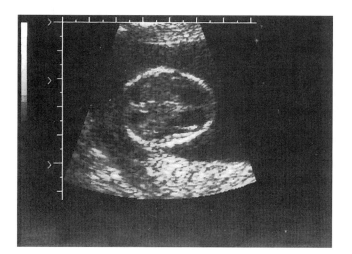
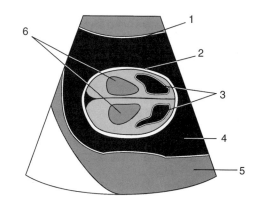

1 _____   4 _____

2 _____   5 _____

3 _____   6 _____

Figure 4-22 F, The ventricles of the fetal brain are _____ (highly echogenic, anechoic, isosonic).

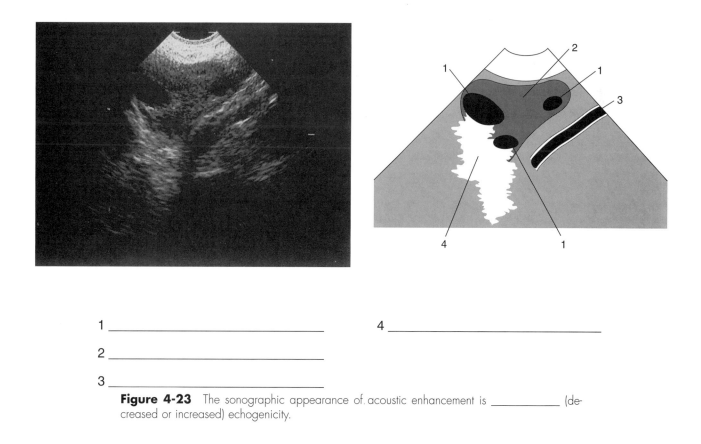

1 _____   4 _____

2 _____

3 _____

Figure 4-23 The sonographic appearance of acoustic enhancement is _____ (decreased or increased) echogenicity.

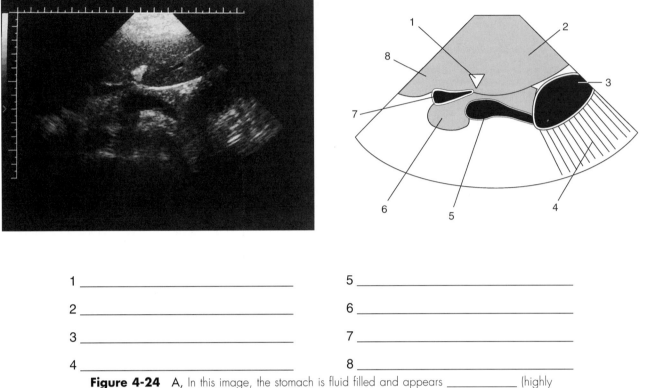

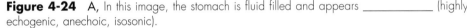

1 _____   5 _____

2 _____   6 _____

3 _____   7 _____

4 _____   8 _____

Figure 4-24 A, In this image, the stomach is fluid filled and appears _____ (highly echogenic, anechoic, isosonic).

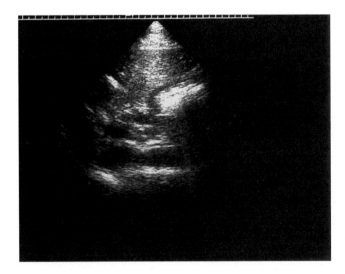

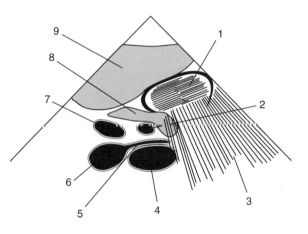

1 _____   6 _____

2 _____   7 _____

3 _____   8 _____

4 _____   9 _____

5 _____

Figure 4-24 B, In this image, the stomach lumen is filled with gas or air and appears _____ (highly echogenic, anechoic, isosonic). The stomach wall is _____ (hyperechoic, hypoechoic) compared with the stomach lumen.

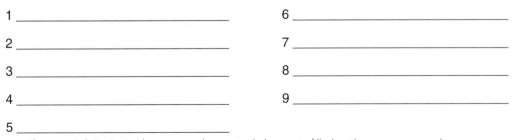

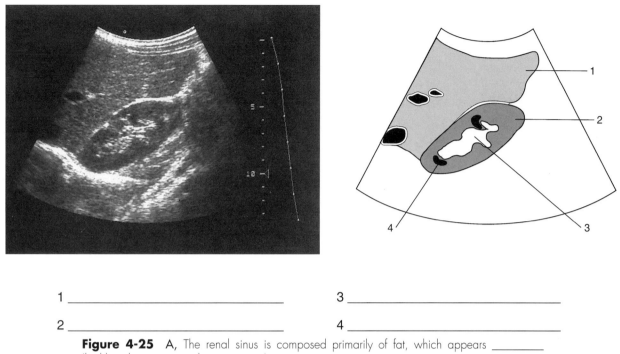

1 _____   3 _____

2 _____   4 _____

Figure 4-25 A, The renal sinus is composed primarily of fat, which appears _____ (highly echogenic, anechoic, isosonic).

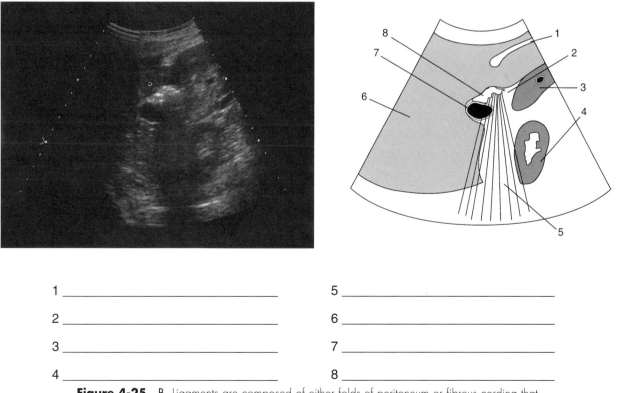

1 _____   5 _____

2 _____   6 _____

3 _____   7 _____

4 _____   8 _____

Figure 4-25 B, Ligaments are composed of either folds of peritoneum or fibrous cording that appears _____ (highly echogenic, anechoic, isosonic).

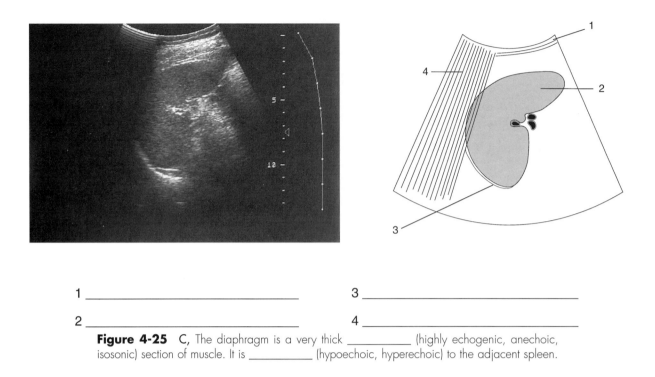

1 _____   3 _____

2 _____   4 _____

Figure 4-25 C, The diaphragm is a very thick _____ (highly echogenic, anechoic, isosonic) section of muscle. It is _____ (hypoechoic, hyperechoic) to the adjacent spleen.

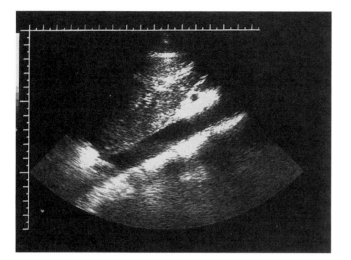
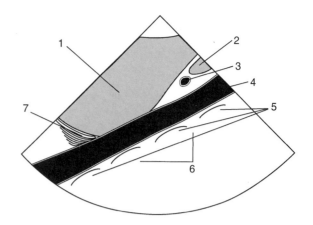

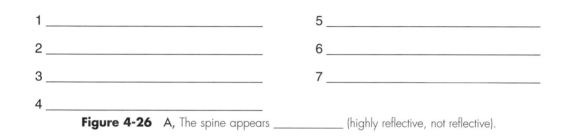

1 _____   5 _____

2 _____   6 _____

3 _____   7 _____

4 _____

Figure 4-26 A, The spine appears _____ (highly reflective, not reflective).

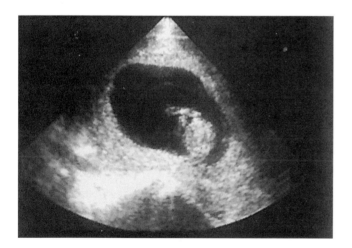
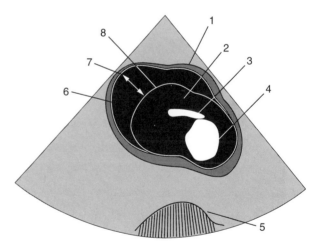

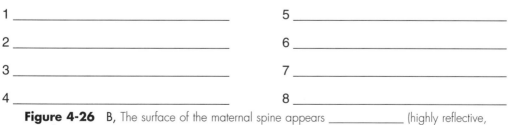

1 _____   5 _____

2 _____   6 _____

3 _____   7 _____

4 _____   8 _____

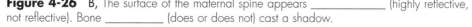

Figure 4-26 B, The surface of the maternal spine appears _____ (highly reflective, not reflective). Bone _____ (does or does not) cast a shadow.

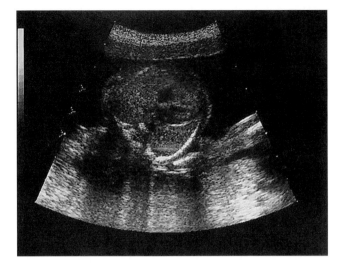
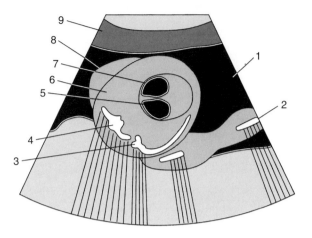

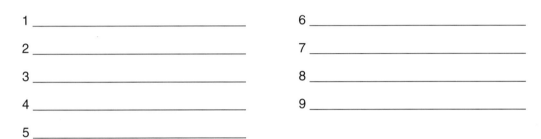

1 _____   6 _____

2 _____   7 _____

3 _____   8 _____

4 _____   9 _____

5 _____

Figure 4-26 C, Fetal bones are easily recognized because of their _____ (highly reflective, not reflective) appearance and _____ (shadowing or nonshadowing) characteristic.

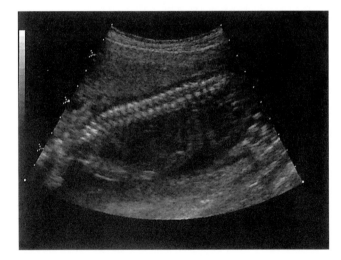
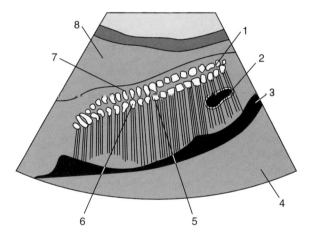

1 _____   5 _____

2 _____   6 _____

3 _____   7 _____

4 _____   8 _____

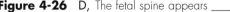
Figure 4-26 D, The fetal spine appears _____.

CHAPTER 5

The Abdominal Aorta

REVIEW QUESTIONS

1. The normal aorta _____ in diameter as it progresses inferiorly.
   a. increases
   b. decreases
   c. remains the same
   d. turns into a vein

2. The common hepatic artery branches from the
   a. proper hepatic artery
   b. left hepatic artery
   c. right hepatic artery
   d. celiac axis

3. The normal aorta should not exceed _____ in diameter.
   a. 3 cm
   b. 4 cm
   c. 2 cm
   d. 1.5 cm

4. The abdominal aorta cannot be imaged in the _____ plane.
   a. sagittal
   b. transverse
   c. longitudinal
   d. thoracic

5. The celiac artery is a branch of the
   a. aorta
   b. iliac artery
   c. gonadal artery
   d. common hepatic artery

6. Arteriography is used to determine
   a. arterial wall thickness
   b. arterial stenosis
   c. arterial flow rate
   d. plethysmography

7. The inferior mesenteric artery is demonstrated with sonography
   a. most of the time
   b. none of the time
   c. infrequently
   d. consistently

8. The three branches of the celiac artery are
   a. left gastric artery, splenic artery, common hepatic artery
   b. left gastric artery, splenic artery, proper hepatic artery
   c. right gastric artery, splenic artery, proper hepatic artery
   d. right gastric artery, common and proper hepatic arteries

9. The structure(s) that receive(s) blood from the superior mesenteric artery include(s) the
   a. brain
   b. head and neck
   c. intestines and pancreas
   d. intestines and kidney

10. Computed tomography (compared with sonography) has the disadvantage of
    a. being portable
    b. producing radiation

    c. being very inaccurate

    d. using magnetic waves to produce an image

11. The aorta is considered the abdominal aorta after it passes through the

    a. diaphragm

    b. first thoracic vertebra

    c. sacrum

    d. second cervical vertebra

12. The right and left renal arteries come off the aorta on either side immediately distal to the

    a. inferior mesenteric artery

    b. celiac artery

    c. superior mesenteric artery

    d. testicular/ovarian artery

13. The right renal artery travels _____ to the inferior vena cava and is _____ than the left renal artery.

    a. posterior/longer

    b. anterior/longer

    c. posterior/shorter

    d. anterior/shorter

14. The celiac artery comes off the aorta _____ to the superior mesenteric artery.

    a. distal

    b. lateral

    c. superficial

    d. superior

15. Distally, the aorta bifurcates into the

    a. gonadal/ovarian arteries

    b. common iliac arteries

    c. inferior phrenic arteries

    d. medial and lateral sacral arteries

16. The common hepatic artery branches into the

    a. proper hepatic and right gastric arteries

    b. proper hepatic and gastroduodenal arteries

    c. gastroduodenal and right gastric arteries

    d. gastroduodenal and left gastric arteries

17. The proper hepatic artery branches into vessels that perfuse the

    a. liver and large intestine

    b. liver and small intestine

    c. liver and urinary bladder

    d. liver and gallbladder

18. The wall of the aorta has _____ layers

    a. 3

    b. 1

    c. 4

    d. 2

19. Sonographically, the normal aorta should have an _____ lumen with _____ walls.

    a. echogenic/anechoic

    b. anechoic/anechoic

    c. echogenic/echogenic

    d. anechoic/echogenic

20. Ultrasound of the aorta is primarily used to identify aneurysms and stenosis.

    a. true

    b. false

21. Name the three types of aneurysms that can affect the aorta.

22. Name the layers of the wall of the aorta.

Identify the structures indicated in the following illustrations. These figures duplicate those found in *Sonography: Introduction to Normal Structure and Function.* Refer to the textbook if you need help.

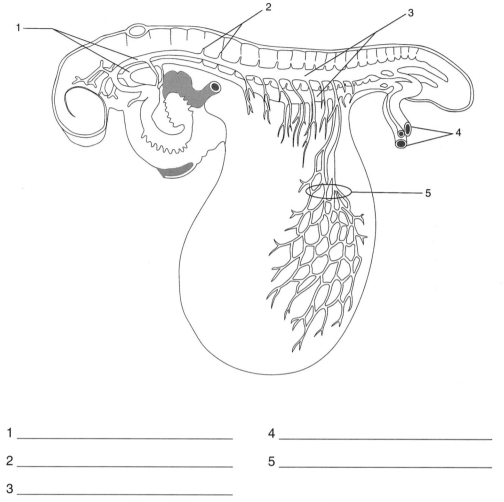

1 _____   4 _____

2 _____   5 _____

3 _____

Figure 5-1 Aortic embryologic development.

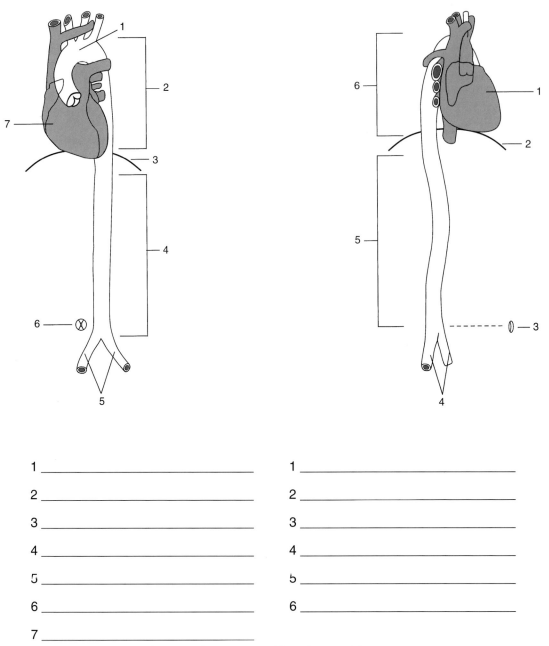

1 _____   1 _____

2 _____   2 _____

3 _____   3 _____

4 _____   4 _____

5 _____   5 _____

6 _____   6 _____

7 _____

Figure 5-2 Anterior and lateral views of the aorta.

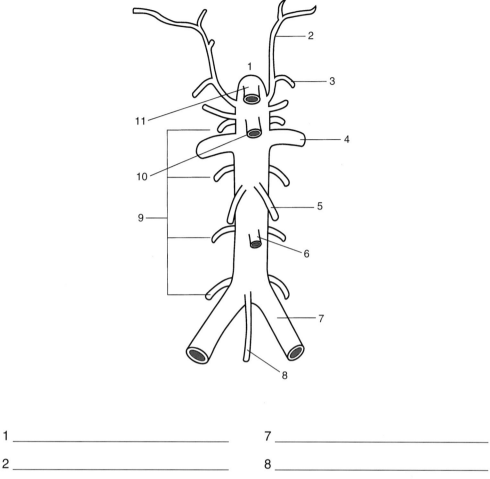

1 _____   7 _____

2 _____   8 _____

3 _____   9 _____

4 _____   10 _____

5 _____   11 _____

6 _____

Figure 5-3 Initial branches of the abdominal aorta.

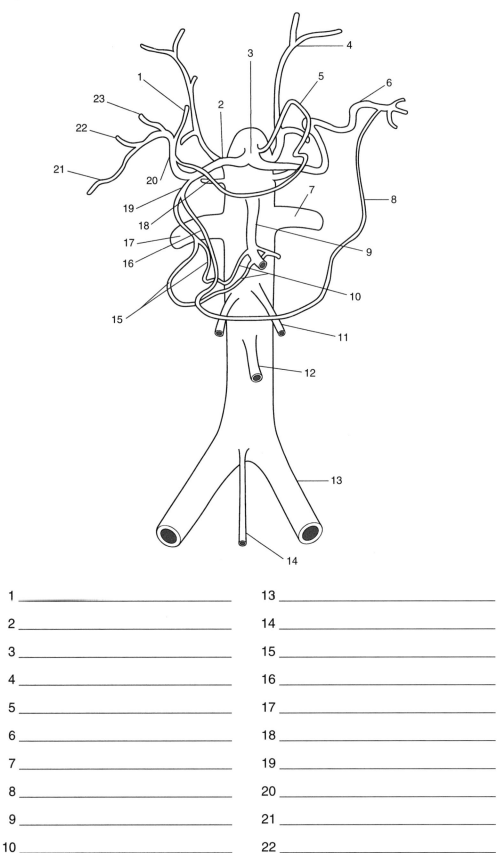

1 _____   13 _____

2 _____   14 _____

3 _____   15 _____

4 _____   16 _____

5 _____   17 _____

6 _____   18 _____

7 _____   19 _____

8 _____   20 _____

9 _____   21 _____

10 _____   22 _____

11 _____   23 _____

12 _____

Figure 5-4 Branches of the abdominal aorta.

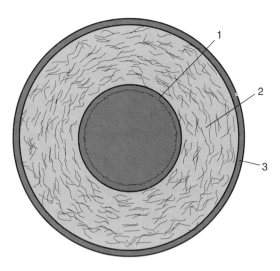

1 _____

2 _____

3 _____

Figure 5-5 Cross-section of an arterial wall.

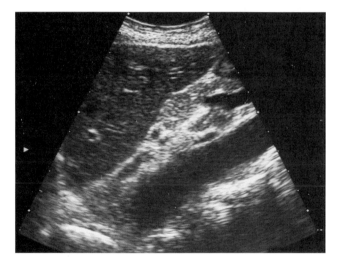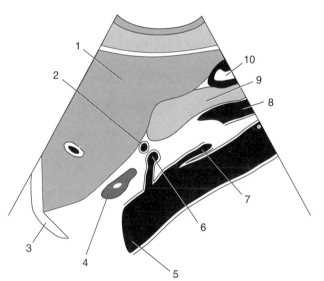

1 _____   6 _____

2 _____   7 _____

3 _____   8 _____

4 _____   9 _____

5 _____   10 _____

Figure 5-6 Longitudinal section of the proximal aorta.

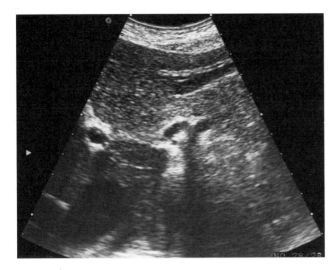
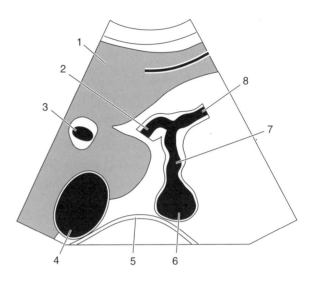

1 _____   5 _____

2 _____   6 _____

3 _____   7 _____

4 _____   8 _____

Figure 5-7 Transverse section of the aorta.

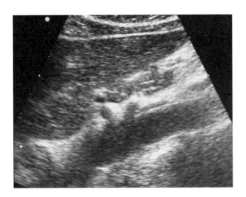
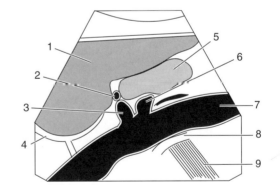

1 _____   6 _____

2 _____   7 _____

3 _____   8 _____

4 _____   9 _____

5 _____

Figure 5-8 Longitudinal section of the mid aorta.

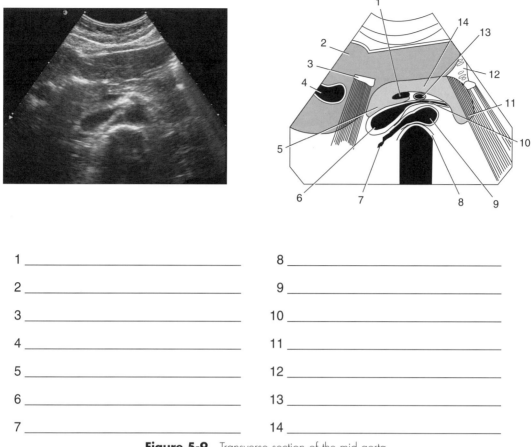

Figure 5-9   Transverse section of the mid aorta.

1 _____	8 _____
2 _____	9 _____
3 _____	10 _____
4 _____	11 _____
5 _____	12 _____
6 _____	13 _____
7 _____	14 _____

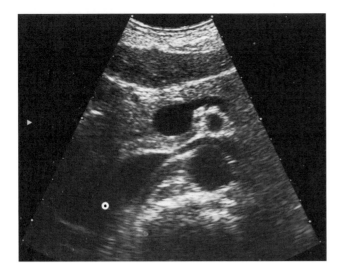
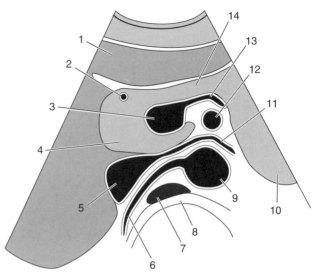

1 _____   8 _____

2 _____   9 _____

3 _____   10 _____

4 _____   11 _____

5 _____   12 _____

6 _____   13 _____

7 _____   14 _____

Figure 5-10 Transverse section of the mid aorta.

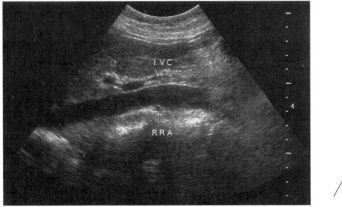
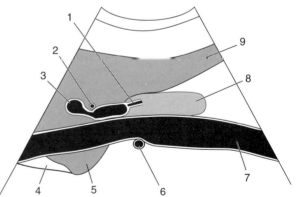

1 _____   6 _____

2 _____   7 _____

3 _____   8 _____

4 _____   9 _____

5 _____

Figure 5-11 Longitudinal section of the inferior vena cava.

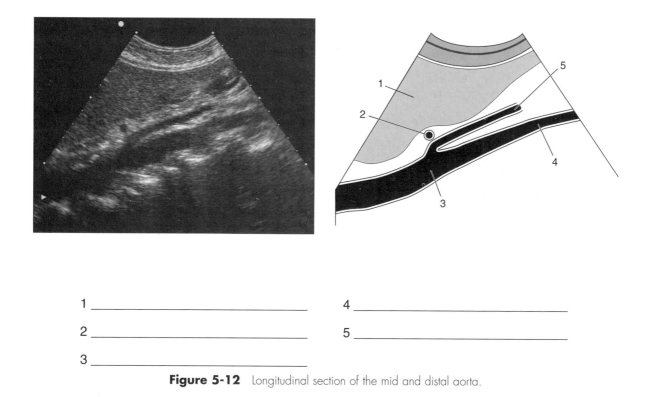

1 _____   4 _____

2 _____   5 _____

3 _____

Figure 5-12 Longitudinal section of the mid and distal aorta.

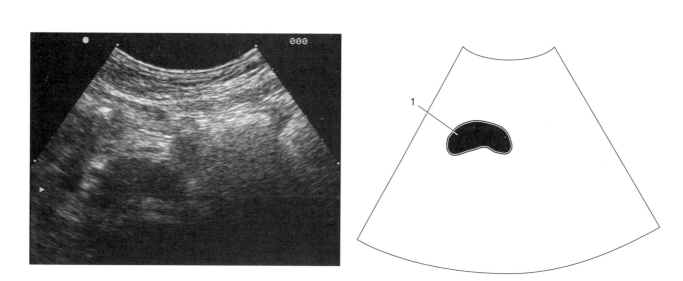

1 _____

Figure 5-13 Transverse section of the distal aorta.

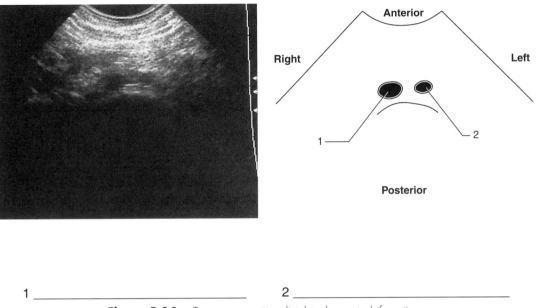

1 _____ 2 _____

Figure 5-14   Transverse section distal to the aorta bifurcation.

CHAPTER 6

The Inferior Vena Cava

REVIEW QUESTIONS

1. The normal venous system is a _____ pressure system.
   a. low
   b. high
   c. medium
   d. no

2. The left gonadal vein empties into the
   a. inferior vena cava
   b. right renal vein
   c. left renal vein
   d. right gonadal vein

3. The right gonadal vein empties into the
   a. inferior vena cava
   b. right renal vein
   c. left renal vein
   d. left gonadal vein

4. _____ is the gold standard when evaluating veins.
   a. Magnetic resonance imaging
   b. Computed tomography
   c. Venography
   d. B-mode sonography

5. The superior mesenteric vein empties into the
   a. inferior vena cava
   b. portal vein
   c. right renal vein
   d. splenic vein

6. The primary function of the IVC is to
   a. carry deoxygenated blood to the heart
   b. carry deoxygenated blood from the heart
   c. regulate heat dissipation from organs
   d. act as a lymph drainage channel

7. Blood flow in veins should be _____ and _____.
   a. spontaneous/phasic
   b. spontaneous/nonphasic
   c. nonspontaneous/phasic
   d. nonspontaneous/nonphasic

8. The inferior vena cava has _____ tunica media than the aorta.
   a. a thicker
   b. a thinner
   c. the same size
   d. a more echogenic

9. The left renal vein has a(n) _____ course compared with the right renal vein.
   a. longer
   b. shorter
   c. wider
   d. identical

10. The lumen of all normal veins should appear without echoes except for
    a. thrombus
    b. valves and slow-moving blood
    c. tumors
    d. aggregated red blood cells

11. Because of the complex formation of the IVC, many possible variations are possible.
    a. true
    b. false

12. Possible congenital variations in IVC formation include
    a. double IVC
    b. left-sided IVC
    c. absence of certain portions of IVC
    d. all of the above
    e. no variations are possible

13. Venous valves
    a. allow blood to move in both directions
    b. help prevent the lumen from overdistension
    c. prevent backflow of blood
    d. are remnants of earlier structures and serve no purpose

14. During real-time sonographic evaluation, the IVC displays significant variation in diameter; however, it should not exceed _____ in diameter.
    a. 1.0 cm
    b. 3.7 cm
    c. 2.5 cm
    d. 0.5 cm

15. The _____ veins drain the lower extremities and pelvis and join to form the IVC.
    a. common iliac veins
    b. inferior phrenic veins
    c. lumbar veins
    d. gonadal veins

16. The left renal vein passes _____ to the aorta and _____ to the superior mesenteric artery as it travels from the left kidney to the IVC.
    a. anterior/anterior
    b. posterior/posterior

    c. anterior/posterior
    d. posterior/anterior

17. Normally the diameter of the IVC will _____ during a Valsalva maneuver or inspiration.
    a. increase
    b. decrease
    c. stay the same
    d. collapse

18. The _____ vein(s) and _____ vein(s) are not consistently imaged.
    a. left hepatic/right hepatic
    b. right renal/left renal
    c. left iliac/right iliac
    d. gonadal/lumbar

19. The IVC and its visible branches are sonographically evaluated for evidence of
    a. intraluminal thrombosis
    b. tumor invasion
    c. a and b
    d. none of the above

20. Vascular surgeons generally treat patients with disorders of the venous system, but other physicians are often involved depending on the other organs involved and the need for treatment other than surgery.
    a. true
    b. false

21. Name three of the common diagnostic tests that may be used to evaluate the venous system.

Identify the structures indicated in the following illustrations. These figures duplicate those found in *Sonography: Introduction to Normal Structure and Function.* Refer to the textbook if you need help.

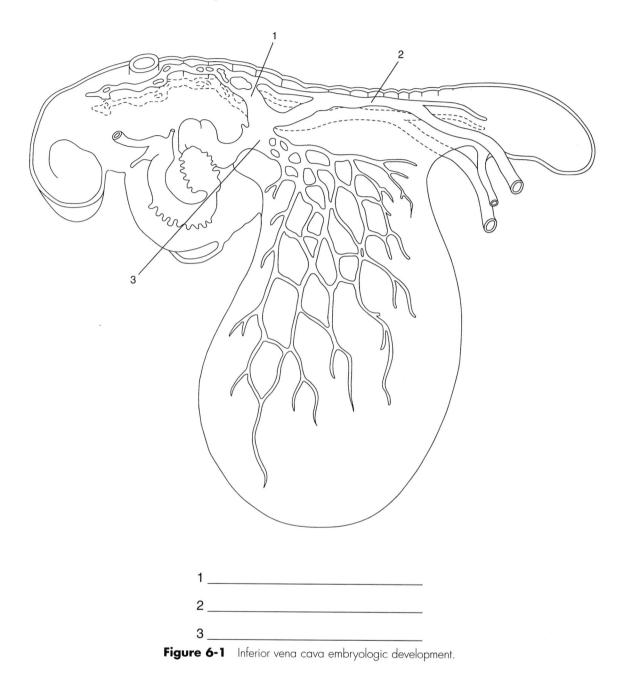

1 _____

2 _____

3 _____

Figure 6-1 Inferior vena cava embryologic development.

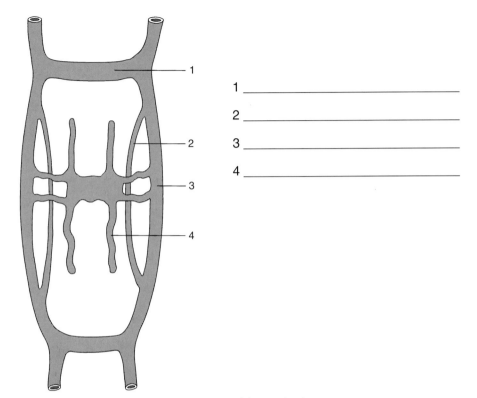

1 _____
2 _____
3 _____
4 _____

Figure 6-2   Anterior view of the cardinal venous system.

1 _____
2 _____
3 _____
4 _____
5 _____

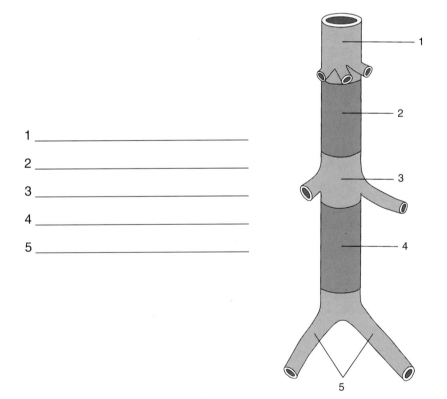

Figure 6-3   Inferior vena cava sections.

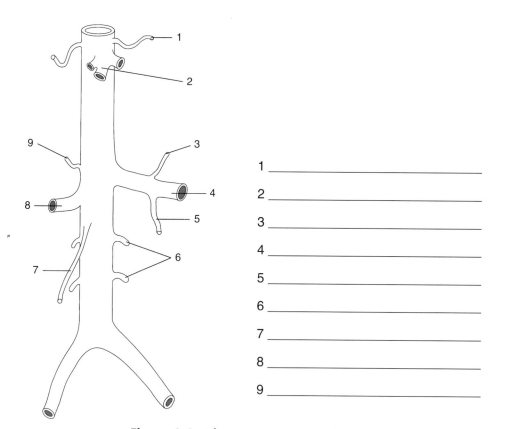

Figure 6-4 Inferior vena cava major tributaries.

1 _____

2 _____

3 _____

4 _____

5 _____

6 _____

7 _____

8 _____

9 _____

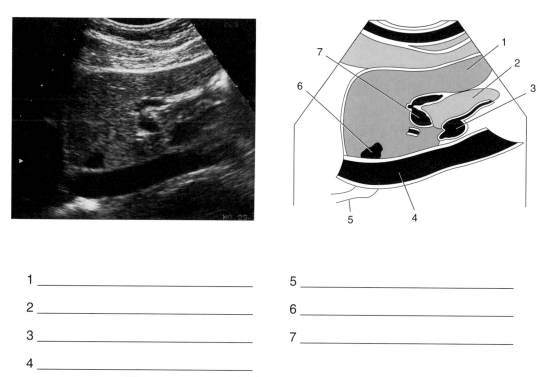

1 _____   5 _____

2 _____   6 _____

3 _____   7 _____

4 _____

Figure 6-5 Longitudinal section of the inferior vena cava.

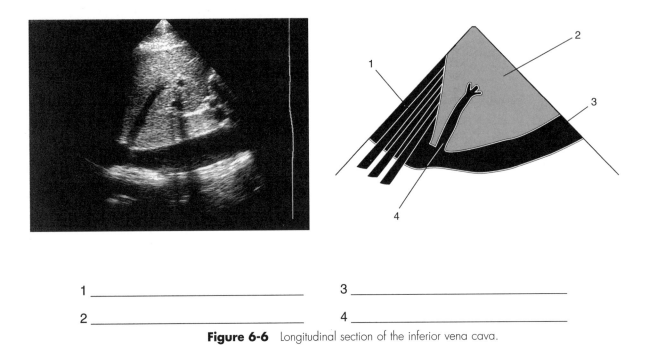

1 _____   3 _____

2 _____   4 _____

Figure 6-6 Longitudinal section of the inferior vena cava.

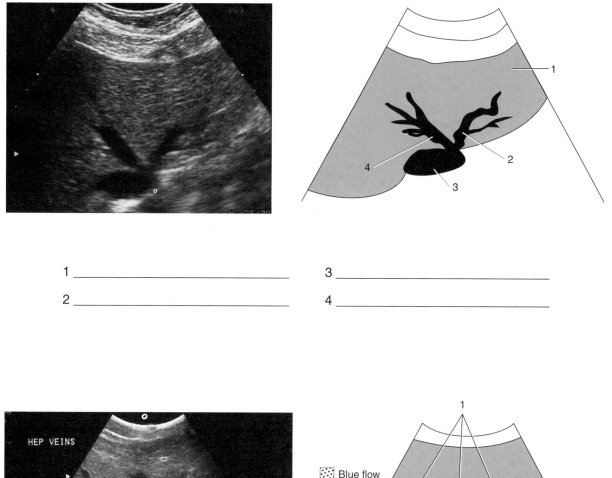

1 _____   3 _____

2 _____   4 _____

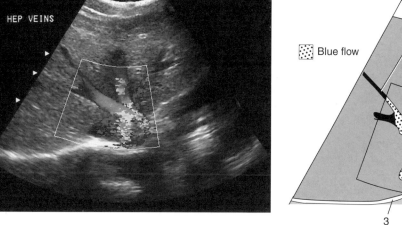

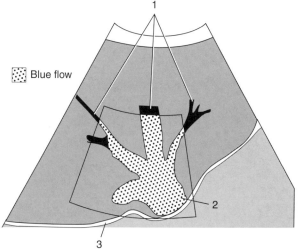

1 _____

2 _____

3 _____

Figure 6-7 Transverse sections of the inferior vena cava.

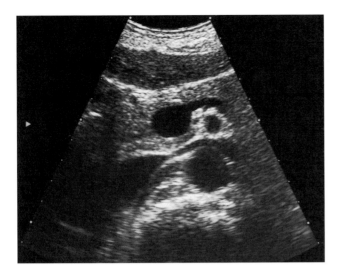
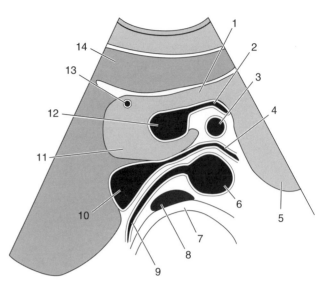

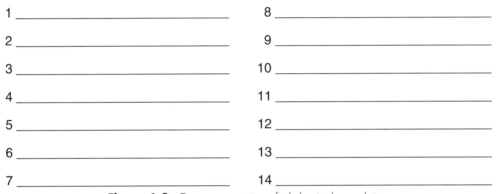

1 _____   8 _____

2 _____   9 _____

3 _____   10 _____

4 _____   11 _____

5 _____   12 _____

6 _____   13 _____

7 _____   14 _____

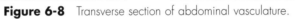

Figure 6-8 Transverse section of abdominal vasculature.

CHAPTER 7

The Portal Venous System

REVIEW QUESTIONS

1. The portal vein supplies the liver with
   a. arterial blood
   b. venous blood
   c. oxygenated blood
   d. venous blood rich in nutrients

2. The portal vein empties blood from
   a. the liver
   b. the gastrointestinal system
   c. the kidneys
   d. the upper body trunk

3. The portal vein should
   a. measure up to 13 mm
   b. measure slightly more than 13 mm
   c. not be easily seen with sonography
   d. be seen with sonography only when the patient is supine

4. The _____ and _____ join to form the portal vein.
   a. superior mesenteric vein/splenic vein
   b. inferior mesenteric vein/splenic vein
   c. superior mesenteric vein/inferior mesenteric vein
   d. inferior vena cava/superior mesenteric vein

5. The right portal vein branches into _____ and _____
   a. anterior/posterior
   b. right/left
   c. anterior/right
   d. medial/lateral

6. The superior mesenteric vein and inferior mesenteric vein empty the
   a. liver
   b. spleen
   c. intestine
   d. gallbladder

7. The portal veins are distinguished on a sonogram by their
   a. highly echogenic walls
   b. anechoic walls
   c. echofree walls
   d. bright red walls when color Doppler is applied

8. The medial branch of the left portal vein feeds the
   a. traditional left lobe of the liver
   b. medial segment of the left lobe of the liver
   c. right lobe of the liver
   d. caudate lobe of the liver

9. The left main portal vein divides into _____ and _____
   a. anterior/posterior
   b. medial/lateral
   c. right/anterior
   d. anterior/left

10. Blood traveling from the spleen to the liver must pass through the
    a. main portal vein
    b. inferior mesenteric vein
    c. superior mesenteric vein
    d. portal artery

11. The function of the portal vein is to deliver blood from the spleen and gastrointestinal tract to the liver for _____ and _____.

a. culling/pitting

b. cholelithiasis/blastocytosis

c. vasodilation/retroflexion

d. metabolism/detoxification

12. Flow should be toward the liver from the portal vein. This flow should be _____ in response to respiration.

a. high pressure

b. phasic

c. nonphasic

d. bigeminy

13. In addition to evaluation of the portal vein for tumor invasion and thrombosis, the most common reason is to uncover portal vein

a. collapse

b. distension

c. hypertension

d. necrosis

14. Pathologies that affect other abdominal organs are often the reason for portal vein pathology.

a. true

b. false

Identify the structures indicated in the following illustrations. These figures duplicate those found in *Sonography: Introduction to Normal Structure and Function.* Refer to the textbook if you need help.

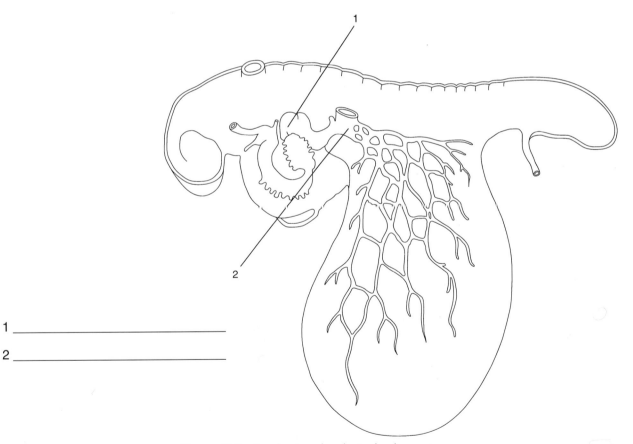

1 _____

2 _____

Figure 7-1 Portal vein embryologic development.

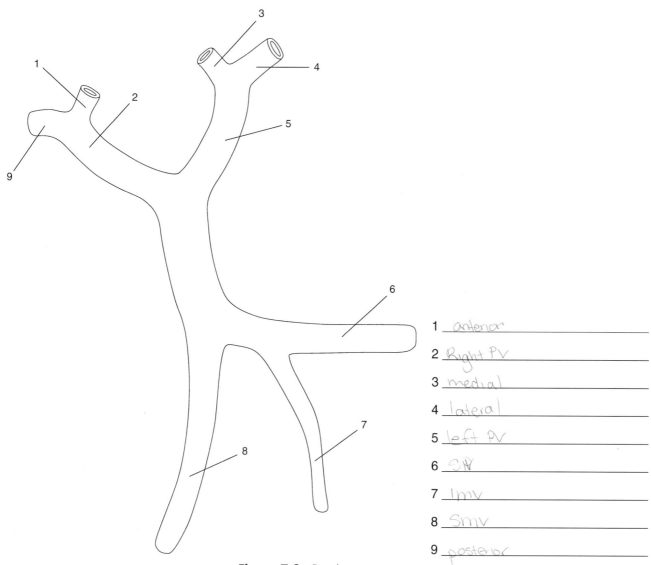

1 _anterior_____

2 _Right PV_____

3 _medial_____

4 _lateral_____

5 _left PV_____

6 _SV_____

7 _Imv_____

8 _Smv_____

9 _posterior_____

Figure 7-2 Portal venous system.

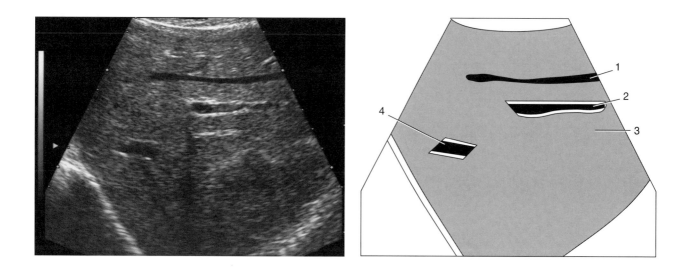

1 _____ 3 _____

2 _____ 4 _____

Figure 7-3 Liver vasculature.

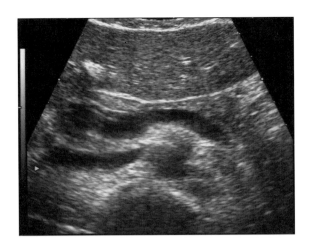
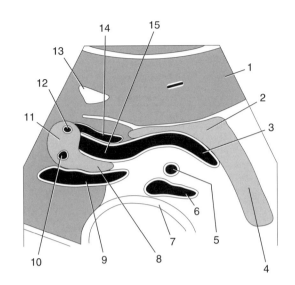

1 _____   9 _____

2 _____   10 _____

3 _____   11 _____

4 _____   12 _____

5 _____   13 _____

6 _____   14 _____

7 _____   15 _____

8 _____

Figure 7-4 Epigastric transverse scan.

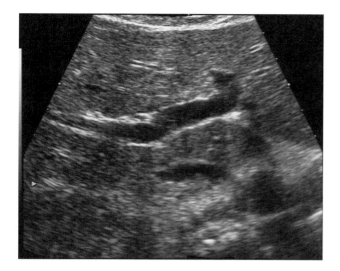

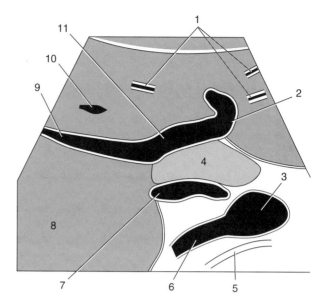

1 _____

2 _____

3 _____

4 _____

5 _____

6 _____

7 _____

8 _____

9 _____

10 _____

11 _____

Figure 7-5 Epigastric transverse scan.

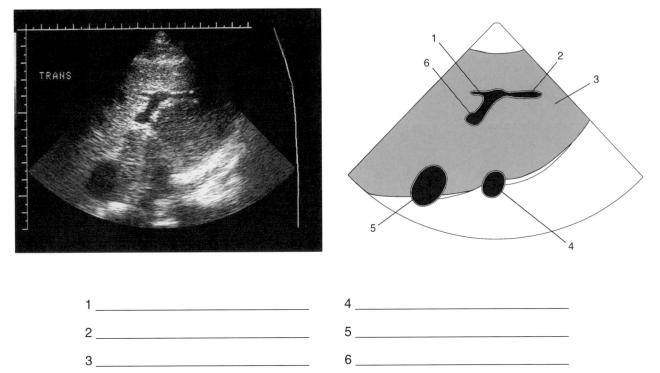

1 _____   4 _____

2 _____   5 _____

3 _____   6 _____

Figure 7-6 Epigastric transverse scan.

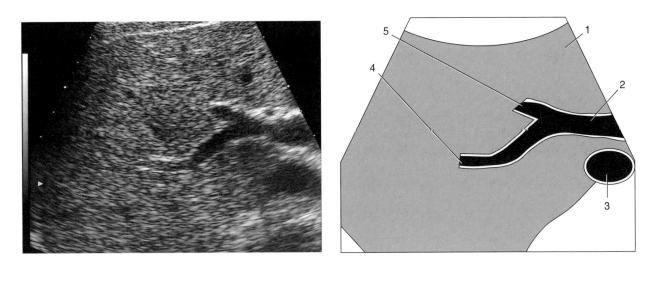

1 _____   4 _____

2 _____   5 _____

3 _____

Figure 7-7 Right liver lobe, transverse scan.

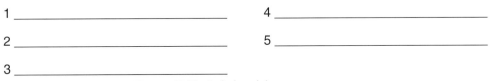

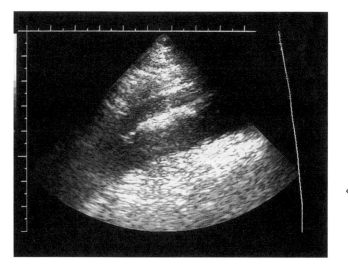
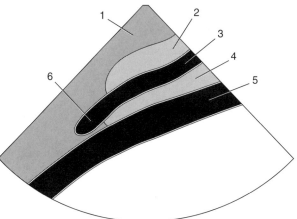

1 _____   4 _____

2 _____   5 _____

3 _____   6 _____

Figure 7-8 Epigastric sagittal scan.

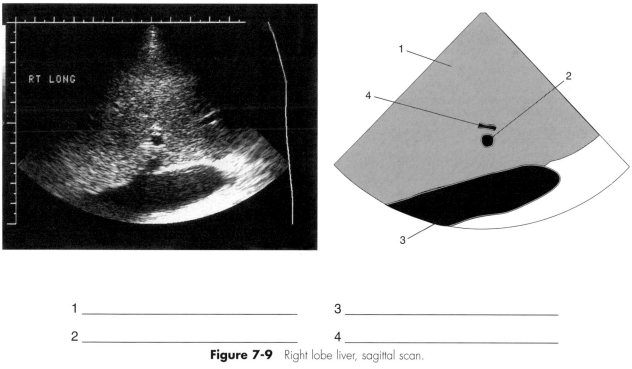

1 _____   3 _____

2 _____   4 _____

Figure 7-9 Right lobe liver, sagittal scan.

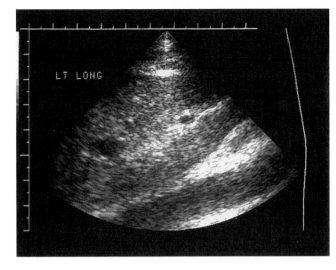

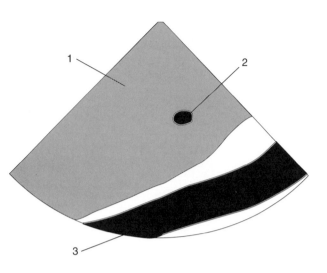

1 _____

2 _____

3 _____

Figure 7-10   Epigastric sagittal scan.

CHAPTER 8

Abdominal Vasculature

REVIEW QUESTIONS

1. Which statement regarding the celiac artery is not true?

   a. the celiac artery feeds organs that have low vascular resistance.

   b. the celiac artery has three branches: the common hepatic, splenic, and left gastric

   c. the celiac artery originates from the posterolateral wall of the abdominal aorta

   d. the superior mesenteric artery and the celiac artery may share a common trunk at their origin

2. Which structure does not border the abdominal aorta anteriorly?

   a. stomach

   b. superior mesenteric artery

   c. celiac axis

   d. portal vein

3. The characteristics of the Doppler spectral waveform from the normal infrarenal abdominal aorta include:

   a. rapid systolic upstroke and rapid deceleration with flow reversal in late systole

   b. rapid systolic upstroke and rapid deceleration with constant forward diastolic flow

   c. rapid systolic upstroke, delayed deceleration, and low diastolic flow

   d. rapid systolic upstroke, reversed late systolic flow, and constant forward diastolic flow

4. The blood flow pattern in the normal renal artery can be characterized as

   a. low resistance with low diastolic flow

   b. high resistance with low diastolic flow

   c. low resistance with high diastolic flow

   d. high resistance with high diastolic flow

5. Which of the following statements best describes the blood flow pattern in the superior mesenteric artery after ingestion of a meal?

   a. peak systolic velocity greater than 200 cm/sec with high diastolic flow

   b. peak systolic velocity less than 200 cm/sec with low diastolic flow

   c. peak systolic velocity greater than 200 cm/sec with low diastolic flow and systolic flow reversal

   d. peak systolic velocity greater than 200 cm/sec, systolic flow reversal, and high diastolic forward flow

6. High-resistance Doppler spectral waveforms recorded throughout the renal medulla and cortex would suggest

   a. proximal renal artery stenosis

   b. flow-limiting disease in the distal renal artery

   c. intrinsic medical renal disease

   d. the presence of accessory renal arteries

7. Which of the following is not a branch of the inferior vena cava?

   a. hepatic vein

   b. portal vein

   c. renal vein

   d. right suprarenal vein

8. Which of the following statements regarding the portal vein is not true?
   a. the portal vein supplies approximately 70% of the oxygenated blood flow to the liver
   b. the portal vein is an intraabdominal vein
   c. the portal vein is formed by the confluence of the umbilical, splenic, and superior mesenteric veins
   d. blood flow in the portal vein is normally hepatopetal in direction

9. The hepatic artery enters the porta hepatis along with the
   a. right hepatic and splenic veins
   b. right hepatic vein and the common bile duct
   c. left portal vein and right branch of the hepatic artery
   d. main portal vein and common bile duct

10. Blood flow in the right, middle, and left hepatic veins is characterized by
    a. four phases of flow: two away from the heart and two toward the heart
    b. three phases of flow: two toward the heart and then a phase of systolic flow reversal
    c. three phases of flow: one toward the heart and then two away from the heart
    d. four phases of flow: two toward the heart followed by two away from the heart

11. Normally flow patterns in the portal vein and its branches are characterized by
    a. continuous, or minimally phasic, disordered flow with low peak and mean velocities
    b. pulsatile, biphasic, disordered flow with low mean velocities
    c. continuous, minimally phasic, disordered flow with high mean velocities
    d. phasic flow with low peak and mean velocities

12. Which of the following does not affect portal venous flow?
    a. posture
    b. dietary state
    c. hematocrit
    d. exercise

13. Which of the following statements is not true regarding the renal arteries?
    a. the renal arteries originate from the lateral wall of the abdominal aorta

b. the proximal renal arteries follow the crus of the diaphragm
c. the right renal artery courses posterior to the inferior vena cava
d. the left renal artery lies superior to the left renal vein

14. The left renal vein serves as a valuable landmark for locating the renal arteries. The left renal vein courses
    a. anterior to the abdominal aorta; posterior to the superior mesenteric artery
    b. posterior to the abdominal aorta; anterior to the left renal artery
    c. posterior to the inferior vena cava; anterior to the abdominal aorta
    d. anterior to the inferior vena cava; anterior to the abdominal aorta

15. Which of the following statements is incorrect?
    a. the inferior mesenteric artery lies anterolateral to the abdominal aorta and enters the pelvis as the superior hemorrhoidal artery
    b. the suprarenal abdominal aortic Doppler velocity waveform is triphasic due to the high resistance vascular bed of the fasting superior mesenteric artery
    c. the kidneys and liver are high resistance end organs
    d. the Doppler time velocity waveform from the postprandial superior mesenteric artery will demonstrate low diastolic flow due to the change in the vascular resistance of the stomach and small intestine that occurs with digestion

16. The Doppler special waveform from the normal renal artery will exhibit constant forward diastolic flow.
    a. true
    b. false

17. Which of the following is an incorrect statement regarding blood flow to the kidney?
    a. the Doppler velocity signal from the interlobar arteries demonstrates significant forward diastolic flow
    b. the spectral waveform from the arcuate vessels of the kidney of a patient in chronic renal failure will exhibit decreased diastolic flow
    c. due to the high metabolic demands of the kidney, flow is forward during diastole
    d. the velocity spectral waveforms from the medulla and cortex of a kidney are normally pulsatile

Identify the structures indicated in the following illustrations. These figures duplicate those found in *Sonography: Introduction to Normal Structure and Function.* Refer to the textbook if you need help.

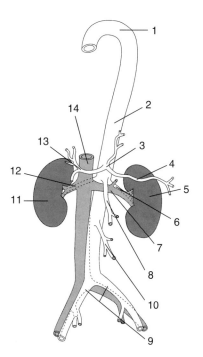

1 _____   8 _____

2 _____   9 _____

3 _____   10 _____

4 _____   11 _____

5 _____   12 _____

6 _____   13 _____

7 _____   14 _____

Figure 8-1 Visceral arterial system.

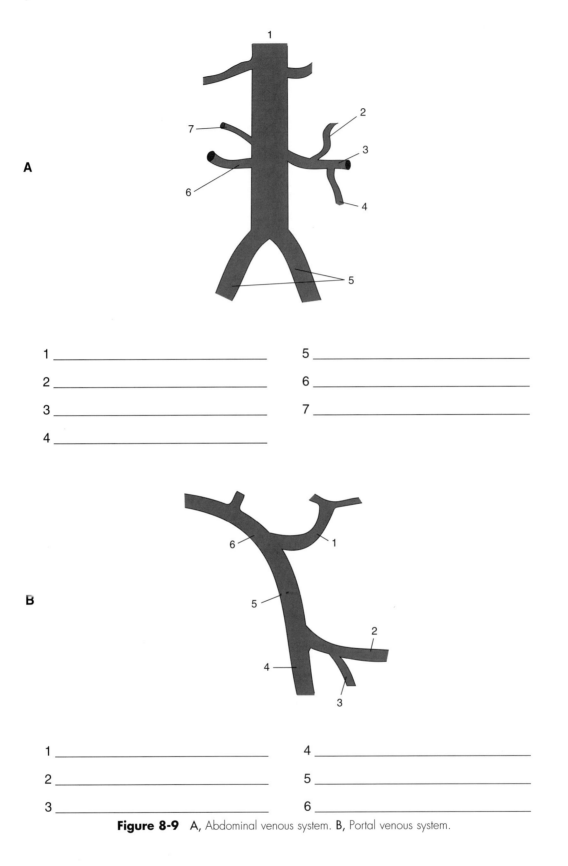

A

1 _____   5 _____

2 _____   6 _____

3 _____   7 _____

4 _____

B

1 _____   4 _____

2 _____   5 _____

3 _____   6 _____

Figure 8-9 **A,** Abdominal venous system. **B,** Portal venous system.

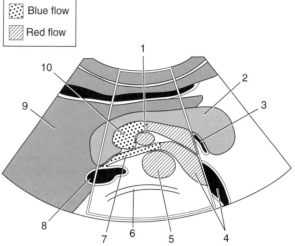

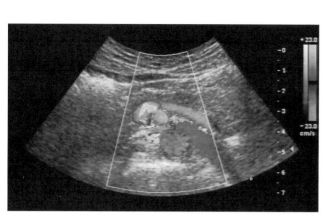

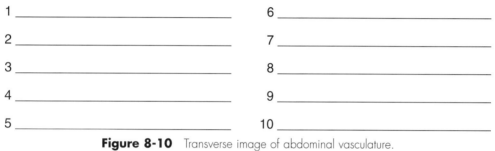

| Blue flow |
| Red flow |

1 _____   6 _____

2 _____   7 _____

3 _____   8 _____

4 _____   9 _____

5 _____   10 _____

Figure 8-10 Transverse image of abdominal vasculature.

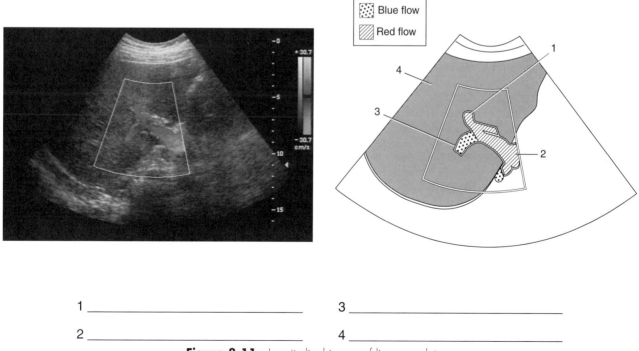

| Blue flow |
| Red flow |

1 _____   3 _____

2 _____   4 _____

Figure 8-11 Longitudinal image of liver vasculature.

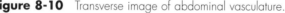
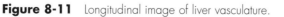

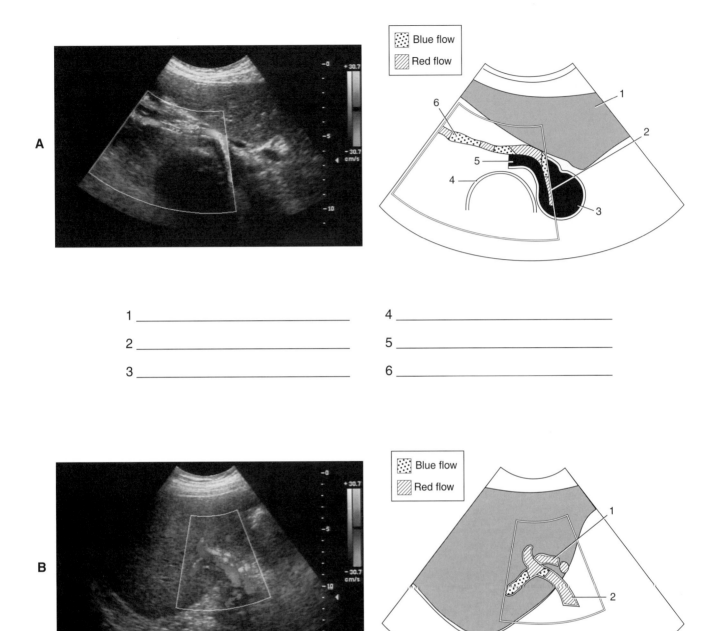

1 _____   4 _____

2 _____   5 _____

3 _____   6 _____

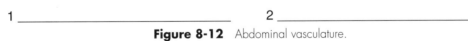

1 _____   2 _____

Figure 8-12 Abdominal vasculature.

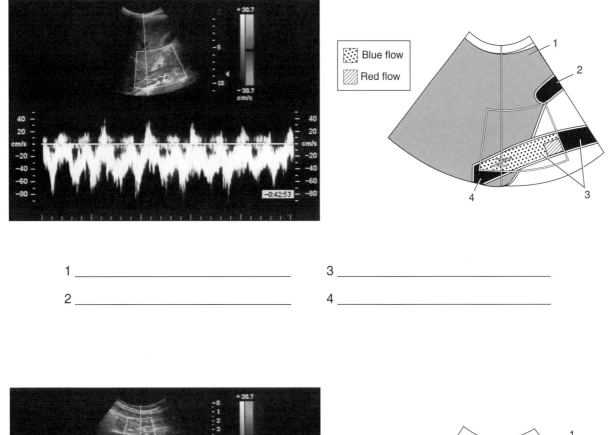

A

Blue flow
Red flow

1 _____   3 _____

2 _____   4 _____

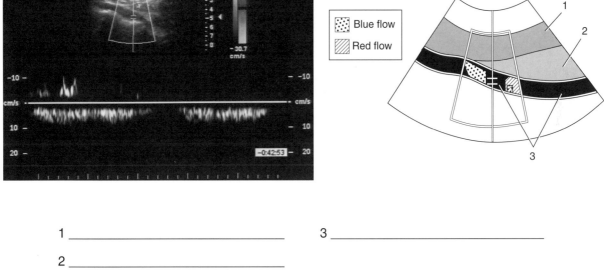

B

Blue flow
Red flow

1 _____   3 _____

2 _____

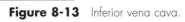

Figure 8-13 Inferior vena cava.

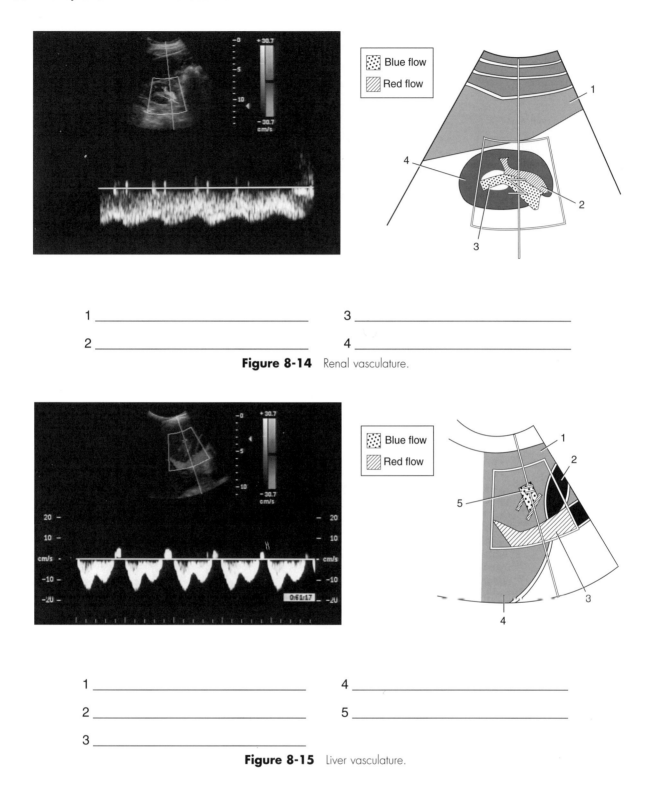

1 _____   3 _____

2 _____   4 _____

Figure 8-14   Renal vasculature.

1 _____   4 _____

2 _____   5 _____

3 _____

Figure 8-15   Liver vasculature.

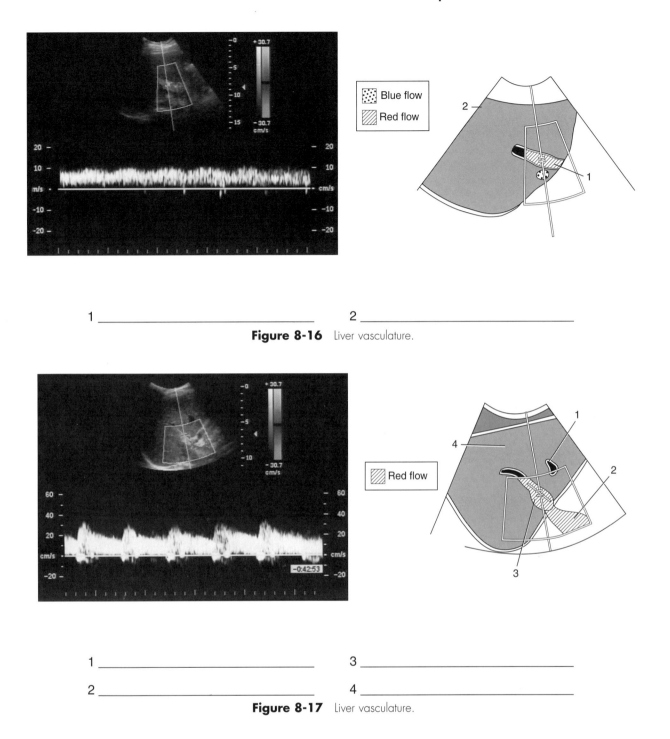

1 _____   2 _____

Figure 8-16 Liver vasculature.

1 _____   3 _____

2 _____   4 _____

Figure 8-17 Liver vasculature.

■ CHAPTER 9

The Liver

REVIEW QUESTIONS

1. The liver originates from which portion of the primitive gut?

   a. foregut

   b. hindgut

   c. midgut

   d. mesentery

2. Any of the following are located within a lobule of the liver, except

   a. hepatocytes

   b. Kupffer cells

   c. portal venules

   d. blood sinuses

3. Hemopoiesis is responsible for _____ of the liver.

   a. hepatocyte formation

   b. the large size

   c. the rapid development

   d. drainage systems

4. Anomalies of the liver include each of those listed, except

   a. situs inversus

   b. hemangioma

   c. extrahepatic biliary stenosis

   d. Reidel's lobe

5. The surface of the liver that rests on the abdominal organs is the _____ surface.

   a. anterior

   b. posterior

   c. superior

   d. inferior

6. The base of the liver pyramid is the _____ surface.

   a. right lateral

   b. superior

   c. left inferior

   d. anterior

7. The caudate lobe of the liver is related to each of the following except the

   a. left portal vein

   b. posterior abdominal wall

   c. splenic vein

   d. inferior vena cava

8. The boundaries of the bare area of the liver include the

   a. lesser sac, hepatoduodenal ligament, and the right kidney

   b. falciform, coronary, and triangular ligaments

   c. inferior vena cava, middle hepatic vein, and main portal vein

   d. left coronary ligament, transverse colon, and stomach antrum

9. The liver occupies a major portion of the _____ region.

   a. hypogastric

   b. umbilical

   c. epigastric

   d. right hypochondriac

10. The inferior surface of the liver is marked by indentations from each of the following, except the
 a. hepatic flexure of the colon
 b. head of the pancreas
 c. right adrenal gland
 d. first part of the duodenum

11. The medial portion of the left lobe of the liver is also referred to as the
 a. Glisson's cap
 b. main lobar fissure
 c. papillary projection
 d. quadrate lobe

12. The left hepatic lobe is _____ size and shape.
 a. fixed in
 b. increased, when compared with the right by
 c. variable in
 d. dependent on the medial lobe for its

13. Which of the following would result in a false statement? The free inferior margin of the left lobe lies adjacent to the
 a. body of the pancreas
 b. splenic vein
 c. hepatic flexure
 d. splenic artery

14. The liver metabolizes
 a. fats, carbohydrates, and proteins
 b. complex sugars, salts, and bile
 c. blood proteins and lymph fluids
 d. none of the above

15. The liver is composed of _____ true lobes.
 a. two
 b. three
 c. four
 d. five

16. The left hepatic vein and the _____ separate the left hepatic lobe from the caudate.
 a. quadrate lobe
 b. intersegmental fissure
 c. bare area
 d. fissure for the ligamentum venosum

17. The hepatic veins are _____ and _____. (Select 2.)
 a. interlobar
 b. intralobar
 c. intrasegmental
 d. intersegmental

18. The portal system supplies what percentage of total blood flow to the liver?
 a. 30
 b. 50
 c. 75
 d. 90

19. The portal confluence has three main tributaries: the inferior mesenteric vein, the superior mesenteric vein, and the
 a. middle hepatic vein
 b. pancreaticoduodenal vein
 c. superior phrenic vein
 d. splenic vein

20. The left portal vein communicates with the _____ in patients with severe portal hypertension.
 a. right portal vein
 b. umbilical vein
 c. splenic artery
 d. left hepatic vein

21. The caudate lobe is supplied with blood flow from the
 a. right portal vein
 b. left portal vein
 c. right and left portal veins
 d. gastroduodenal artery

22. The opening of the liver through which the portal veins and hepatic arteries enter and the hepatic ducts exit is called the
 a. portal duct
 b. foramen of Winslow
 c. porta hepatis
 d. greater omentum

23. The common bile duct and the hepatic artery course _____ to the portal vein within the liver.
 a. anterior
 b. medial
 c. superior
 d. posterior

24. The liver should have a/an _____ sonographic appearance.
    a. anechoic
    b. homogeneous
    c. heterogeneous
    d. low level echogenicity in its

25. The main lobar fissure represents a
    a. landmark for the caudate lobe
    b. divider between the mid and lateral portions of the left lobe
    c. marker for the falciform ligament
    d. boundary between the right and left lobes

26. The left portal vein takes a C-shaped superior course in the liver, proximal to the
    a. falciform ligament
    b. caudate lobe
    c. left hepatic vein
    d. ligamentum venosum

27. A fibrous cord that extends upward from the diaphragm to the anterior wall and was patent before birth may be noted as any of the following except the
    a. round ligament
    b. ligamentum teres
    c. falciform ligament
    d. umbilical vein

28. The hepatic veins _____ in size as they drain toward the IVC.
    a. increase
    b. decrease
    c. do not change

29. Abnormal lesions usually are _____ in echogenicity when compared with the moderate echo strength of the liver parenchyma.
    a. increased
    b. decreased
    c. either increased or decreased
    d. similar

30. Normal variants of the liver include a right lobe that may extend inferiorly to the iliac crest or a left lobe that may extend laterally to the spleen.
    a. true
    b. false

31. In human embryonic circulation, which of the following vessels are responsible for returning blood from the yolk sac to the heart?
    a. ductus venosus
    b. portal veins
    c. umbilical veins
    d. vitelline veins

32. Which of the following vessels develops as a large shunt allowing some blood to bypass the liver and flow directly from the placenta to the fetal heart?
    a. ductus venosus
    b. portal veins
    c. umbilical veins
    d. vitelline veins

33. Figure 9-9 represents the characteristic H pattern of anatomic lobar segmentation. Identify the structures and hepatic lobes represented by the line segments.
    a.   b.

    # H

    c.   d.

34. The crossbar of the H depicts the _____

Determine which type of metabolism is associated most commonly with each of the following. Mark C for carbohydrate metabolism, F for fat metabolism, and P for protein metabolism.

35. _____ ketones
36. _____ gallbladder contraction
37. _____ glucose
38. _____ cholesterol
39. _____ urea
40. _____ hair growth

41. Which of the following may be excluded from an association with bile in the liver?
    a. cholesterol   c. jaundice   e. urea
    b. bilirubin   d. fat

Identify the structures indicated in the following illustrations. These figures duplicate those found in *Sonography: Introduction to Normal Structure and Function*. Refer to the textbook if you need help.

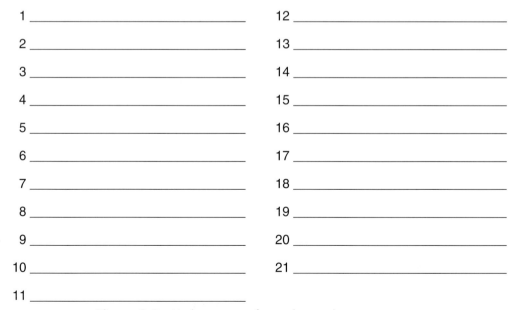
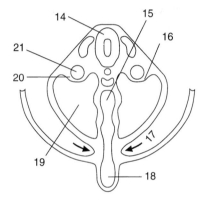
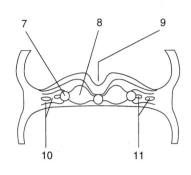
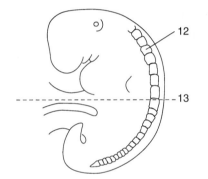

1 _____

2 _____

3 _____

4 _____

5 _____

6 _____

7 _____

8 _____

9 _____

10 _____

11 _____

12 _____

13 _____

14 _____

15 _____

16 _____

17 _____

18 _____

19 _____

20 _____

21 _____

Figure 9-1 Median section of an embryo outlining primitive gut.

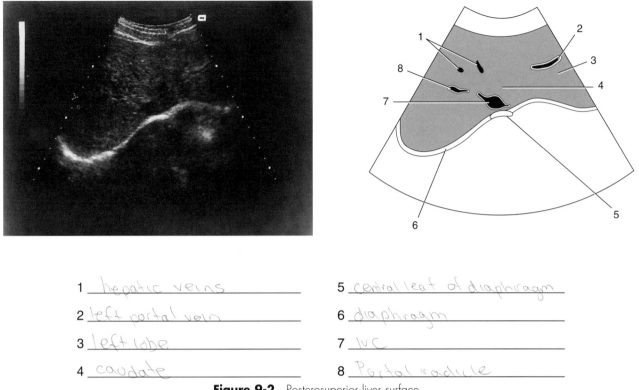

1 _hepatic veins_   5 _central leaf of diaphragm_

2 _left portal vein_   6 _diaphragm_

3 _left lobe_   7 _IVC_

4 _caudate_   8 _portal radicle_

Figure 9-2 Posterosuperior liver surface.

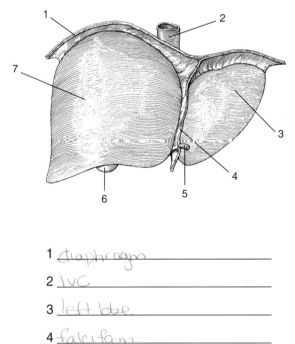

1 _diaphragm_

2 _IVC_

3 _left lobe_

4 _falciform_

5 _round_

6 _fundus of gallbladder_

7 _right lobe_

Figure 9-3 Anterior liver surface.

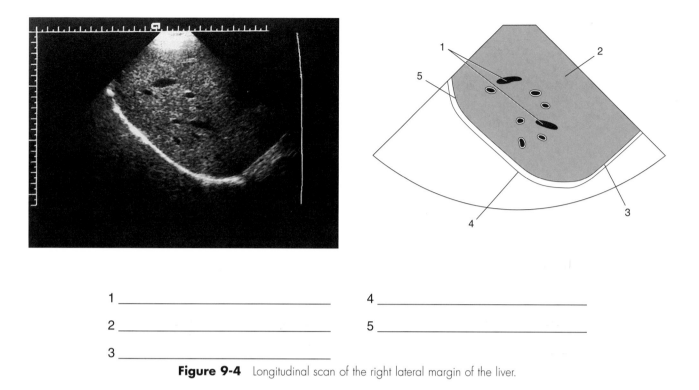

1 _____   4 _____

2 _____   5 _____

3 _____

Figure 9-4 Longitudinal scan of the right lateral margin of the liver.

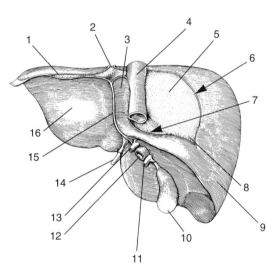

1 _left triangular ligament_   9 _right lobe_

2 _falciform_   10 _gallbladder_

3 _caudate_   11 _hepatic duct_

4 _IVC_   12 _portal vein_

5 _bare area_   13 _hepatic artery_

6 _anterior coronary lig._   14 _round lig_

7 _posterior coronary lig_   15 _lesser omentum_

8 _right triangular ligament_   16 _left lobe_

Figure 9-5 Posterior liver surface.

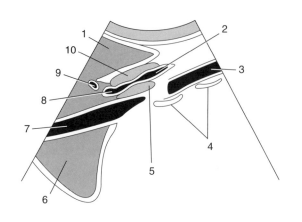

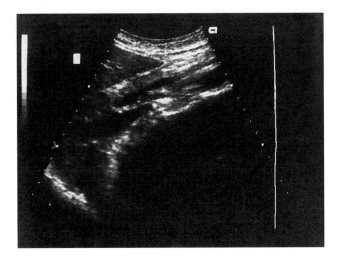

1 <u>liver</u>   6 <u>liver</u>

2 <u>smv</u>   7 <u>IVC</u>

3 <u>IVC</u>   8 <u>portal confluence</u>

4 <u>spine</u>   9 <u>PV</u>

5 <u>uncinate process</u>   10 <u>pancreas</u>

Figure 9-6 Longitudinal image of the left inferior margin of the left lobe.

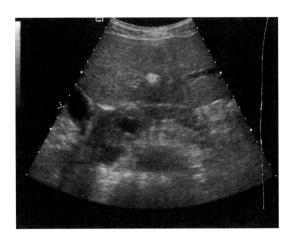

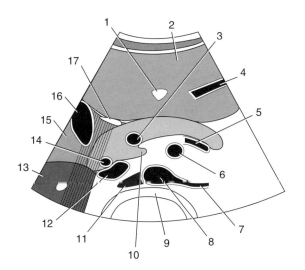

1 _____   10 _____

2 _____   11 _____

3 _____   12 _____

4 _____   13 _____

5 _____   14 _____

6 _____   15 _____

7 _____   16 _____

8 _____   17 _____

9 _____

Figure 9-7 Transverse liver section.

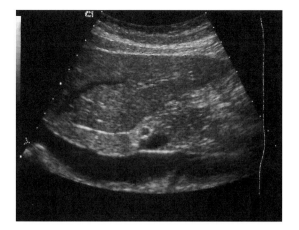
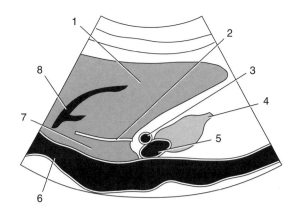

1 <u>left lobe</u>   5 <u>PV</u>

2 <u>lig venosum</u>   6 <u>IVC</u>

3 <u>hepatic artery</u>   7 <u>caudate</u>

4 <u>pancreas</u>   8 <u>Right hepatic vein</u>

Figure 9-8 Longitudinal liver section.

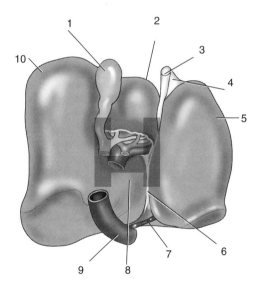
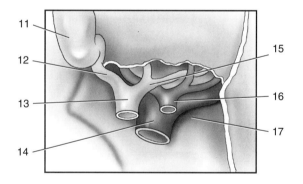

1 <u>gallbladder</u>   10 <u>right lobe</u>

2 <u>quadrate</u>   11 <u>gallbladder</u>

3 <u>lig teres</u>   12 <u>cystic duct</u>

4 <u>falciform</u>   13 <u>CBD</u>

5 <u>left lobe</u>   14 <u>MPV</u>

6 <u>lig venosum</u>   15 <u>CHD</u>

7 <u>hepatic vein</u>   16 <u>hepatic artery</u>

8 <u>caudate</u>   17 <u>porta hepatis</u>

9 <u>IVC</u>

Figure 9-9 Inferior surface of the liver.

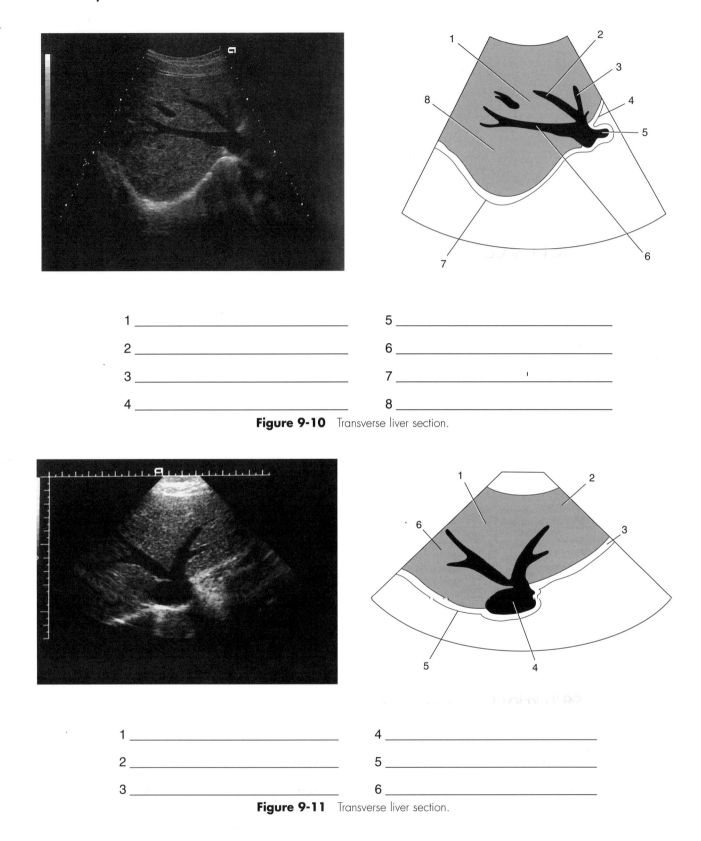

1 _____   5 _____

2 _____   6 _____

3 _____   7 _____

4 _____   8 _____

Figure 9-10   Transverse liver section.

1 _____   4 _____

2 _____   5 _____

3 _____   6 _____

Figure 9-11   Transverse liver section.

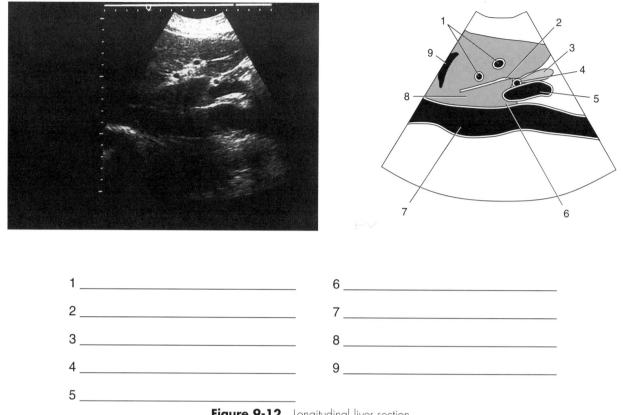

1 _____   6 _____

2 _____   7 _____

3 _____   8 _____

4 _____   9 _____

5 _____

Figure 9-12 Longitudinal liver section.

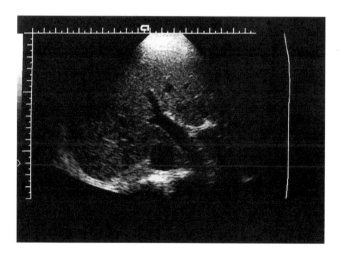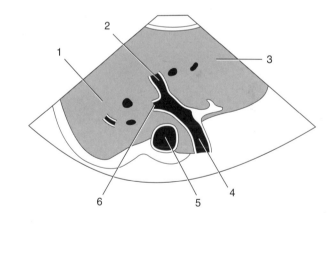

1 _____   4 _____

2 _____   5 _____

3 _____   6 _____

Figure 9-13 Transverse liver section.

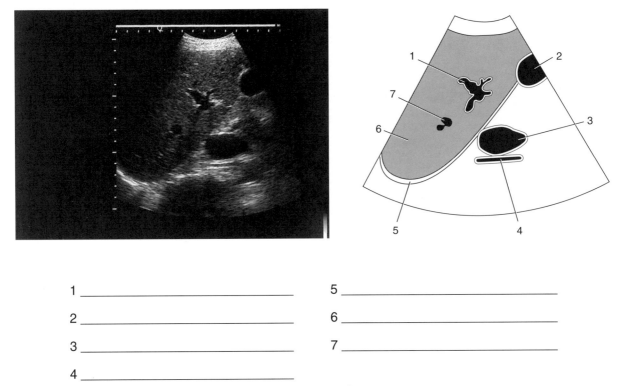

1 _____   5 _____

2 _____   6 _____

3 _____   7 _____

4 _____

Figure 9-14 Transverse liver section.

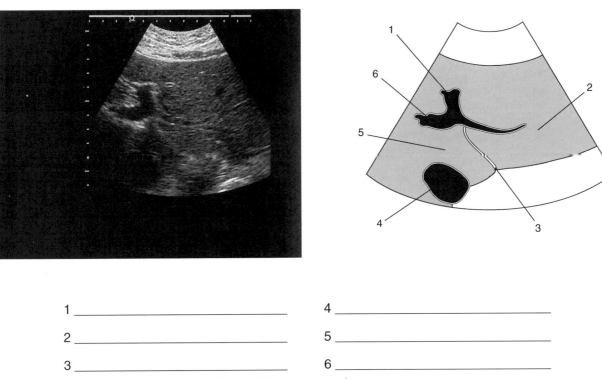

1 _____   4 _____

2 _____   5 _____

3 _____   6 _____

Figure 9-15 Transverse liver section.

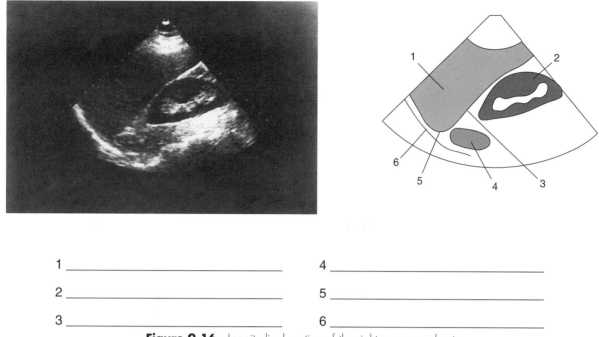

1 _____	4 _____
2 _____	5 _____
3 _____	6 _____

Figure 9-16 Longitudinal section of the right upper quadrant.

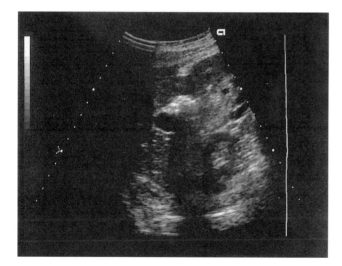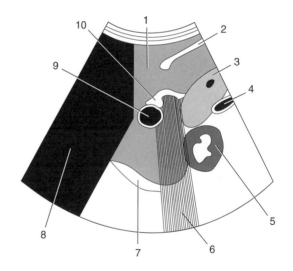

1 _____	6 _____
2 _____	7 _____
3 _____	8 _____
4 _____	9 _____
5 _____	10 _____

Figure 9-17 Longitudinal section of the right upper quadrant.

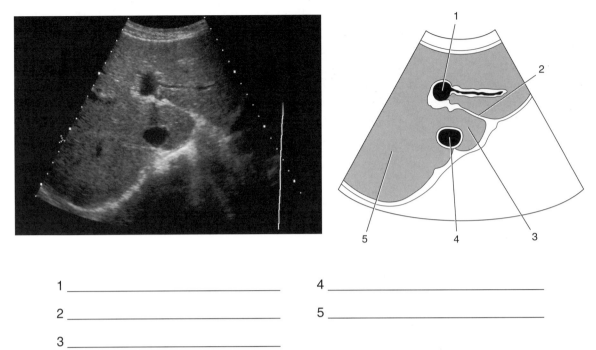

1 _____   4 _____

2 _____   5 _____

3 _____

Figure 9-18 Transverse liver section.

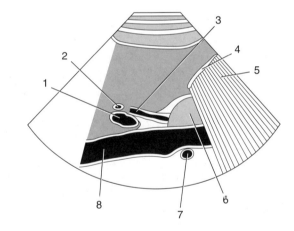

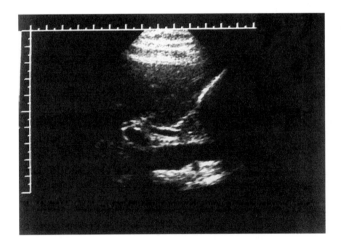

1 _____   5 _____

2 _____   6 _____

3 _____   7 _____

4 _____   8 _____

Figure 9-19 Longitudinal section of the right upper quadrant.

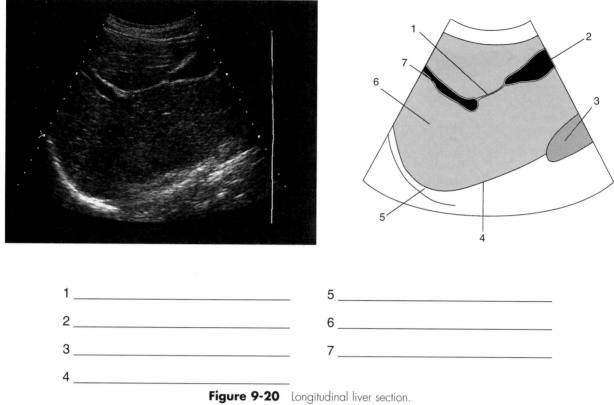

1 _____   5 _____

2 _____   6 _____

3 _____   7 _____

4 _____

Figure 9-20 Longitudinal liver section.

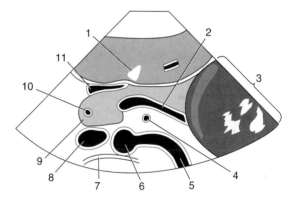

1 _____   7 _____

2 _____   8 _____

3 _____   9 _____

4 _____   10 _____

5 _____   11 _____

6 _____

Figure 9-21 Transverse epigastric section.

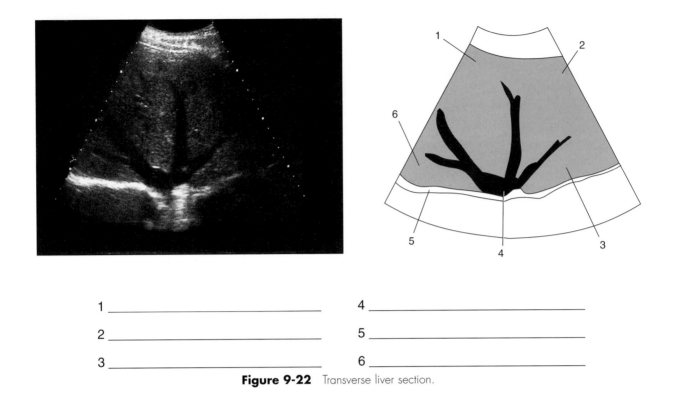

1 _____   4 _____

2 _____   5 _____

3 _____   6 _____

Figure 9-22 Transverse liver section.

CHAPTER 10

The Biliary System

REVIEW QUESTIONS

1. The gallbladder is located _____ and _____ to the liver.
   a. anterior/medial
   b. anterior/right lateral
   c. posterior/inferior
   d. posterior/superior

2. The porta hepatis is
   a. a normal variant of the liver
   b. the hilum or doorway to the liver
   c. the area of the liver that the inferior vena cava passes through
   d. the name of the liver fossa in the right upper quadrant

3. The proximal portion of the biliary duct is the
   a. common hepatic duct
   b. cystic duct
   c. common bile duct
   d. supraduodenal portion of the common bile duct

4. The intrahepatic ducts are the
   a. common hepatic duct and cystic duct
   b. common hepatic duct and common bile duct
   c. cystic duct and common bile duct
   d. right and left hepatic ducts

5. The distal portion of the biliary duct is the
   a. common bile duct
   b. common hepatic duct
   c. cystic duct
   d. main portal vein

6. The portal triad consists of the
   a. portal vein, hepatic vein, and common bile duct
   b. portal vein, hepatic artery, and common bile duct
   c. portal vein, gastroduodenal artery, and common bile duct
   d. portal vein, hepatic vein, and common hepatic duct

7. The range of normal diameter size of the common hepatic and common bile ducts is
   a. 1 to 5 mm
   b. 5 to 10 mm
   c. 1 to 7 mm
   d. 4 to 6 mm

8. The normal thickness of the gallbladder wall is
   a. 0.5 mm
   b. 3 mm or less
   c. 6 mm
   d. 1 mm or less

9. In most patients the fundus of the gallbladder is located _____ to the superior pole of the right kidney.
   a. right lateral
   b. posterior
   c. medial
   d. anterior

10. The bile-filled biliary system can be described sono-graphically as
    a. hyperechoic
    b. anechoic with echogenic walls
    c. hypoechoic
    d. having medium- to low-level echoes with reflective walls

11. The basic function of the biliary system is to
    a. secrete mucus into and absorb water from the stomach
    b. make bile and transport it to the liver
    c. drain bile from the liver and store it until needed
    d. produce hormones that regulate stomach acids

12. The gallbladder may be divided into three major sections
    a. head, neck, body
    b. neck, body, fundus
    c. left, right, middle
    d. superior, medial, inferior

13. The common hepatic duct is formed by the
    a. right and left hepatic ducts
    b. common bile duct and cystic duct
    c. left and right portal veins
    d. cystic duct and right hepatic duct

14. The common bile duct is formed by the joining of the
    a. left hepatic duct and right portal vein
    b. common bile duct and left portal vein
    c. ampulla of Vater and right hepatic duct
    d. cystic duct and common hepatic duct

15. The cystic duct connects the gallbladder to the _____ to form the common bile duct
    a. common hepatic duct
    b. right hepatic vein
    c. left hepatic duct
    d. gastroduodenal bulb

16. The gallbladder is perfused by the
    a. gastroduodenal artery
    b. left gastric artery
    c. proper hepatic artery
    d. cystic artery

17. To help locate the gallbladder, the sonographer can use the right kidney, which is _____ to the gallbladder.
    a. anterior
    b. caudal
    c. coronal
    d. posterior

18. The sphincter of Oddi helps in regulating bile flow into the duodenum.
    a. true
    b. false

19. When closed, the sphincter of Oddi allows bile to flow into the duodenum.
    a. true
    b. false

20. Spiral valves of Heister prevent the cystic duct from overdistending or collapsing.
    a. true
    b. false

21. The most common variation in gallbladder shape is a
    a. bilobed gallbladder
    b. Hartmann's pouch
    c. Phrygian cap
    d. true septated gallbladder

22. The portal triad "Mickey's sign" consists of the
    a. portal vein, hepatic vein, and common bile duct
    b. portal vein, hepatic artery, and common bile duct
    c. portal vein, cystic vein, and common bile duct
    d. portal vein, common hepatic duct, and cystic duct

23. The gallbladder's venous drainage is by means of the cystic veins draining through tributaries of the hepatic/portal vein system.
    a. true
    b. false

Identify the structures indicated in the following illustrations. These figures duplicate those found in *Sonography: Introduction to Normal Structure and Function*. Refer to the textbook if you need help.

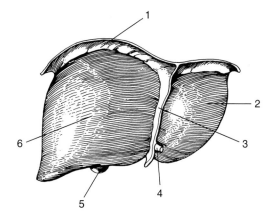

1 _____   4 _____

2 _____   5 _____

3 _____   6 _____

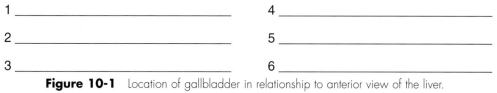

Figure 10-1 Location of gallbladder in relationship to anterior view of the liver.

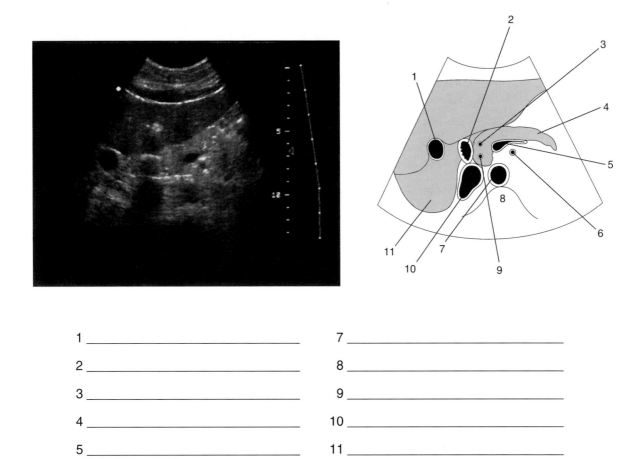

1 _____   7 _____

2 _____   8 _____

3 _____   9 _____

4 _____   10 _____

5 _____   11 _____

6 _____

Figure 10-2 Relationship of gallbladder, duodenum, and pancreas.

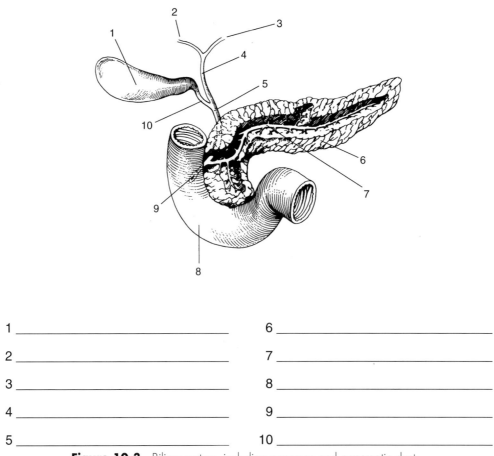

1 _____   6 _____

2 _____   7 _____

3 _____   8 _____

4 _____   9 _____

5 _____   10 _____

Figure 10-3 Biliary system, including pancreas and pancreatic duct.
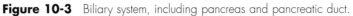
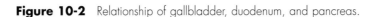

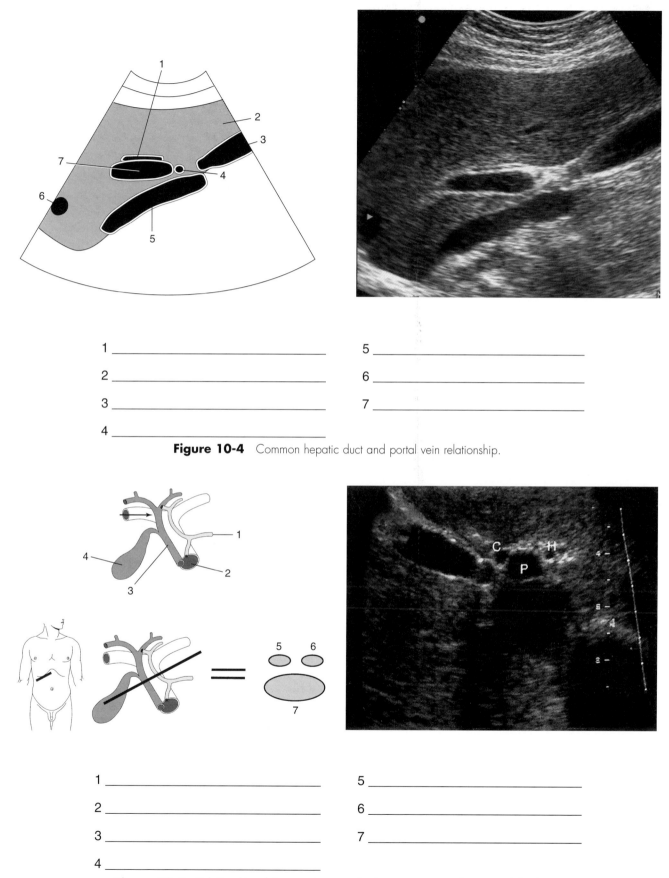

1 _____   5 _____

2 _____   6 _____

3 _____   7 _____

4 _____

Figure 10-4 Common hepatic duct and portal vein relationship.

1 _____   5 _____

2 _____   6 _____

3 _____   7 _____

4 _____

Figure 10-5 Relationship of the portal vein to the hepatic artery and common bile duct.

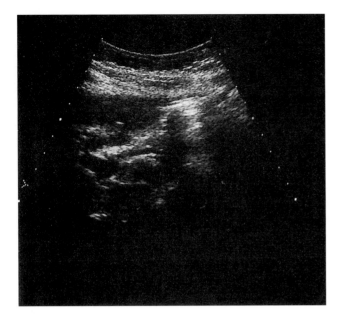

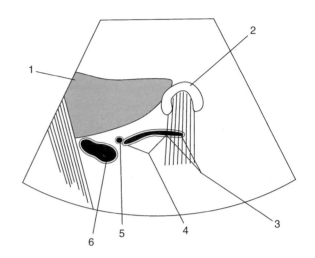

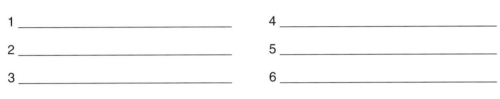

1 _____   4 _____

2 _____   5 _____

3 _____   6 _____

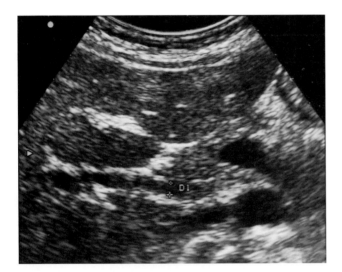

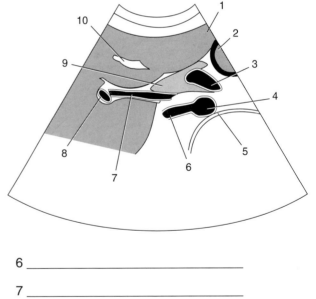

1 _____   6 _____

2 _____   7 _____

3 _____   8 _____

4 _____   9 _____

5 _____   10 _____

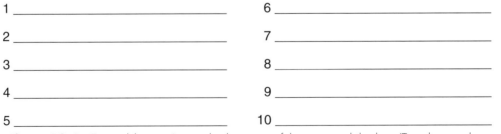

Figure 10-6 *Top* and *bottom*, Longitudinal sections of the common bile duct. (Top ultrasound image courtesy Jeanes Hospital, Philadelphia, PA).

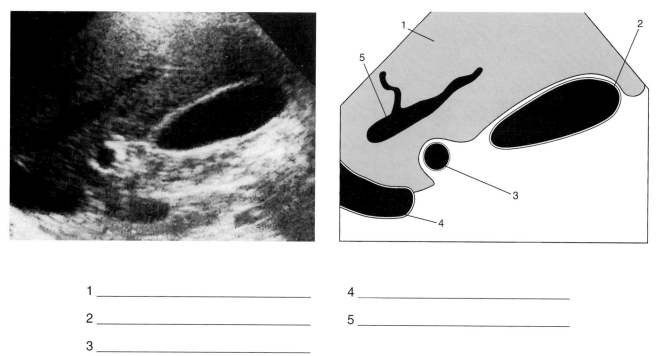

1 _____   4 _____

2 _____   5 _____

3 _____

Figure 10-7 Longitudinal section of gallbladder.

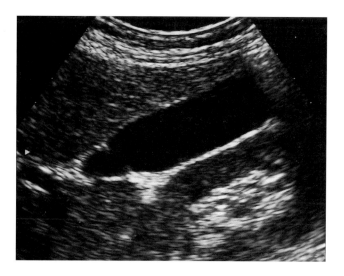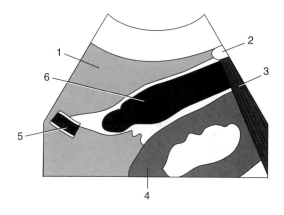

1 _____   4 _____

2 _____   5 _____

3 _____   6 _____

Figure 10-8 Longitudinal section of gallbladder.

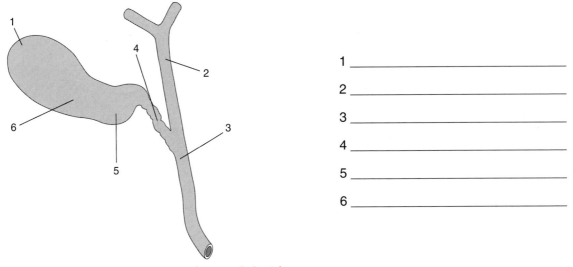

Figure 10-9 Biliary system anatomy.

1 _____

2 _____

3 _____

4 _____

5 _____

6 _____

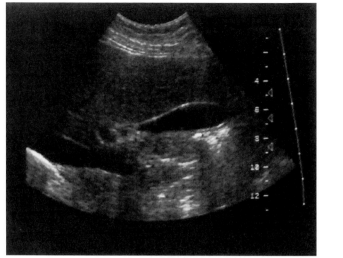

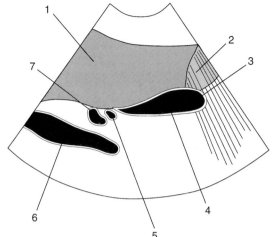

1 _____   5 _____

2 _____   6 _____

3 _____   7 _____

4 _____

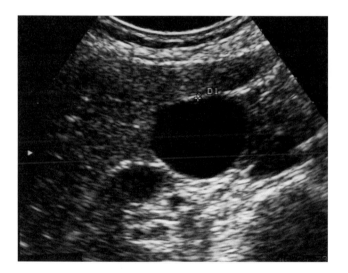

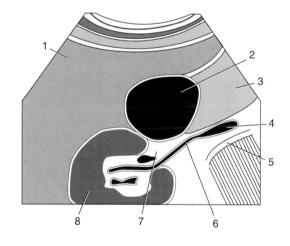

1 _____   5 _____

2 _____   6 _____

3 _____   7 _____

4 _____   8 _____

Figure 10-10 *Left,* Longitudinal section of gallbladder. *Right,* Transverse section of gallbladder.

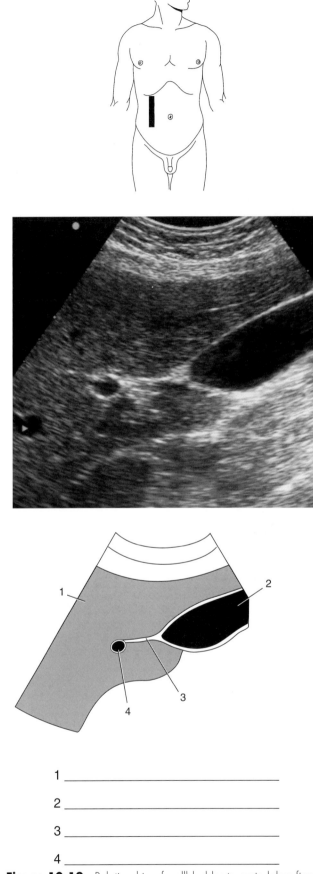

1 _____

2 _____

3 _____

4 _____

Figure 10-12 Relationship of gallbladder to main lobar fissure.

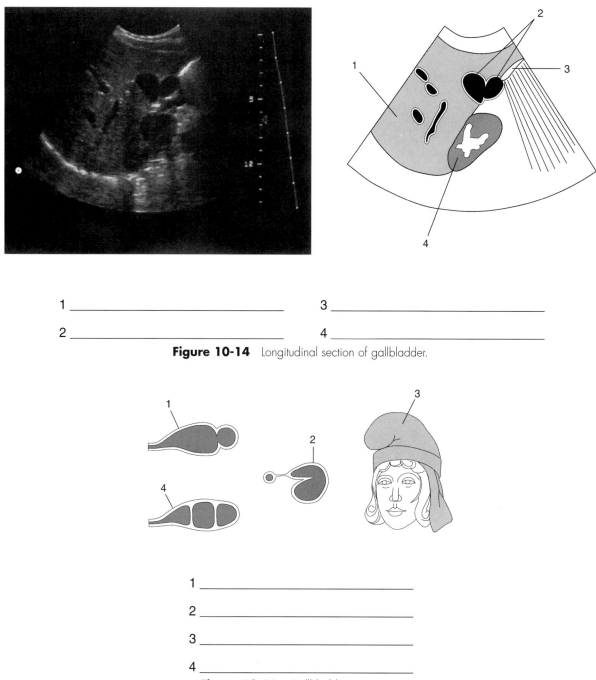

1 _____   3 _____

2 _____   4 _____

Figure 10-14 Longitudinal section of gallbladder.

1 _____

2 _____

3 _____

4 _____

Figure 10-15 Gallbladder variations.

CHAPTER 11

The Pancreas

REVIEW QUESTIONS

1. Name the parts of the pancreas and the vascular anatomy that borders it.

2. Name the blood supply to the pancreas.

3. List three components of pancreatic juice and the food substances they act on.

4. List three hormones produced by the pancreas and their function.

5. List two structures that appear in the head of the pancreas. How can these structures be identified on images?

6. Describe the echogenicity of the pancreas.

7. On a transverse image of the pancreas, what type of section of the pancreas can be obtained?

8. A sagittal image shows the aorta and superior mesenteric artery. What part of the pancreas will be shown?

9. What part of the pancreas is located to the left (toward the aorta) of an imaginary line drawn between the porta/splenic confluence and the inferior vena cava?

10. Describe vessels from the biliary tree and pancreas that enter the duodenum.

11. The pancreas is a _____ (exocrine) and a _____ (endocrine) gland.

12. Where in the abdominal cavity is the pancreas located?

13. As an exocrine gland, the pancreas produces pancreatic juice composed of enzymes. Name these enzymes and tell what they do.

14. Pancreatic juice moves through the _____ and usually meets the common bile duct before both enter the duodenum through the _____.

15. The functional part of the pancreas as an endocrine gland is located in the _____.

16. The _____ is an accessory duct and normal variant that enters the duodenum immediately superior to the main duct.

17. Name the four parts of the pancreas and the structures and vessels near them.
    a. the _____ of the pancreas is cradled in the _____ of the duodenum
    b. the _____ of the pancreas is _____ to the superior mesenteric vein and portal splenic confluence
    c. the _____ of the pancreas is _____ to the superior mesenteric artery
    d. the _____ of the pancreas can be seen near the _____ of the pancreas

18. The _____ vein lies just posterior to the body and tail of the pancreas.

19. What is the uncinate process?

20. What is the normal size of the pancreas, and why is it important to assess the glandular contour?

21. What two vessels can be seen in the head of the pancreas?

22. The _____ artery perfuses the head of the pancreas, and the _____ artery supplies the body and tail of the pancreas.

23. The sonographic appearance of the pancreas is a little more _____ than the normal liver, but less _____.

24. Sagittal views of the pancreas show the organ in _____ sections. Transverse views of the pancreas show the organ in its _____ axis.

Identify the structures indicated in the following illustrations. These figures duplicate those found in *Sonography: Introduction to Normal Structure and Function.* Refer to the textbook if you need help.

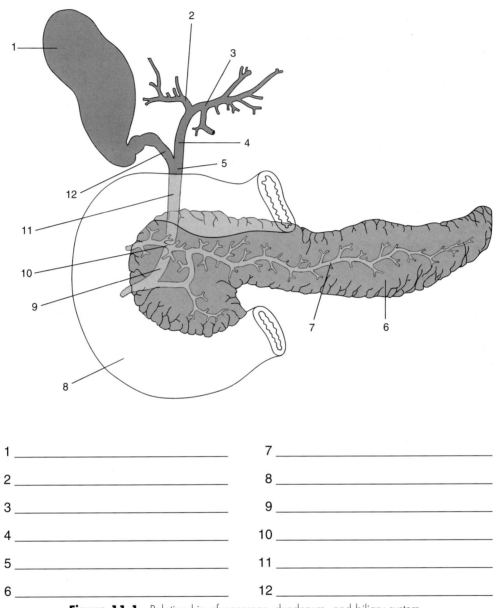

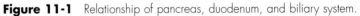

1 _____   7 _____

2 _____   8 _____

3 _____   9 _____

4 _____   10 _____

5 _____   11 _____

6 _____   12 _____

Figure 11-1   Relationship of pancreas, duodenum, and biliary system.

1 _____

2 _____

3 _____

4 _____

5 _____

6 _____

7 _____

8 _____

9 _____

10 _____

11 _____

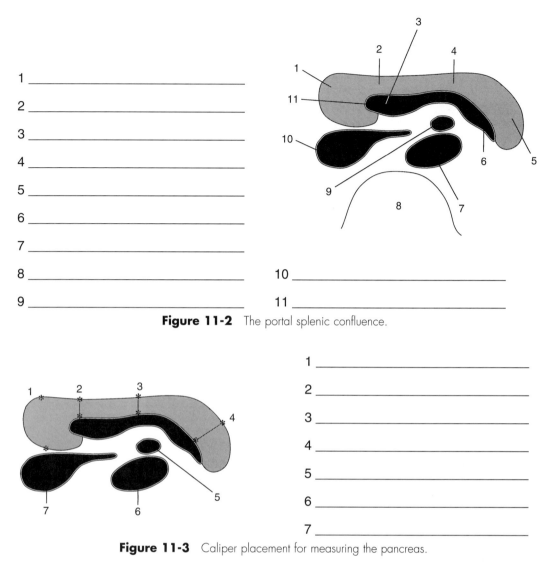

Figure 11-2 The portal splenic confluence.

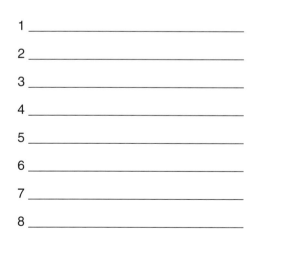

1 _____

2 _____

3 _____

4 _____

5 _____

6 _____

7 _____

Figure 11-3 Caliper placement for measuring the pancreas.

1 _____

2 _____

3 _____

4 _____

5 _____

6 _____

7 _____

8 _____

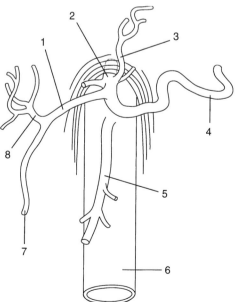

Figure 11-4 Celiac axis and branches.

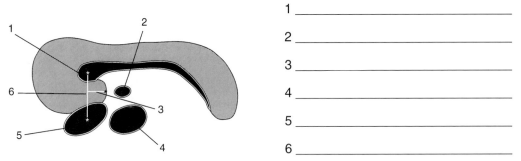

1 _____

2 _____

3 _____

4 _____

5 _____

6 _____

Figure 11-5 Transverse section of the pancreas.

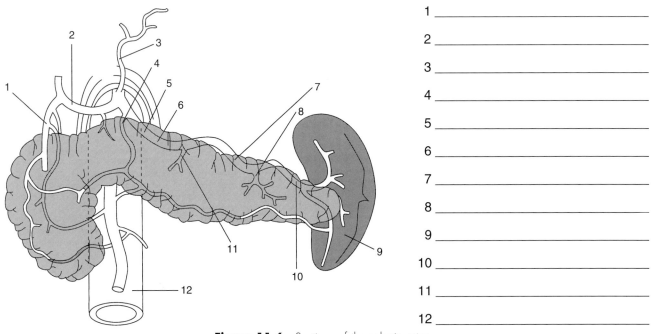

1 _____

2 _____

3 _____

4 _____

5 _____

6 _____

7 _____

8 _____

9 _____

10 _____

11 _____

12 _____

Figure 11-6 Sections of the splenic artery.

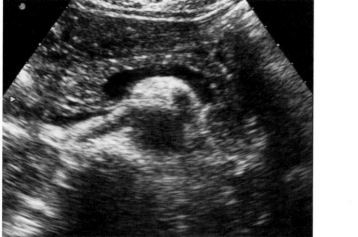
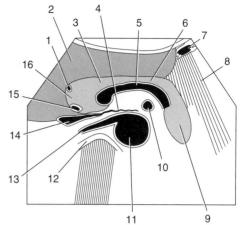

1 _____   9 _____

2 _____   10 _____

3 _____   11 _____

4 _____   12 _____

5 _____   13 _____

6 _____   14 _____

7 _____   15 _____

8 _____   16 _____

Figure 11-7 Transverse image of the pancreas.

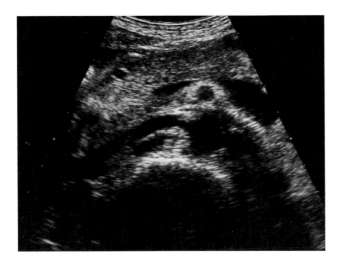
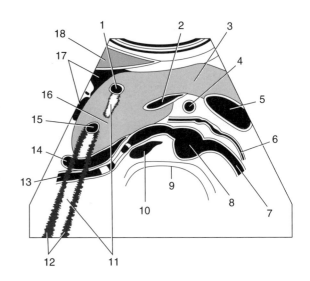

1 _____

2 _____

3 _____

4 _____

5 _____

6 _____

7 _____

8 _____

9 _____

10 _____

11 _____

12 _____

13 _____

14 _____

15 _____

16 _____

17 _____

18 _____

Figure 11-8 Transverse image of the pancreas.

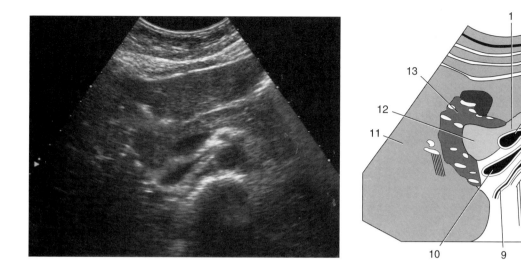

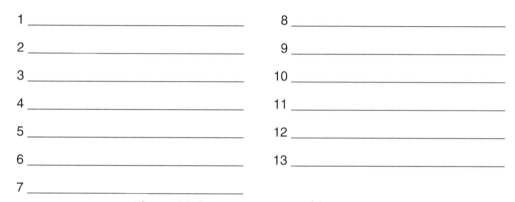

1 _____	8 _____
2 _____	9 _____
3 _____	10 _____
4 _____	11 _____
5 _____	12 _____
6 _____	13 _____
7 _____	

Figure 11-9 Transverse image of the pancreas.

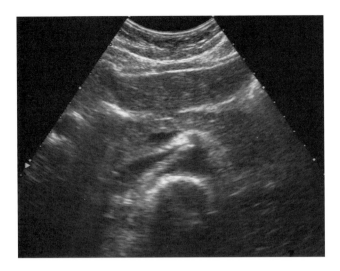

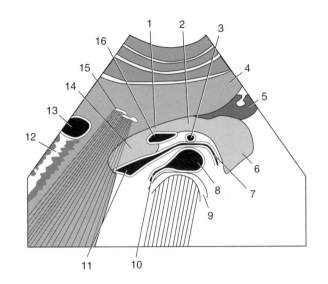

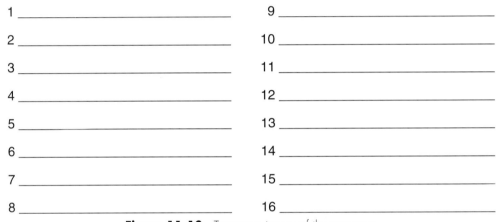

1 _____	9 _____
2 _____	10 _____
3 _____	11 _____
4 _____	12 _____
5 _____	13 _____
6 _____	14 _____
7 _____	15 _____
8 _____	16 _____

Figure 11-10 Transverse image of the pancreas.

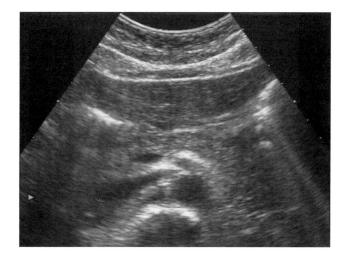
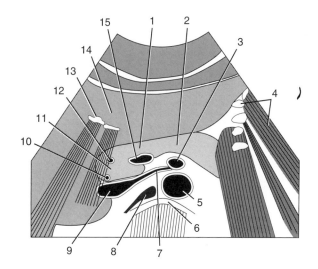

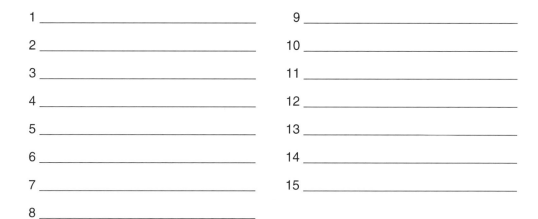

1 _____   9 _____

2 _____   10 _____

3 _____   11 _____

4 _____   12 _____

5 _____   13 _____

6 _____   14 _____

7 _____   15 _____

8 _____

Figure 11-11 Transverse image of the pancreas.

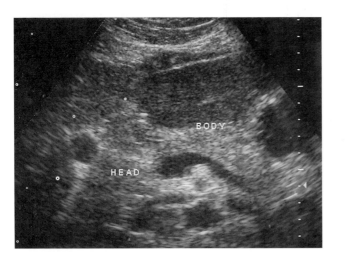 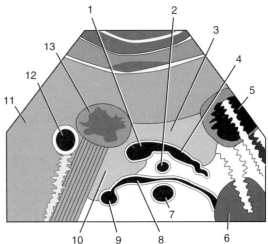

1 _____   8 _____

2 _____   9 _____

3 _____   10 _____

4 _____   11 _____

5 _____   12 _____

6 _____   13 _____

7 _____

Figure 11-12 Transverse image of the pancreas.

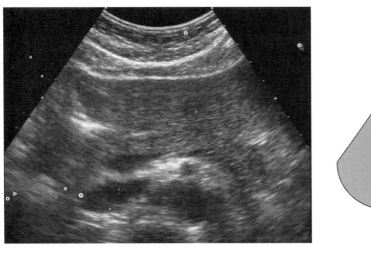 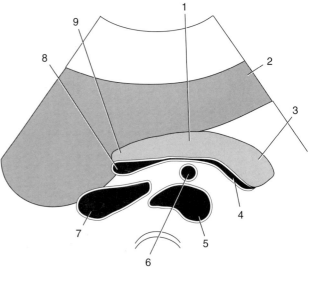

1 _____   6 _____

2 _____   7 _____

3 _____   8 _____

4 _____   9 _____

5 _____

Figure 11-13 Transverse image of the pancreas.

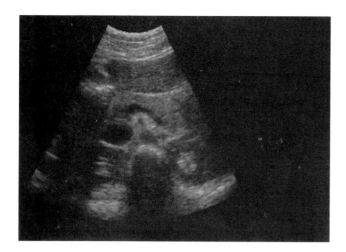
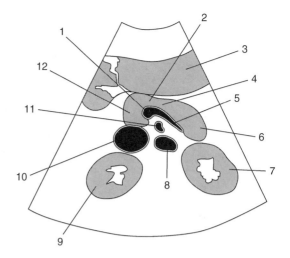

1 _____	7 _____
2 _____	8 _____
3 _____	9 _____
4 _____	10 _____
5 _____	11 _____
6 _____	12 _____

Figure 11-14 Transverse image of the pancreas. (Image courtesy Jeanes Hospital, Philadelphia, PA.)

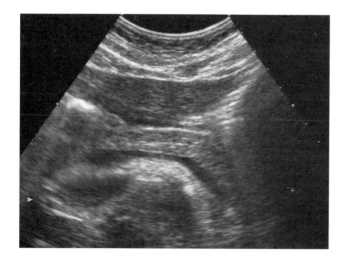
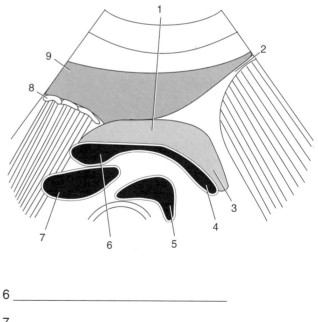

1 _____	6 _____
2 _____	7 _____
3 _____	8 _____
4 _____	9 _____
5 _____	

Figure 11-15 Transverse image of the pancreas.

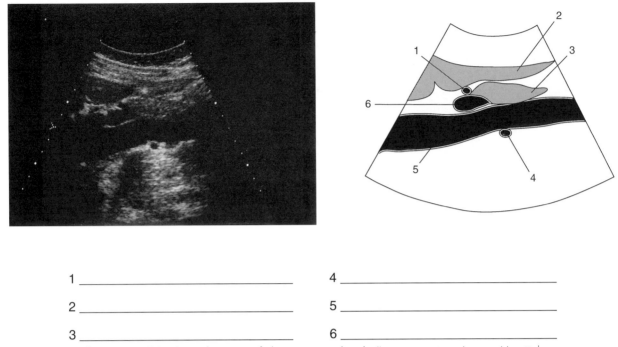

1 _____   4 _____

2 _____   5 _____

3 _____   6 _____

Figure 11-16 Sagittal image of the pancreas head. (Image courtesy Jeanes Hospital, Philadelphia, PA.)

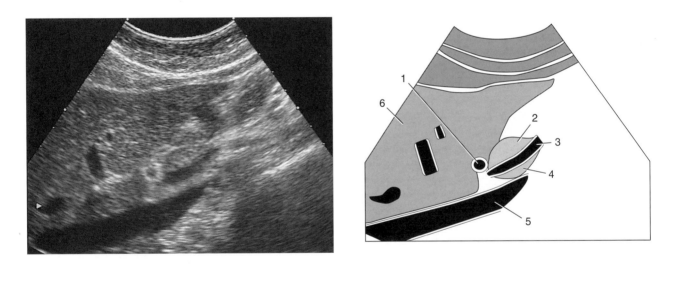

1 _____   4 _____

2 _____   5 _____

3 _____   6 _____

Figure 11-17 Sagittal image of the pancreas head and uncinate.

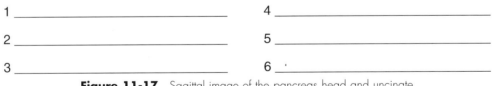

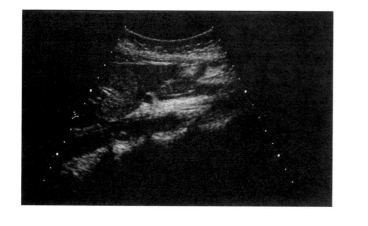
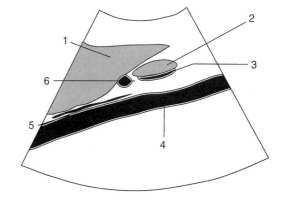

1 _____   4 _____

2 _____   5 _____

3 _____   6 _____

Figure 11-18 Sagittal image of the pancreas neck. (Image courtesy Jeanes Hospital, Philadelphia, PA.)

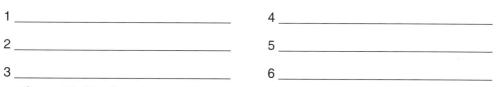
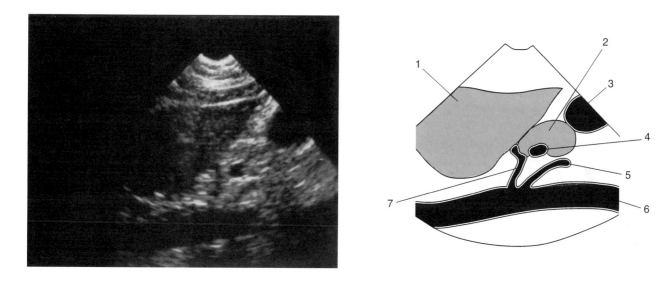

1 _____   5 _____

2 _____   6 _____

3 _____   7 _____

4 _____

Figure 11-19 Sagittal image of the pancreas body.

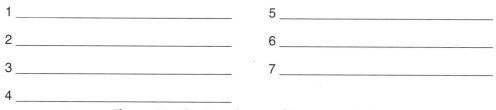
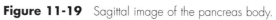

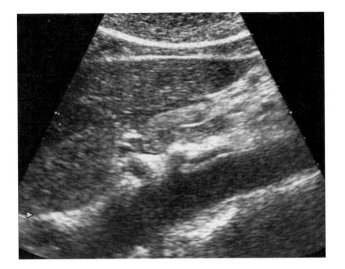
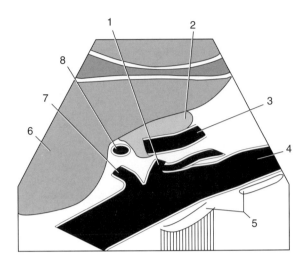

1 _____   5 _____

2 _____   6 _____

3 _____   7 _____

4 _____   8 _____

Figure 11-20   Sagittal image of the pancreas body.

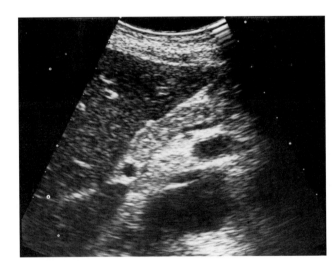
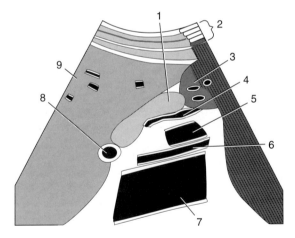

1 _____   6 _____

2 _____   7 _____

3 _____   8 _____

4 _____   9 _____

5 _____

Figure 11-21   Sagittal image of the pancreas body.

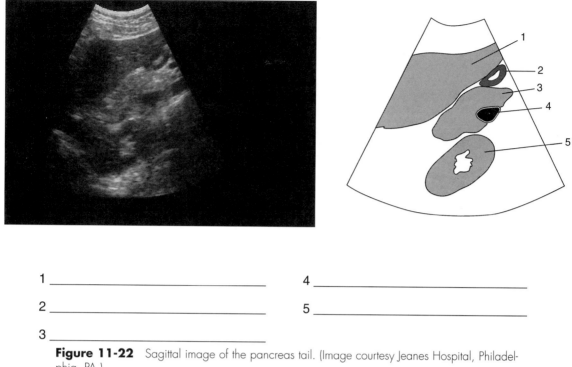

1 _____   4 _____

2 _____   5 _____

3 _____

Figure 11-22 Sagittal image of the pancreas tail. (Image courtesy Jeanes Hospital, Philadelphia, PA.)

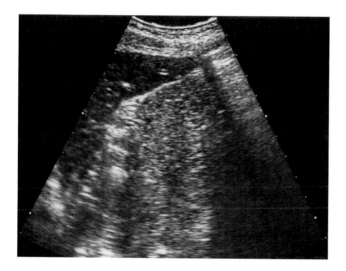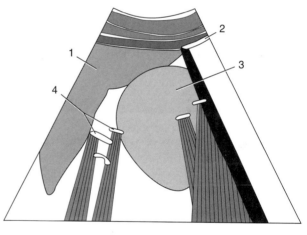

1 _____   3 _____

2 _____   4 _____

Figure 11-23 Sagittal image of the pancreas tail.

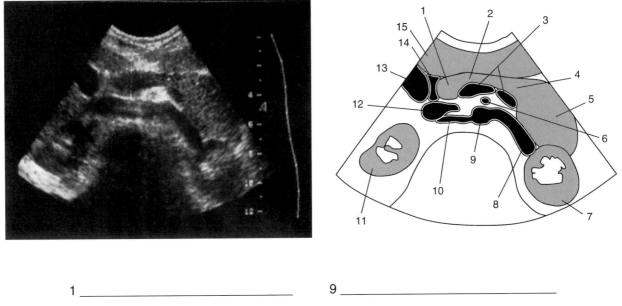

1 _____   9 _____

2 _____   10 _____

3 _____   11 _____

4 _____   12 _____

5 _____   13 _____

6 _____   14 _____

7 _____   15 _____

8 _____

Figure 11-24   Transverse image of the pancreas.

CHAPTER 12

The Urinary System

REVIEW QUESTIONS

1. Describe the function of the urinary system.

2. The kidneys are anterior to which structures?

3. The right kidney is posterior to which structures?

4. The left kidney is posterior to which structures?

5. Describe the location of the ureters.

6. Describe the location of the urinary bladder.

7. List the normal sizes of the urinary system structures.

8. Describe urine development by the kidneys.

9. Describe the parts of the urinary system and their sonographic appearance.

10. List the reasons why ultrasound is used to evaluate the urinary system.

11. Describe the normal variants of the urinary system that are recognized by ultrasound.

12. Name three types of physicians who diagnose or treat the urinary system and define what they do.

13. Name and define two diagnostic tests other than ultrasound that are commonly used to evaluate the urinary system.

14. What are the normal laboratory values for BUN and Cr, and what do these values represent?

15. Name and define the hormones that affect the kidneys.

16. The purpose of the urinary system is
   a. to transport nutrients to the cells
   b. aiding in the digestion of fats
   c. regulation of oil and sweat glands
   d. chemical equilibrium of the body

151

17. Name the organs of the urinary system.

18. The kidneys, ureter, and bladder are all located in the
   a. peritoneum
   b. retroperitoneum
   c. mediastinum
   d. thoracic cavity

19. What is the size of the normal adult kidney?
   a. 9-12 cm L $\times$ 2.5-4 cm D $\times$ 4-6 cm Dia
   b. 12-14 cm L $\times$ 4-6 cm D $\times$ 6-8 cm Dia
   c. 6-9 cm L $\times$ 1-3 cm D $\times$ 2-4 cm Dia
   d. any size is normal

20. What is the size of the normal neonatal kidney?
   a. any size is normal as long as it functions
   b. 1.5-3.3 cm L $\times$ 0.5-1.5 cm D $\times$ 1.0-2 cm Dia
   c. 4.0-6.5 cm L $\times$ 3.3-4.5 cm D $\times$ 3.5-5.5 cm Dia
   d. 3.3-5.0 cm L $\times$ 1.5-2.5 cm D $\times$ 2.0-3.0 cm Dia

21. Define the following renal structures, explain their location, and describe their sonographic appearance.
true capsule:

cortex:

arcuate vessels:

medullae:

renal sinus:

22. What is the renal hilum?

23. Describe the urinary bladder, its location, and sonographic appearance.

24. What are ureteral jets and where do they enter the bladder?

25. The functional unit of the kidney is
   a. Gerota's fascia
   b. the nephron
   c. the corpus spongiosum
   d. the tunica adventitia

Identify the structures indicated in the following illustrations. These figures duplicate those found in *Sonography: Introduction to Normal Structure and Function*. Refer to the textbook if you need help.

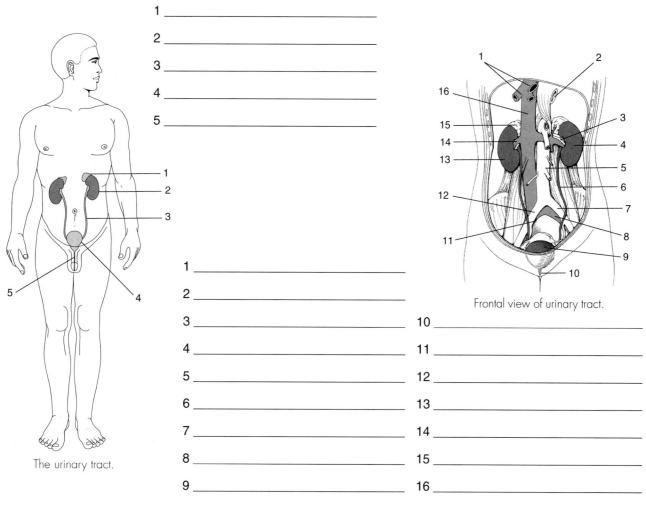

1 _____
2 _____
3 _____
4 _____
5 _____

The urinary tract.

Frontal view of urinary tract.

1 _____
2 _____
3 _____
4 _____
5 _____
6 _____
7 _____
8 _____
9 _____

10 _____
11 _____
12 _____
13 _____
14 _____
15 _____
16 _____

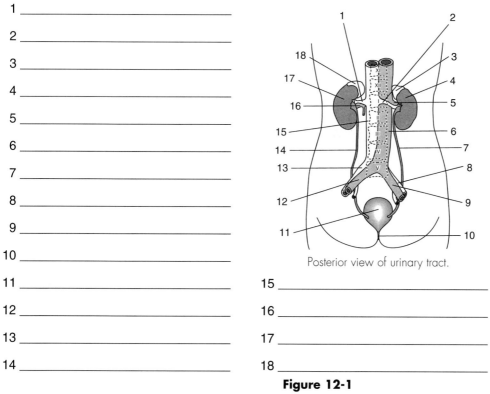

Posterior view of urinary tract.

1 _____
2 _____
3 _____
4 _____
5 _____
6 _____
7 _____
8 _____
9 _____
10 _____
11 _____
12 _____
13 _____
14 _____

15 _____
16 _____
17 _____
18 _____

Figure 12-1

1 _____

2 _____

3 _____

4 _____

5 _____

6 _____

7 _____

8 _____

9 _____

10 _____

11 _____

12 _____

13 _____

14 _____

15 _____

16 _____

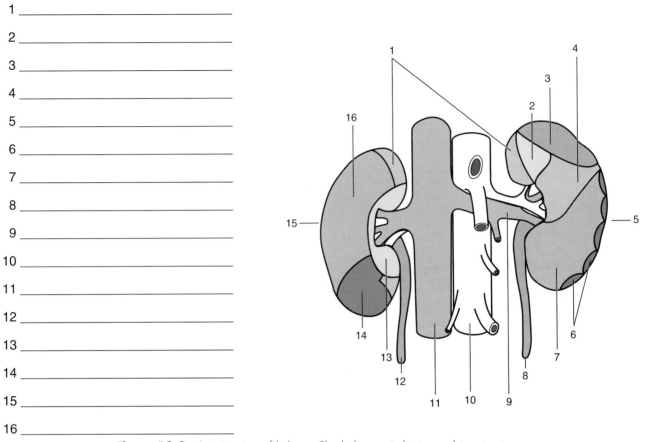

Figure 12-2 Anterior view of kidneys. Shaded areas indicate overlying structures.

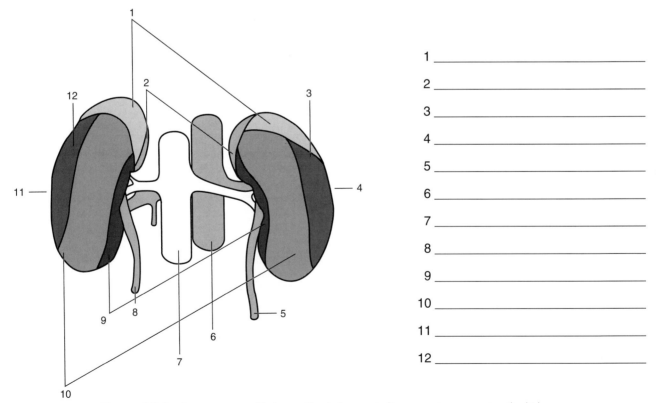

1 _____

2 _____

3 _____

4 _____

5 _____

6 _____

7 _____

8 _____

9 _____

10 _____

11 _____

12 _____

Figure 12-3 Posterior view of kidneys. Shaded areas indicate structures covering the kidneys from behind.

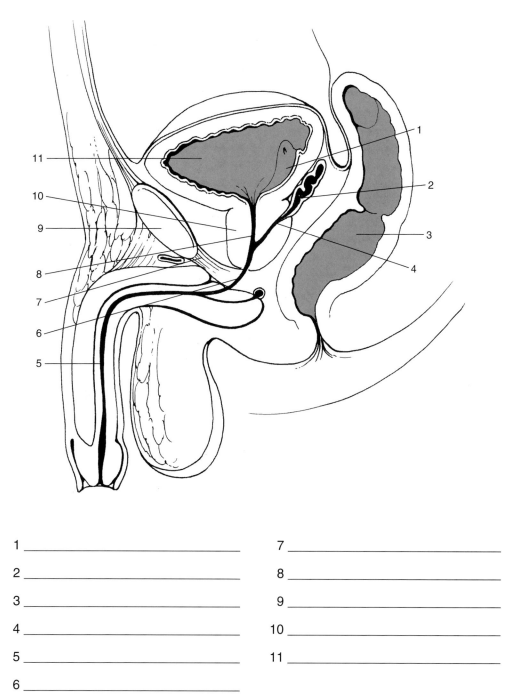

1 _____   7 _____

2 _____   8 _____

3 _____   9 _____

4 _____   10 _____

5 _____   11 _____

6 _____

Figure 12-4 Lower urinary tract in the male.

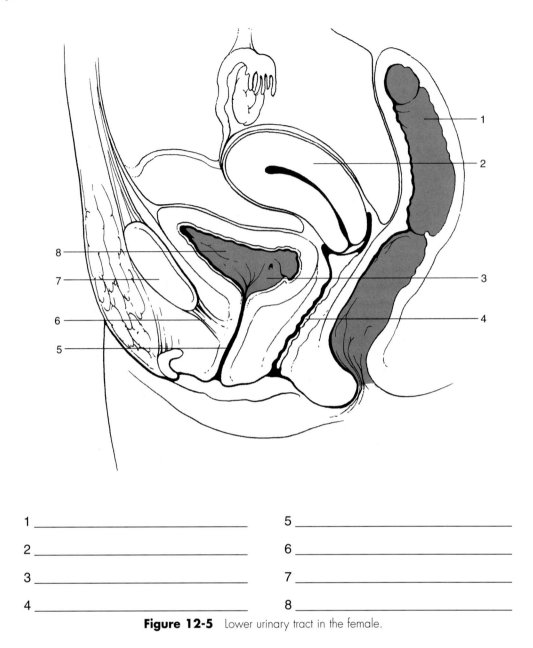

1 _____   5 _____

2 _____   6 _____

3 _____   7 _____

4 _____   8 _____

Figure 12-5 Lower urinary tract in the female.

1 _____

2 _____

3 _____

4 _____

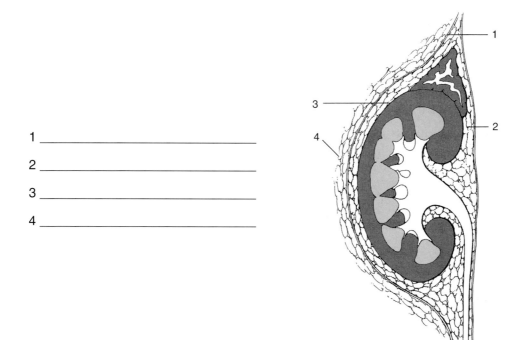

Figure 12-6 Layers surrounding the kidney.

1 _____

2 _____

3 _____

4 _____

5 _____

6 _____

7 _____

8 _____

9 _____

10 _____

11 _____

12 _____

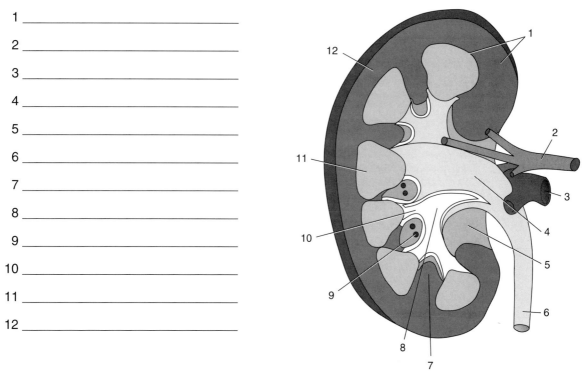

Figure 12-7 Section of internal kidney anatomy.

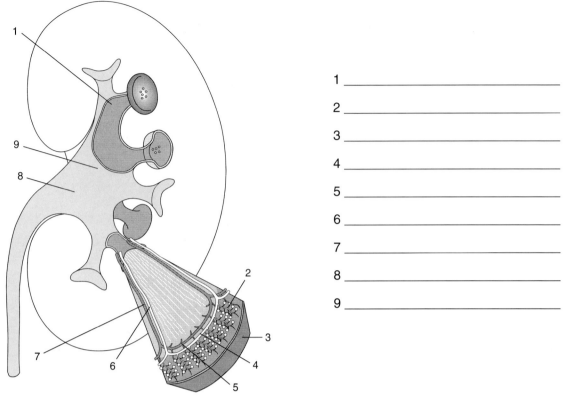

1 _____

2 _____

3 _____

4 _____

5 _____

6 _____

7 _____

8 _____

9 _____

Figure 12-8 Renal lobe.

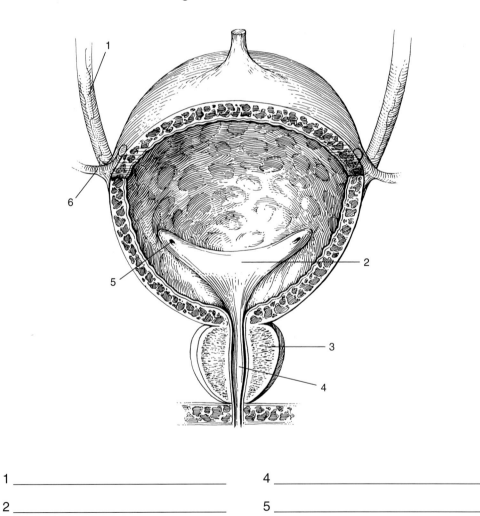

1 _____   4 _____

2 _____   5 _____

3 _____   6 _____

Figure 12-9 Urinary bladder.

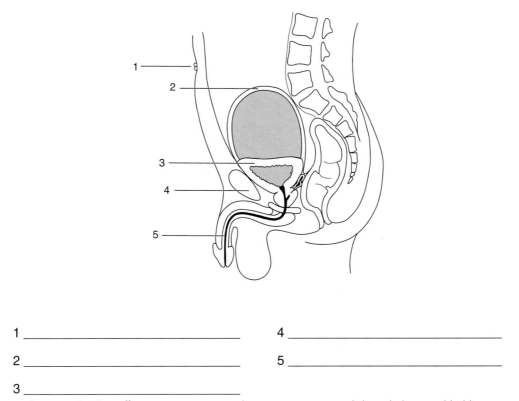

1 _____   4 _____

2 _____   5 _____

3 _____

Figure 12-10 Difference in appearance between an empty and distended urinary bladder.

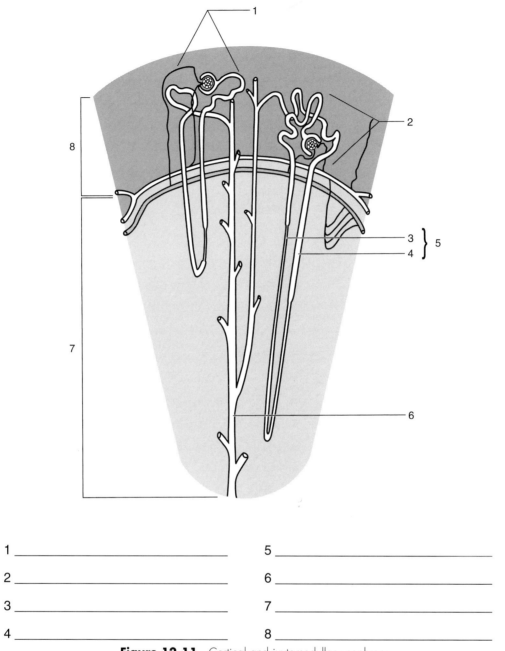

1 _____   5 _____

2 _____   6 _____

3 _____   7 _____

4 _____   8 _____

Figure 12-11 Cortical and juxtamedullary nephrons.

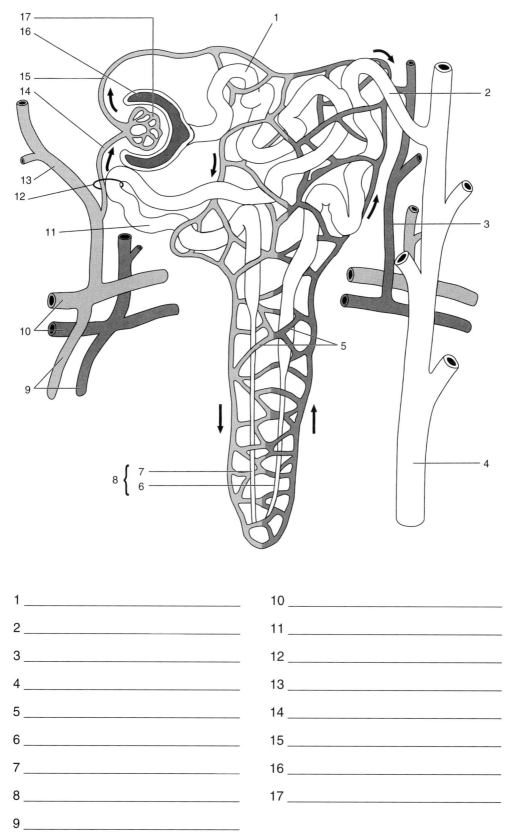

Figure 12-12 A nephron.

1 _____   10 _____

2 _____   11 _____

3 _____   12 _____

4 _____   13 _____

5 _____   14 _____

6 _____   15 _____

7 _____   16 _____

8 _____   17 _____

9 _____

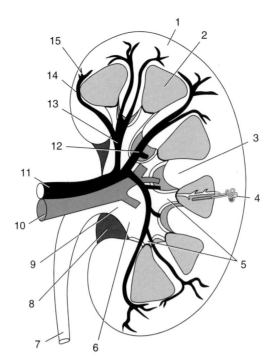

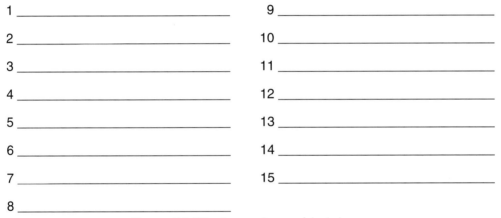

1 _____   9 _____

2 _____   10 _____

3 _____   11 _____

4 _____   12 _____

5 _____   13 _____

6 _____   14 _____

7 _____   15 _____

8 _____

Figure 12-13   Dissected view of the kidney.

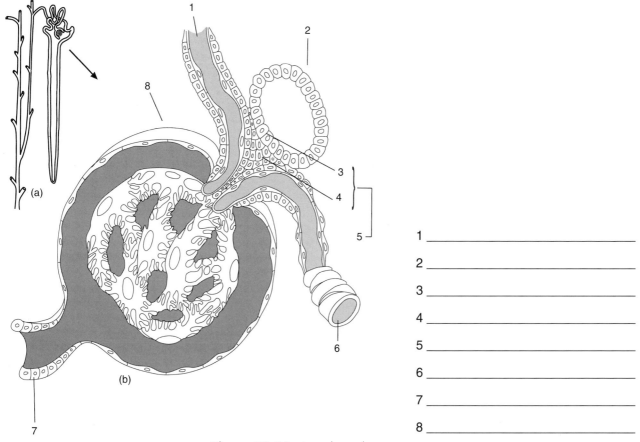

1 _____

2 _____

3 _____

4 _____

5 _____

6 _____

7 _____

8 _____

Figure 12-14 Juxtaglomerular apparatus.

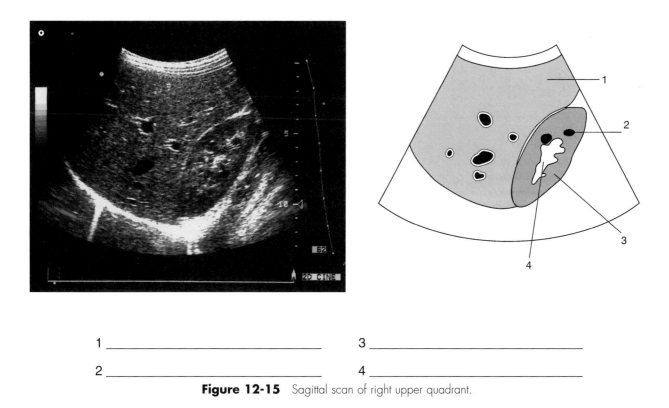

1 _____   3 _____

2 _____   4 _____

Figure 12-15 Sagittal scan of right upper quadrant.

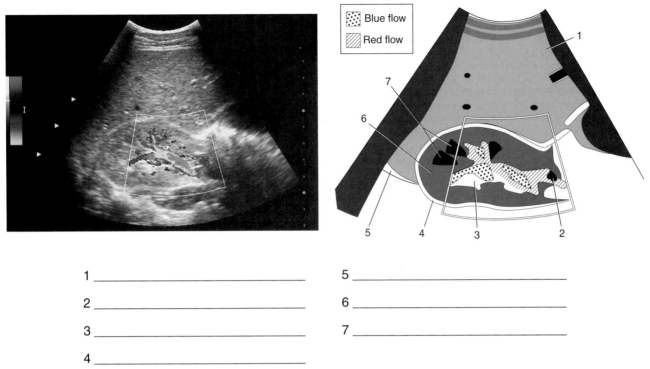

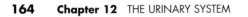

Blue flow

Red flow

1 _____   5 _____

2 _____   6 _____

3 _____   7 _____

4 _____

Figure 12-16 Transverse scan of right upper quadrant.

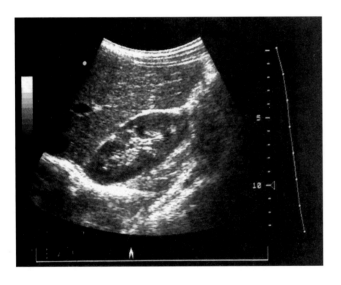

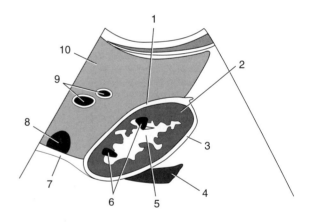

1 _____   6 _____

2 _____   7 _____

3 _____   8 _____

4 _____   9 _____

5 _____   10 _____

Figure 12-17 Longitudinal kidney section.

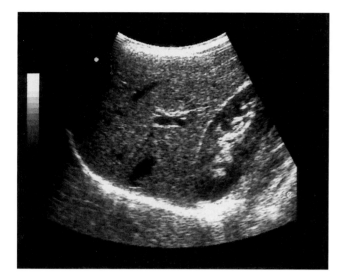
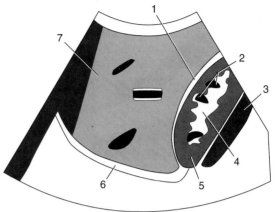

1 _____   5 _____

2 _____   6 _____

3 _____   7 _____

4 _____

Figure 12-18 Sagittal scan of right upper quadrant.

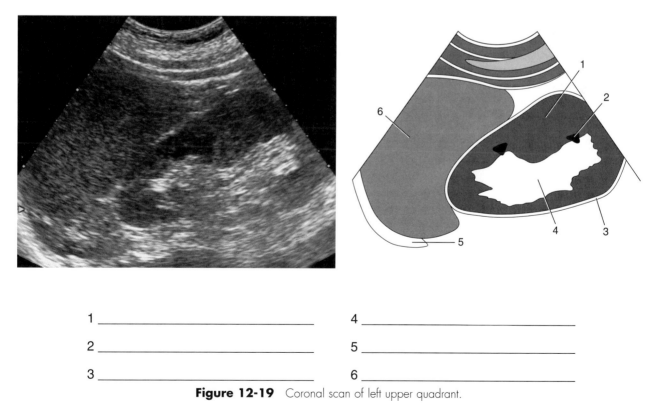

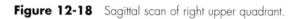

1 _____   4 _____

2 _____   5 _____

3 _____   6 _____

Figure 12-19 Coronal scan of left upper quadrant.

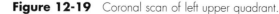

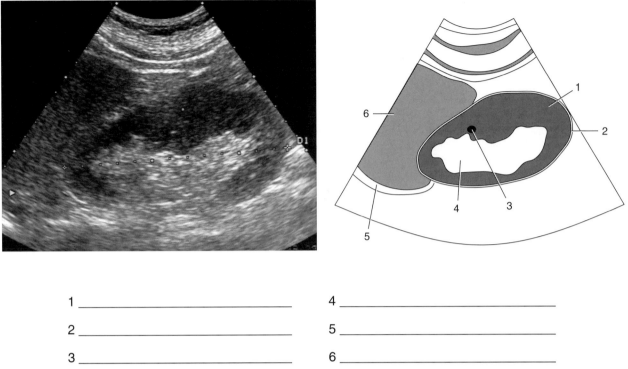

1 _____   4 _____

2 _____   5 _____

3 _____   6 _____

Figure 12-20 Coronal scan of left upper quadrant.

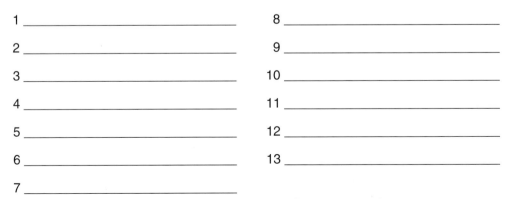

1 _____   8 _____

2 _____   9 _____

3 _____   10 _____

4 _____   11 _____

5 _____   12 _____

6 _____   13 _____

7 _____

Figure 12-21 Transverse section of right upper quadrant.

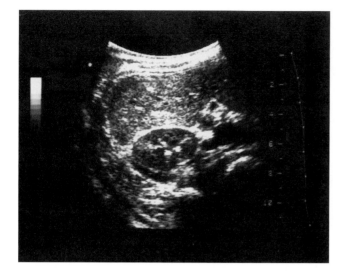
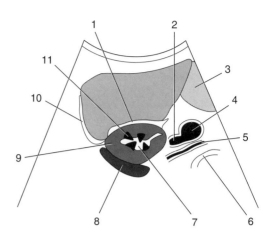

1 _____   7 _____

2 _____   8 _____

3 _____   9 _____

4 _____   10 _____

5 _____   11 _____

6 _____

Figure 12-22 Transverse section of right upper quadrant.

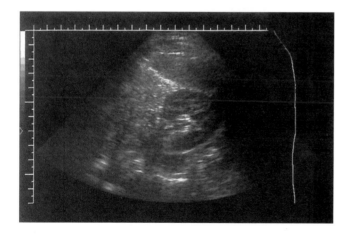
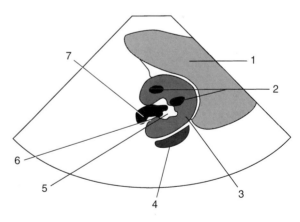

1 _____   5 _____

2 _____   6 _____

3 _____   7 _____

4 _____

Figure 12-23 Transverse section of left upper quadrant.

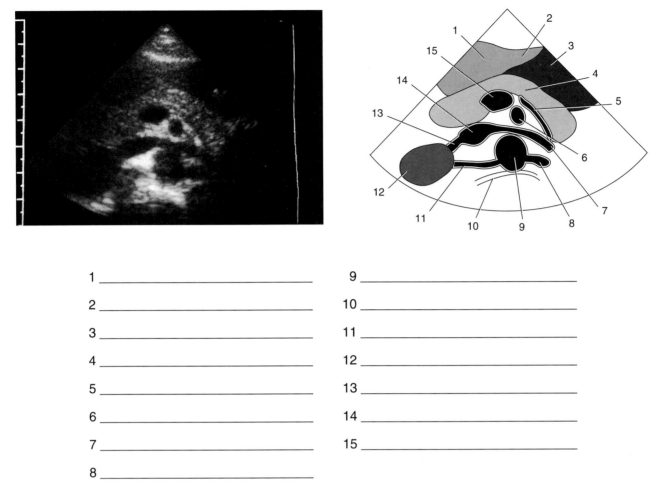

1 _____   9 _____

2 _____   10 _____

3 _____   11 _____

4 _____   12 _____

5 _____   13 _____

6 _____   14 _____

7 _____   15 _____

8 _____

Figure 12-25 Transverse epigastric section.

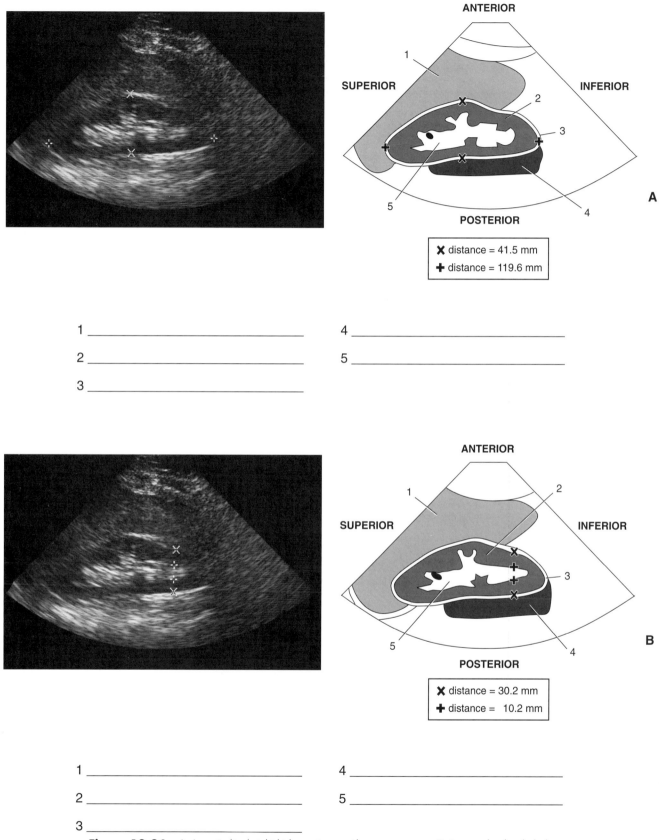

1 _____   4 _____

2 _____   5 _____

3 _____

1 _____   4 _____

2 _____   5 _____

3 _____

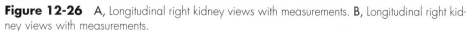

Figure 12-26 A, Longitudinal right kidney views with measurements. B, Longitudinal right kidney views with measurements.

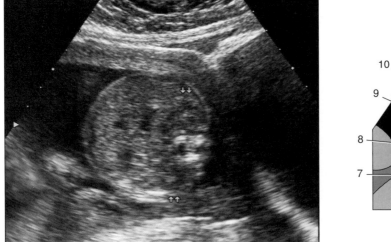

A

1 _____	6 _____
2 _____	7 _____
3 _____	8 _____
4 _____	9 _____
5 _____	10 _____

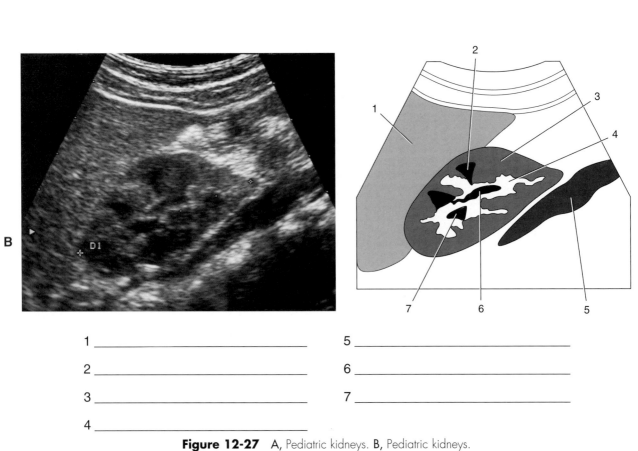

B

1 _____	5 _____
2 _____	6 _____
3 _____	7 _____
4 _____	

Figure 12-27 A, Pediatric kidneys. B, Pediatric kidneys.

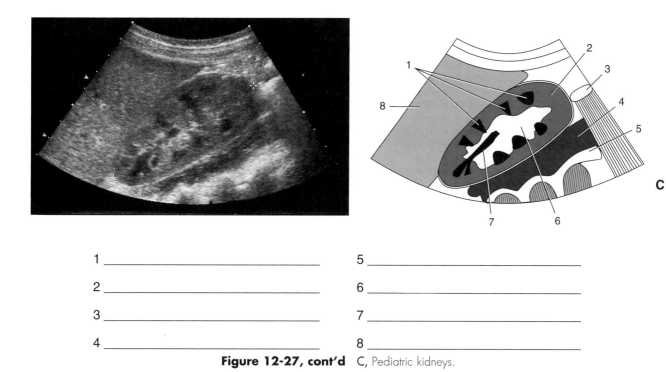

1 _____   5 _____

2 _____   6 _____

3 _____   7 _____

4 _____   8 _____

Figure 12-27, cont'd C, Pediatric kidneys.

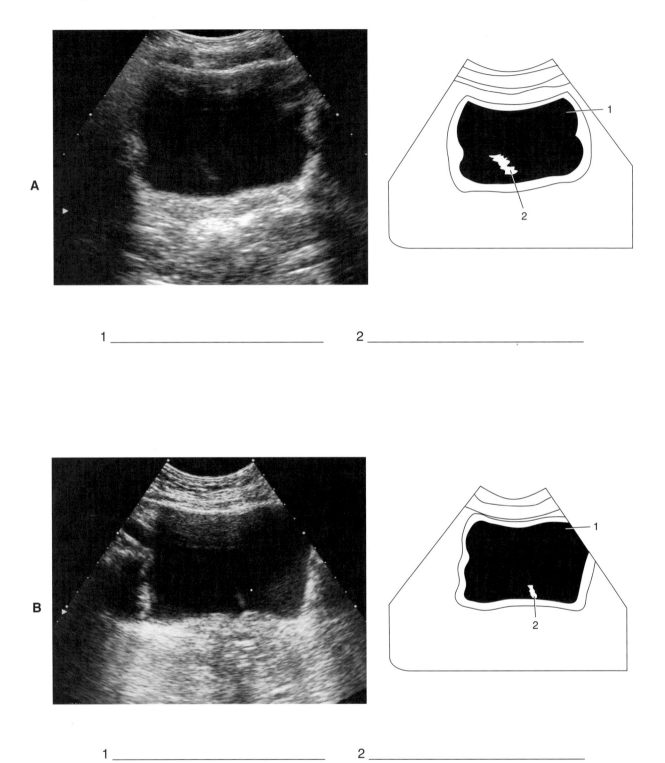

A

1 _____   2 _____

B

1 _____   2 _____

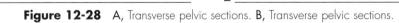

Figure 12-28   A, Transverse pelvic sections. B, Transverse pelvic sections.

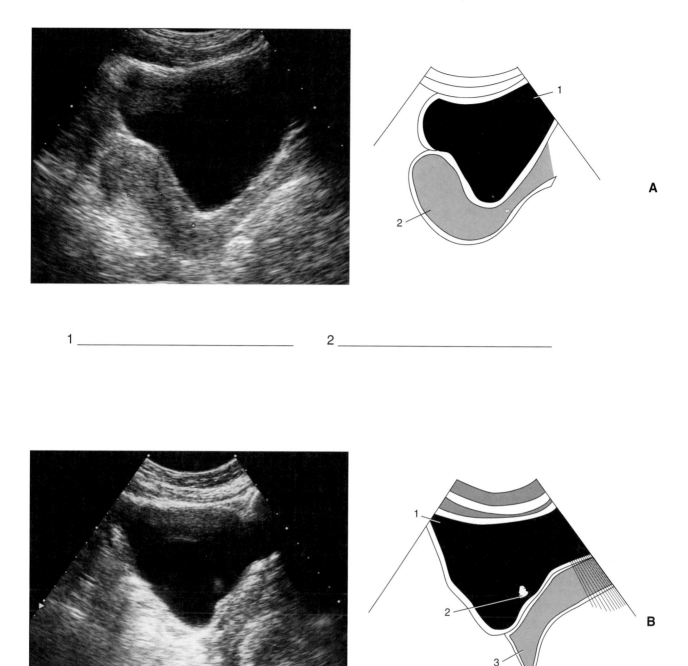

1 _____   2 _____

1 _____   3 _____

2 _____

Figure 12-29 A, Longitudinal pelvic views. B, Longitudinal pelvic views.

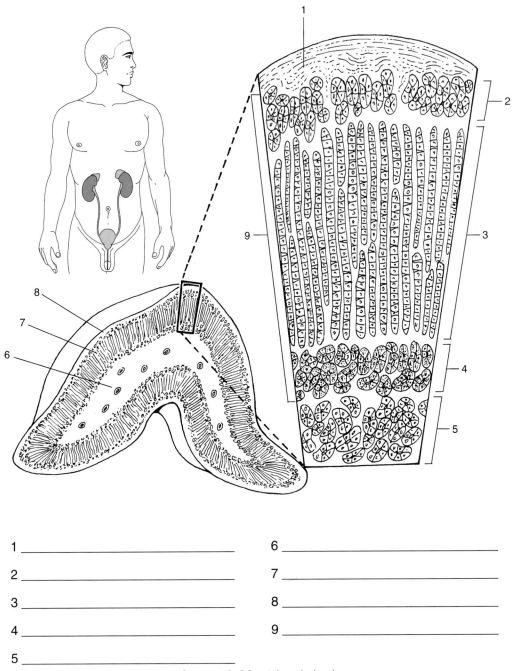

1 _____   6 _____

2 _____   7 _____

3 _____   8 _____

4 _____   9 _____

5 _____

Figure 12-30 Adrenal gland.

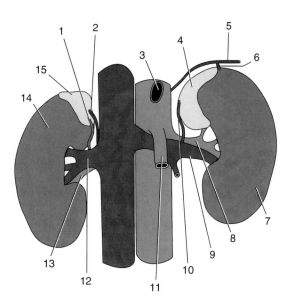

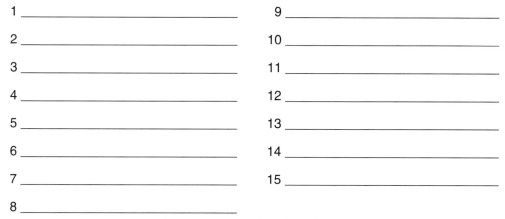

1 _____

2 _____

3 _____

4 _____

5 _____

6 _____

7 _____

8 _____

9 _____

10 _____

11 _____

12 _____

13 _____

14 _____

15 _____

Figure 12-31 Adrenal vasculature.

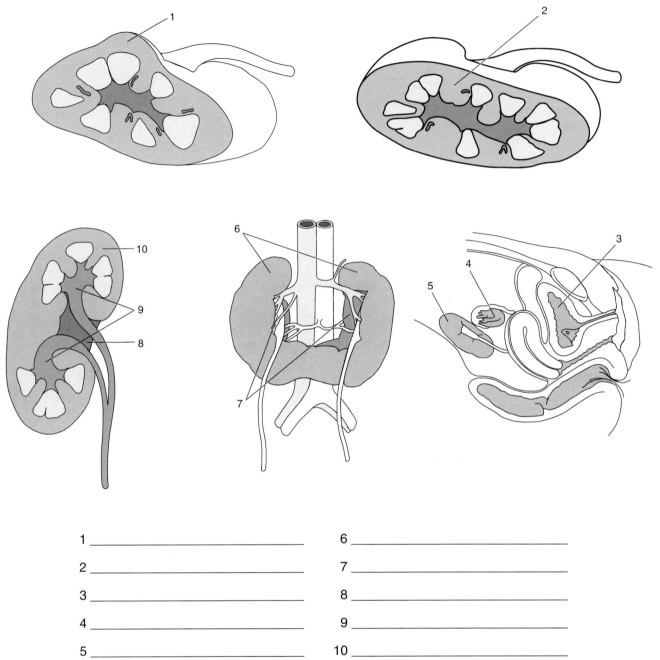

1	_____		6	_____
2	_____		7	_____
3	_____		8	_____
4	_____		9	_____
5	_____		10	_____

Figure 12-32 Renal variants.

CHAPTER 13

The Spleen

REVIEW QUESTIONS

1. Which of the following is not a reticuloendothelial function of the spleen?
   a. the storage of iron
   b. the production of lymphocytes
   c. the production of antibodies
   d. pitting function

2. The spleen arises from which embryologic tissue?
   a. ectoderm
   b. mesoderm
   c. endoderm

3. The spleen begins to develop during the _____ week of gestation.
   a. fifth
   b. tenth
   c. fifteenth
   d. near term

4. Which function of the spleen ends shortly after birth?
   a. pitting function
   b. hematopoiesis
   c. culling function
   d. reservoir function

5. The upper limit of normal for the superior to inferior length of the spleen is _____ cm.
   a. 5-6
   b. 7-8
   c. 9-10
   d. 12-13

6. The spleen is essential to sustain life.
   a. true
   b. false

7. Which of the following describes a decrease in the number of platelets within the circulation?
   a. leukopenia
   b. hyalinization
   c. erythrocytosis
   d. thrombocytopenia

8. The spleen is a(n) _____ organ.
   a. retroperitoneal
   b. intraperitoneal

9. The cells within the spleen that perform the primary lymphocytic functions of the spleen are the
   a. red pulp
   b. white pulp
   c. malpighian corpuscles
   d. splenic sinuses

10. Phagocytosis of degenerating red blood cells occurs within which portion of the spleen?
    a. white pulp
    b. red pulp
    c. malpighian corpuscles
    d. splenic arteries

11. The spleen lies _____ to the tail of the pancreas.
    a. anterior
    b. inferior
    c. medial
    d. lateral

12. The left kidney lies _____ to the spleen.
    a. anterior
    b. posterior
    c. superior
    d. lateral

13. The most common splenic pigment is
    a. amyloid
    b. anthrotic
    c. malarial
    d. hemosiderin

14. The malpighian corpuscles are found within which portion of the spleen?
    a. splenic hilum
    b. red pulp
    c. white pulp
    d. splenic cords

15. Which of the following statements best describes the sonographic appearance of the spleen?
    a. a homogeneous organ with an echogenicity pattern similar to that of liver
    b. a heterogeneous echo pattern
    c. more echogenic than the pancreas
    d. very echogenic due to its high volume of blood

16. Letter A on the following figure represents which correct orientation?
    a. superior
    b. inferior
    c. anterior
    d. lateral

A

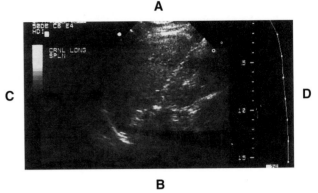

C · · · · · · · · · · · · · D

B

17. Letter C on the above figure represents which correct orientation?
    a. superior
    b. inferior
    c. anterior
    d. lateral

18. Letter D on the above figure represents which correct orientation?
    a. superior
    b. inferior
    c. anterior
    d. lateral

19. Letter D on the figure below represents which correct orientation?
    a. superior
    b. lateral
    c. medial
    d. posterior

20. Letter B on the figure below represents which correct orientation?
    a. superior
    b. lateral
    c. medial
    d. posterior

A

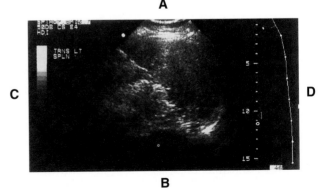

C · · · · · · · · · · · · · D

B

21. The spleen is considered to be a part of which body system?
    a. digestive system
    b. cardiovascular system
    c. reticuloendothelial system
    d. endocrine system

22. The reticuloendothelial system is primarily responsible for
    a. producing nerve tissue
    b. activating the clotting factor in the blood
    c. phagocytosis of pathogens and damaged or worn red blood cells
    d. balancing electrolytes

23. Lymphocytes are able to differentiate themselves into
    a. red blood cells and plasma
    b. memory cells and red blood cells
    c. white blood cells and red blood cells
    d. plasma cells and memory cells

24. Plasma cells identify and produce antibodies to destroy invading microorganisms.
    a. true
    b. false

25. Memory cells "remember" microorganisms that have previously attacked the body and enable antibodies to be activated more quickly.
    a. true
    b. false

26. The average adult splenic volume is about
    a. 350 ml
    b. 200 ml
    c. 500 ml
    d. 150 ml

27. In cases of severe hemorrhage, the spleen is able to give the body a "self-transfusion" of blood.
    a. true
    b. false

28. In the adult, the spleen never produces red blood cells.
    a. true
    b. false

29. What is the most common use of sonographic imaging of the spleen?
    a. splenic masses
    b. asplenia
    c. splenic rupture or hemorrhage
    d. to detect splenic enlargement

30. Asplenia is incompatible with life.
    a. true
    b. false

Identify the structures indicated in the following illustrations. These figures duplicate those found in *Sonography: Introduction to Normal Structure and Function*. Refer to the textbook if you need help.

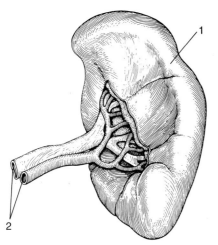

Figure 13-1 Splenic anatomy.

1 _____

2 _____

3 _____

4 _____

5 _____

6 _____

7 _____

8 _____

9 _____

10 _____

11 _____

12 _____

13 _____

14 _____

15 _____

16 _____

17 _____

18 _____

19 _____

20 _____

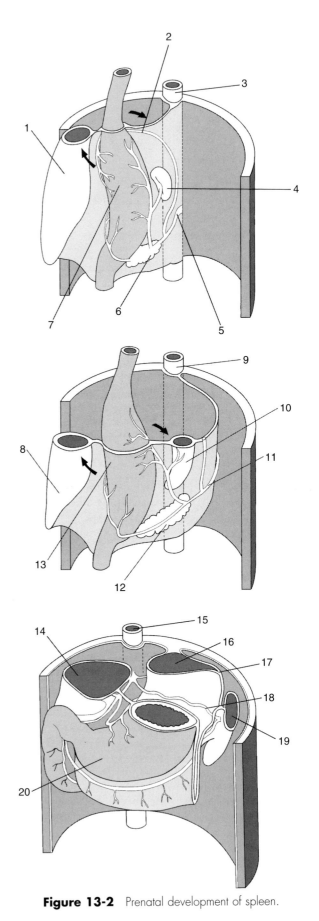

Figure 13-2 Prenatal development of spleen.

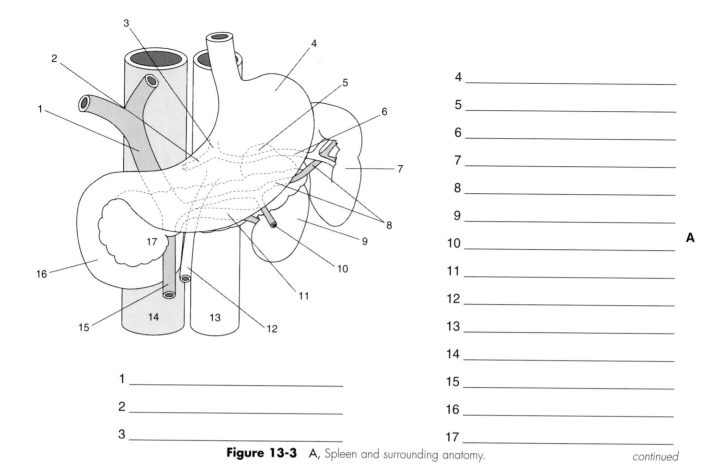

Figure 13-3 A, Spleen and surrounding anatomy.

continued

1 _____

2 _____

3 _____

4 _____

5 _____

6 _____

7 _____

8 _____

9 _____

10 _____

11 _____

12 _____

13 _____

14 _____

15 _____

16 _____

17 _____

A

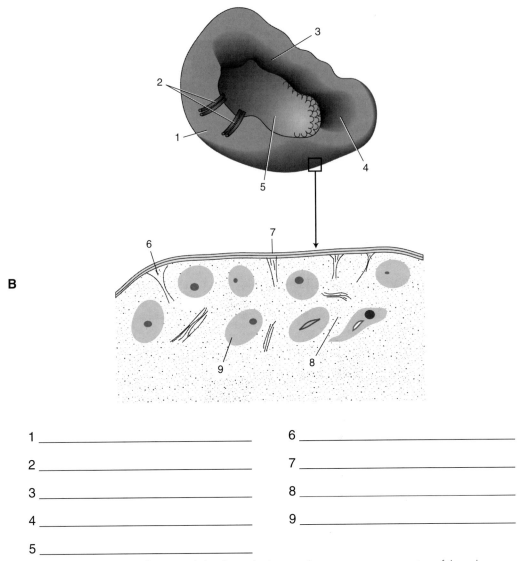

B

1 _____	6 _____
2 _____	7 _____
3 _____	8 _____
4 _____	9 _____
5 _____	

Figure 13-3, cont'd   B, Medial surface of spleen and microscopic organization of the spleen.

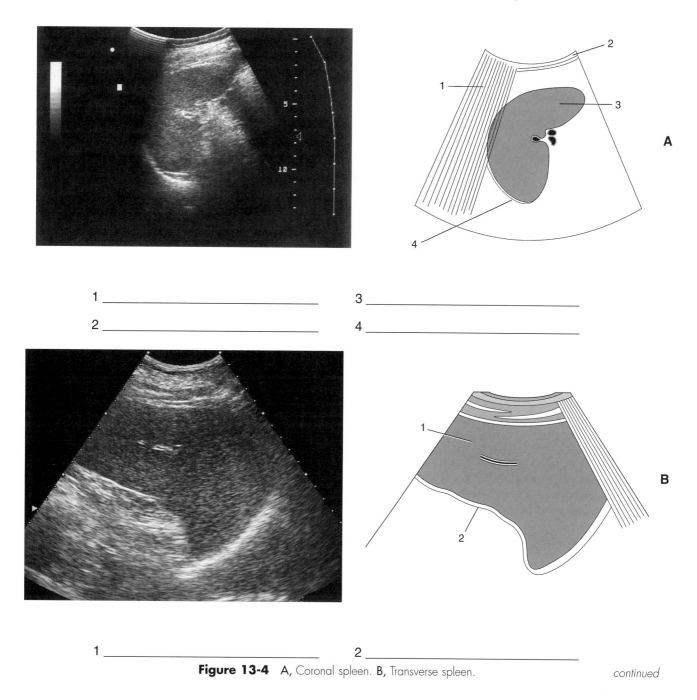

1 _____ 3 _____

2 _____ 4 _____

1 _____ 2 _____

Figure 13-4 A, Coronal spleen. B, Transverse spleen.

continued

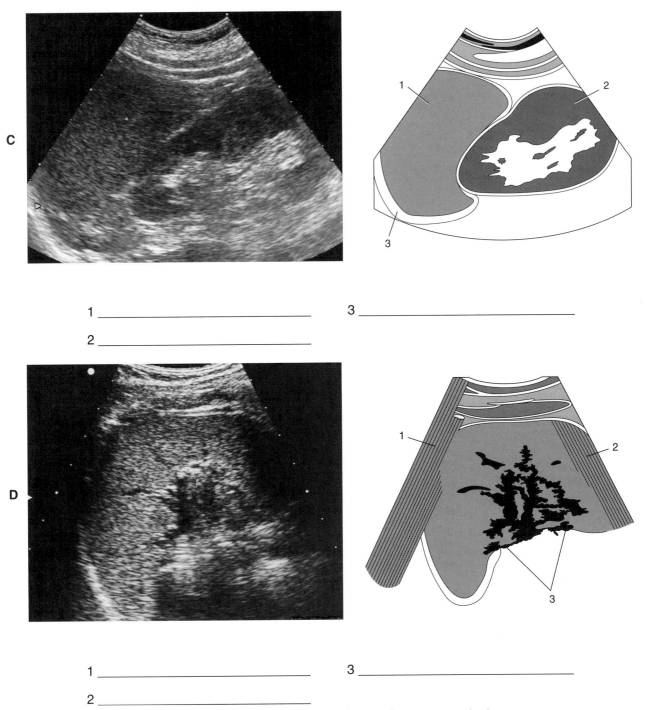

C

1 _____   3 _____

2 _____

D

1 _____   3 _____

2 _____

Figure 13-4, cont'd C, Spleen/kidney interface. D, Coronal spleen.

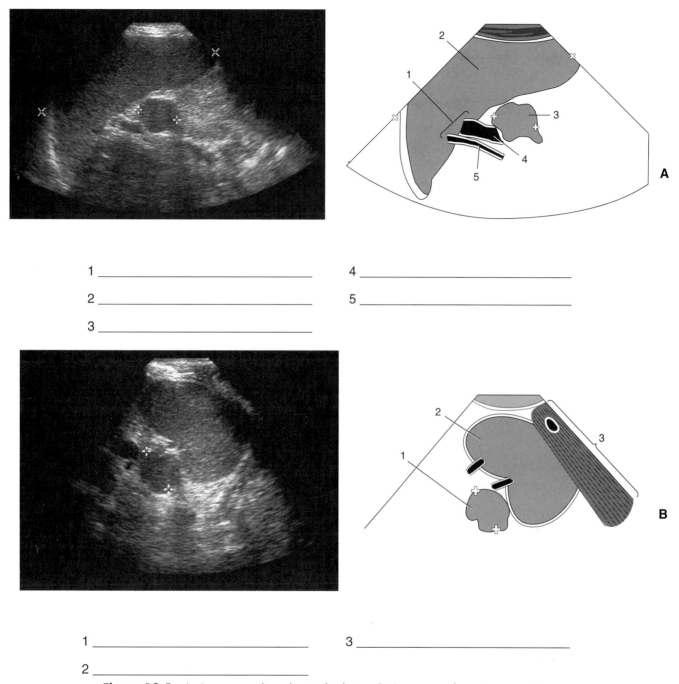

1 _____   4 _____

2 _____   5 _____

3 _____

1 _____   3 _____

2 _____

Figure 13-5 A, Accessory spleen, longitudinal view. B, Accessory spleen, transverse view.

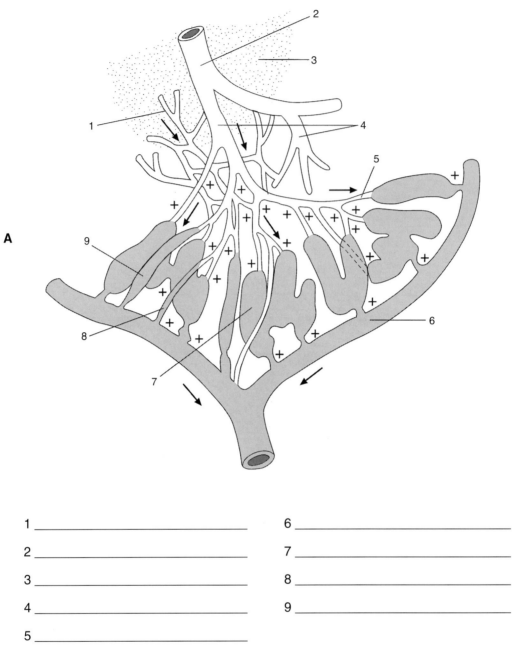

A

1 _____   6 _____

2 _____   7 _____

3 _____   8 _____

4 _____   9 _____

5 _____

Figure 13-6 A, Vascular anatomy of spleen.

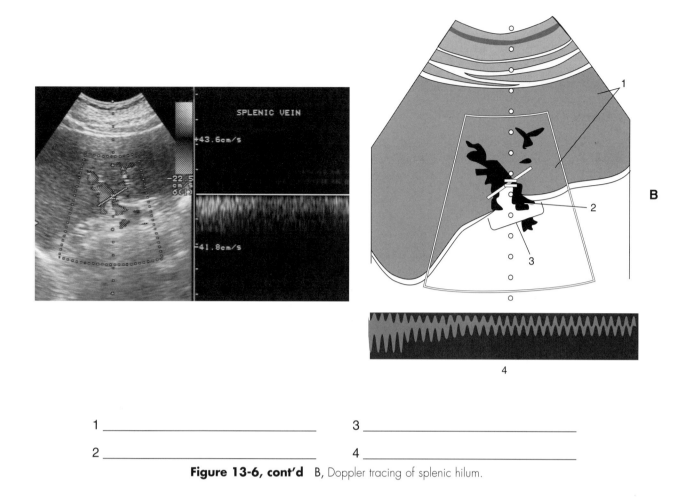

B

Figure 13-6, cont'd   B, Doppler tracing of splenic hilum.

1 _____   3 _____

2 _____   4 _____

CHAPTER 14

The Gastrointestinal System

REVIEW QUESTIONS

1. The majority of the digestive processes of the GI tract take place in which portion of the tract?
   a. mouth
   b. stomach
   c. small bowel
   d. colon

2. Each of the following substances is digested and absorbed in the GI tract except
   a. fats
   b. proteins
   c. carbohydrates
   d. vitamins
   e. water
   f. there are no exceptions

Select the region that best approximates the location of each item.

3. _____ stomach   a. foregut
4. _____ proximal duodenum b. midgut
5. _____ superior mesenteric c. hindgut
6. _____ sigmoid   d. tailgut
7. _____ ascending colon
8. _____ resorbed
9. _____ celiac
10. _____ inferior mesenteric

11. The final position of the stomach is the result of
    a. midgut
    b. two rotations
    c. division of the ventral mesentery
    d. fixation of the mesenteric root

12. Midgut herniation out of and back into the abdominal cavity occurs during embryogenesis.
    a. true
    b. false.

13. The terminal part of the esophagus connects with which portion of the stomach?
    a. antrum
    b. pylorus
    c. fundus
    d. cardiac

14. The stomach is located within each of the following regions except
    a. left upper quadrant
    b. left inguinal
    c. epigastric
    d. left hypochondrium

15. The stomach is separated from the pleura of the left lung and the apex of the heart by the
    a. left hemidiaphragm
    b. cardiac orifice
    c. the left lobe of the liver
    d. the falciform ligament

16. The posterior surface of the stomach is related to each of the following except the
    a. diaphragm
    b. superior pole of the left kidney
    c. left lobe of the liver
    d. anterior surface of the pancreas
    e. gastric surface of the spleen

17. The stomach is located within the retroperitoneum.
    a. true
    b. false

18. The small bowel is divided into three portions, including each of those shown below except
    a. cecum
    b. jejunum
    c. duodenum
    d. ileum

19. The duodenum contains portions located both in the peritoneal cavity and within the retroperitoneum.
    a. true
    b. false

20. The duodenal bulb is supported by the hepatoduodenal ligament and passes _____ to the common bile duct, the head of the pancreas, and the gastroduodenal artery.
    a. medial
    b. lateral
    c. anterior
    d. posterior

21. The portion of duodenum that receives the common bile duct via the ampulla of Vater is the
    a. first (superior)
    b. second (descending)
    c. third (transverse)
    d. fourth (ascending)

22. The large intestine begins in which of the following regions?
    a. right hypochondrium
    b. umbilical
    c. left hypogastric
    d. right inguinal

23. The ascending colon bends at the
    a. splenic flexure
    b. duodenojejunal flexure
    c. hepatic flexure
    d. ligament of Treitz

24. The smallest, widest, and most fixed portion of the small intestine is the
    a. duodenum
    b. ileum
    c. ampulla of Vater
    d. jejunum

25. The pylorus of the stomach is subdivided into three regions, including each of the following except
    a. antrum
    b. body
    c. canal
    d. sphincter

26. Which of the following is not a part of the large intestine?
    a. appendix
    b. cecum
    c. rectum
    d. ileum
    e. right and left flexures

27. The colon is divided into segments called
    a. rugae
    b. alveoli
    c. valvulae conniventes (valves of Kerckring)
    d. haustra

28. The hormone that is released by the presence of fat in the intestine and that regulates gallbladder contraction and gastric emptying is
    a. gastrin
    b. secretin
    c. cholecystokinin
    d. lipase

29. After the major food products are mixed with digestive secretions and enzymes, carbohydrates are reduced to monosaccharides and disaccharides, proteins to amino acids and peptides, and fats to monoglycerides and fatty acids. These nutrients are then
    a. absorbed through intestinal mucosa into the bloodstream
    b. propelled into the duodenum for digestion
    c. released into the large bowel for elimination
    d. transported into the portal system via intestinal lymphatics

30. Visualization of the bowel is impeded by
    a. fluid
    b. air
    c. gas
    d. all of the above
    e. b and c

31. The layers of the bowel wall create a characteristic sonographic appearance called a "gut signature." Up to _____ layers can be visualized.
    a. three
    b. four
    c. five
    d. six

32. The majority of the bowel wall layers recognizable on sonographic images are
    a. anechoic
    b. echogenic
    c. hypoechoic
    d. isoechoic

33. Each of the following may demonstrate a target appearance (bull's eye pattern) on sonographic images of the GI tract with the exception of
    a. EG junction
    b. inflamed appendix
    c. stomach antrum
    d. ileus
    e. there are no exceptions

34. The ascending colon is anterolateral to the
    a. tail of the pancreas
    b. neck of the gallbladder
    c. left iliac crest
    d. lower pole of the right kidney

35. Abnormal bowel loops demonstrate peristalsis and are compressible, and normal loops are noncompressible.
    a. true
    b. false

36. The splenic flexure refers to
    a. the inferior border of the stomach as it empties into the pylorus, anterior to the body of the pancreas
    b. the curvature of the transverse colon as it crosses the abdomen anterior to the duodenum, below the transpyloric plane
    c. that portion of the ascending colon in the epigastric region that courses toward the right side of the body from the region of the splenic hilum
    d. the colon bending to descend on the left, inferior to the spleen into the left iliac fossa

37. Which of the following muscles is unlikely to be penetrated by the rectum as it travels inferiorly to become the anal canal?
    a. levator ani
    b. pubococcygeus
    c. iliococcygeus
    d. obturator internus

38. The stomach originates as a
    a. fusiform dilatation of the caudal foregut
    b. dorsal wall of the mesentery
    c. bulge growing into the ventral mesentery
    d. herniation of the midgut

39. The esophagus begins at the level of the
    a. cricoid cartilage of the neck
    b. sixth cervical vertebra
    c. both a and b are correct
    d. neither a nor b is correct

40. The juncture of the greater and lesser curvatures of the stomach occurs at the
    a. cardiac orifice
    b. esophageal orifice
    c. entrance of the esophagus into the stomach
    d. each of the above is correct
    e. none of the above are correct

41. The lesser curvature of the stomach marks the _____ border of the organ.
    a. right
    b. left
    c. anterior
    d. posterior

42. The greater curvature of the stomach marks the _____ border of the organ.
    a. right
    b. left
    c. anterior
    d. posterior

43. The stomach would not be normally visualized on ultrasound to the right of midline.
    a. true
    b. false

44. The middle third of the descending duodenum is crossed anteriorly by the _____ portion of the colon.
    a. ascending
    b. descending
    c. transverse
    d. sigmoid

45. The esophageal wall normally measures _____ at the esophagogastric (EG) junction.
    a. 2 cm
    b. 3 mm
    c. 5 mm
    d. 10 mm

46. On transverse scans of the thyroid gland, the esophagus is normally visualized
    a. as a hypoechoic density with posterior acoustic enhancement, medial to the sternocleidomastoid muscle
    b. as a high echogenic mass proximal to the superior parathyroid gland on the left
    c. as a target lesion inferior to the lower pole of the right lobe
    d. posterior to the gland on the left, with a bull's eye appearance

Identify the structures indicated in the following illustrations. These figures duplicate those found in *Sonography: Introduction to Normal Structure and Function*. Refer to the textbook if you need help.

1 _____

2 _____

3 _____

4 _____

5 _____

6 _____

7 _____

8 _____

9 _____

10 _____

11 _____

12 _____

13 _____

14 _____

15 _____

16 _____

17 _____

18 _____

19 _____

20 _____

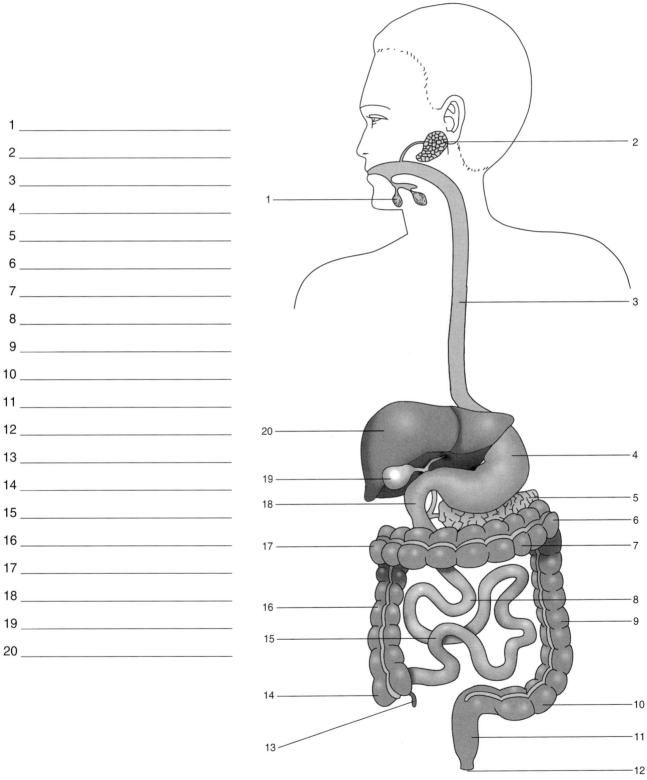

Figure 14-1 GI tract.

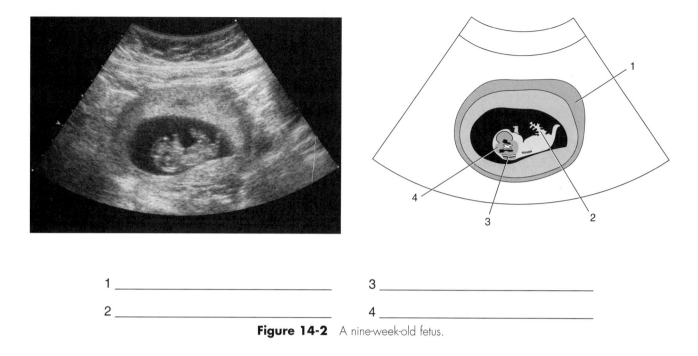

1 _____   3 _____

2 _____   4 _____

Figure 14-2 A nine-week-old fetus.

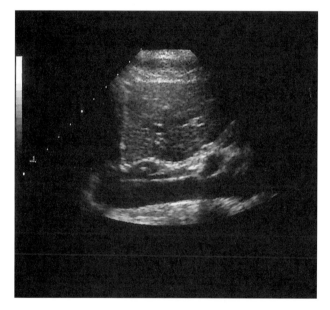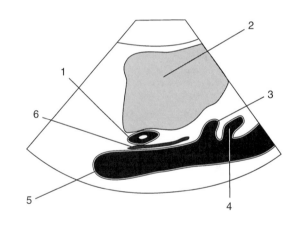

1 _____   4 _____

2 _____   5 _____

3 _____   6 _____

Figure 14-3 Longitudinal abdomen section.

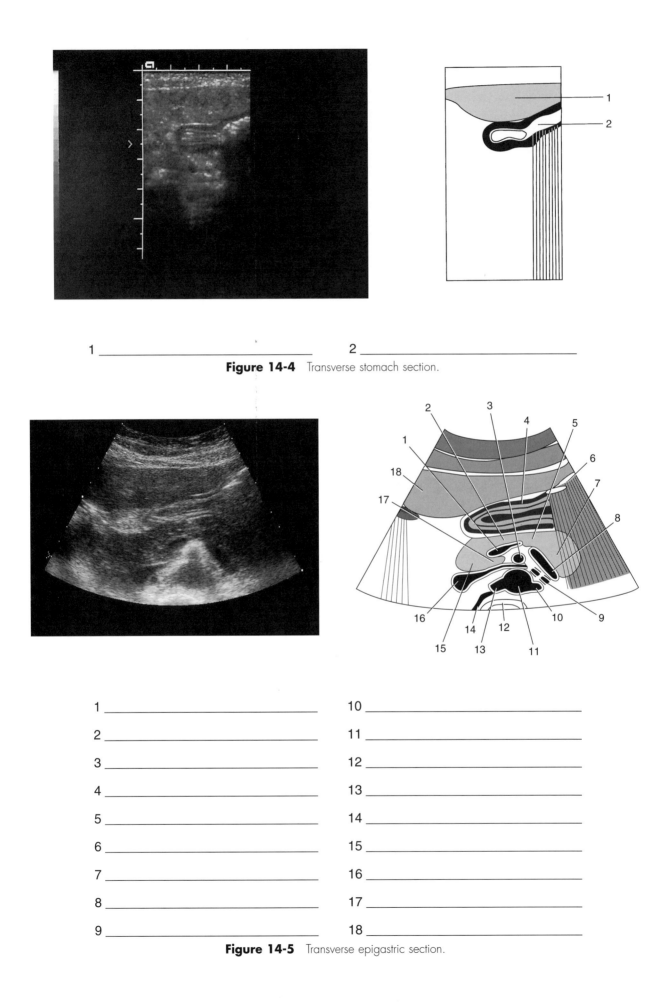

1 _____   2 _____

Figure 14-4 Transverse stomach section.

1 _____   10 _____

2 _____   11 _____

3 _____   12 _____

4 _____   13 _____

5 _____   14 _____

6 _____   15 _____

7 _____   16 _____

8 _____   17 _____

9 _____   18 _____

Figure 14-5 Transverse epigastric section.

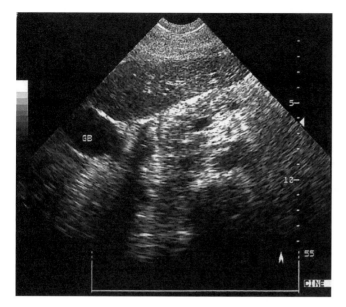

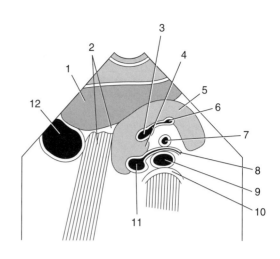

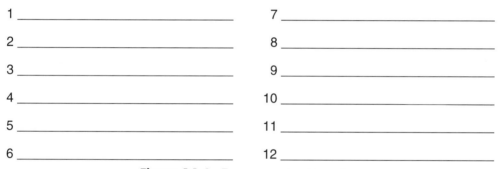

1 _____   7 _____

2 _____   8 _____

3 _____   9 _____

4 _____   10 _____

5 _____   11 _____

6 _____   12 _____

Figure 14-6 Transverse epigastric section.

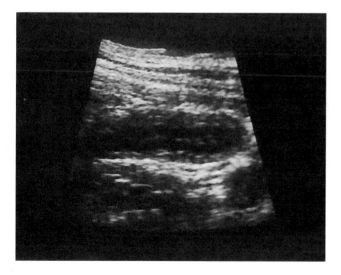

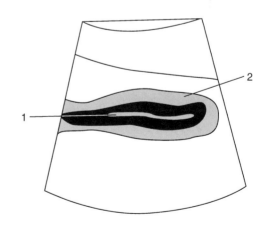

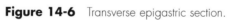

1 _____   2 _____

Figure 14-7 Right lower quadrant section.

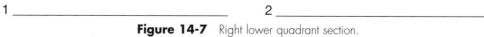

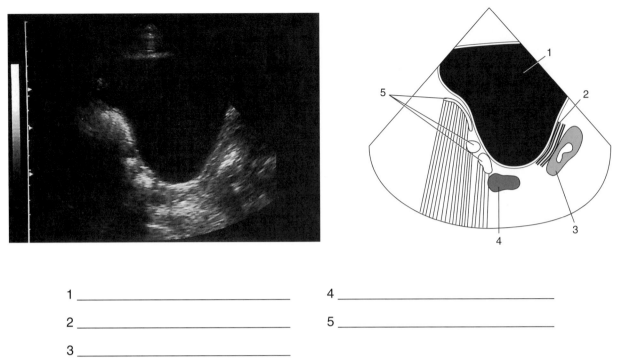

1 _____   4 _____

2 _____   5 _____

3 _____

Figure 14-8 Sagittal scan of the female pelvis.

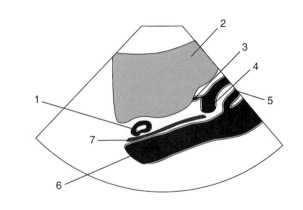
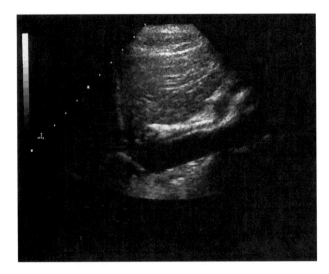

1 _____   5 _____

2 _____   6 _____

3 _____   7 _____

4 _____

Figure 14-9 Longitudinal abdomen section.

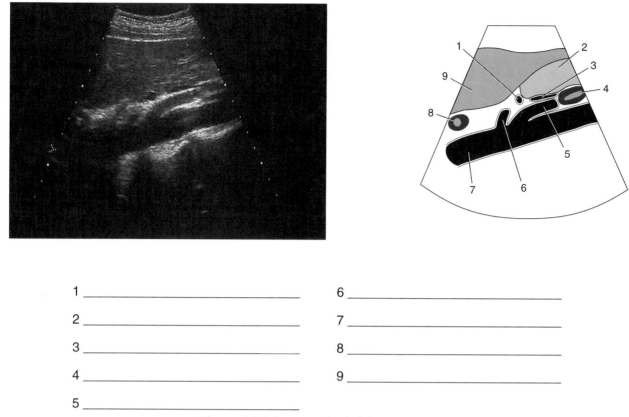

1 _____ 6 _____

2 _____ 7 _____

3 _____ 8 _____

4 _____ 9 _____

5 _____

Figure 14-10 Longitudinal abdomen section.

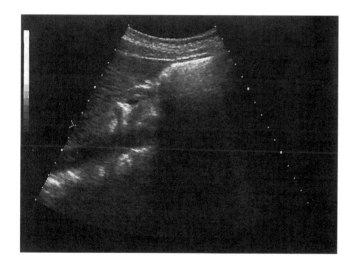
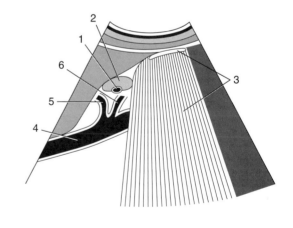

1 _____ 4 _____

2 _____ 5 _____

3 _____ 6 _____

Figure 14-11 Longitudinal abdomen section.

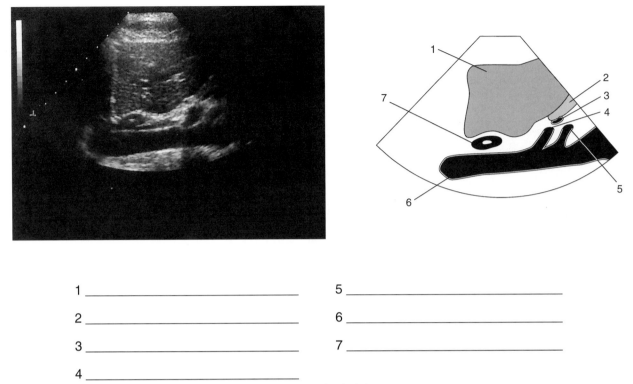

1 _____	5 _____
2 _____	6 _____
3 _____	7 _____
4 _____	

Figure 14-12 Longitudinal abdomen section.

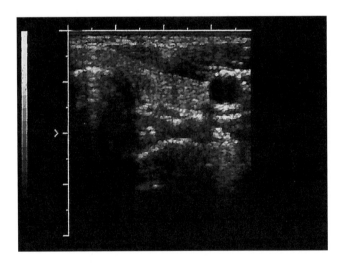
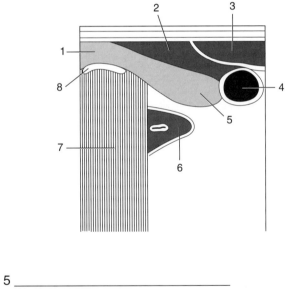

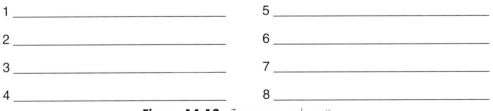

1 _____	5 _____
2 _____	6 _____
3 _____	7 _____
4 _____	8 _____

Figure 14-13 Transverse neck section.

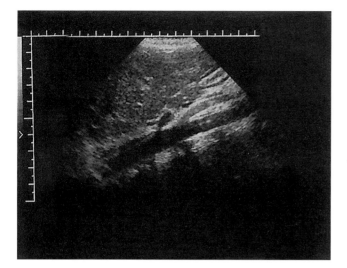
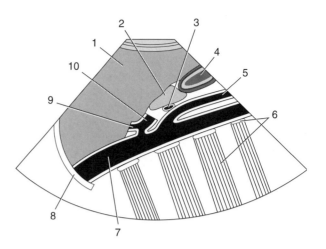

1 _____   6 _____

2 _____   7 _____

3 _____   8 _____

4 _____   9 _____

5 _____   10 _____

Figure 14-14 Longitudinal abdomen section.

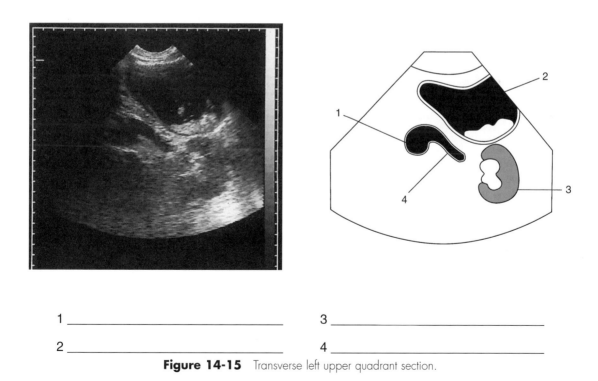
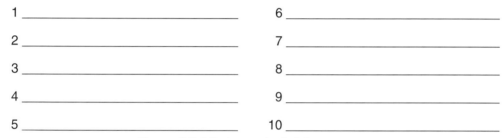
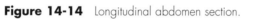

1 _____   3 _____

2 _____   4 _____

Figure 14-15 Transverse left upper quadrant section.

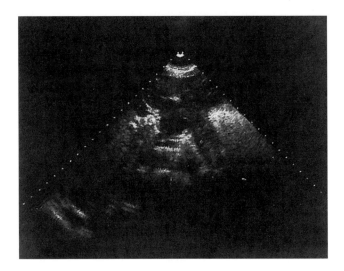
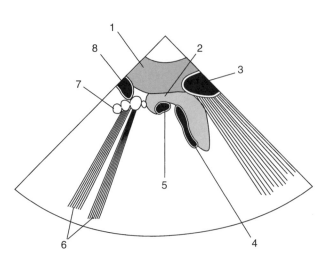

1 _____	5 _____
2 _____	6 _____
3 _____	7 _____
4 _____	8 _____

Figure 14-16 Transverse epigastric section.

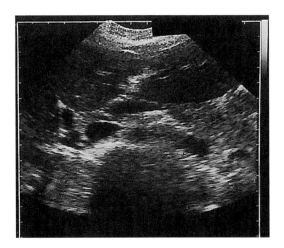
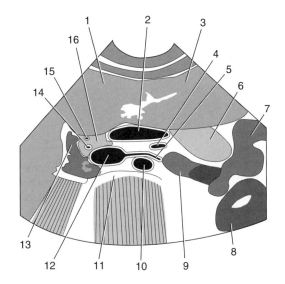

1 _____	9 _____
2 _____	10 _____
3 _____	11 _____
4 _____	12 _____
5 _____	13 _____
6 _____	14 _____
7 _____	15 _____
8 _____	16 _____

Figure 14-17 Transverse epigastric section.

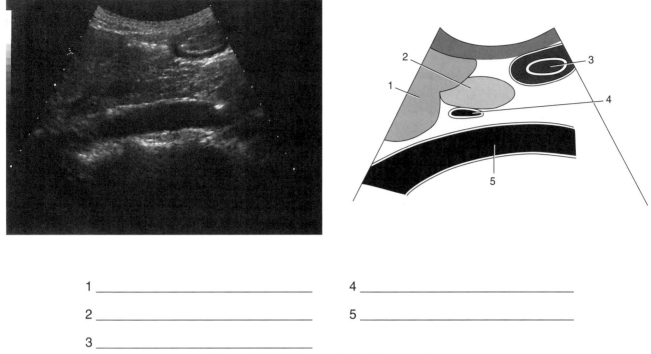

1 _____	4 _____
2 _____	5 _____
3 _____	

Figure 14-18 Longitudinal abdomen section.

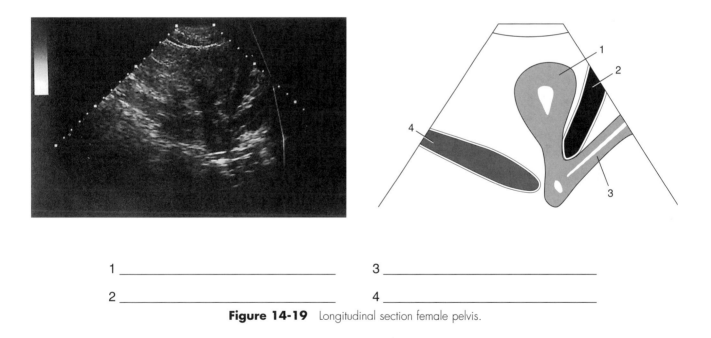

| 1 _____ | 3 _____ |
| 2 _____ | 4 _____ |

Figure 14-19 Longitudinal section female pelvis.

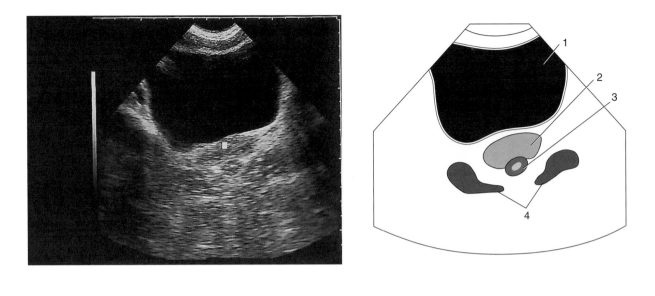

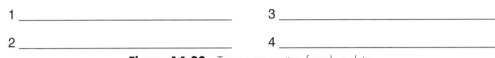

1 _____   3 _____

2 _____   4 _____

Figure 14-20 Transverse section female pelvis.

CHAPTER 15

The Male Pelvis

REVIEW QUESTIONS

1. Sex is determined by the presence or absence of the Y chromosome. The normal male fetus is identified as having the 46XY karyotype.

    a. true

    b. false

2. The maximum diameter of the seminal vesicles is normally greater than 1 cm.

    a. true

    b. false

3. Which of the following is not found within each testis?

    a. ductus epididymis

    b. seminiferous tubules

    c. rete testis

    d. straight tubules

4. The left testicular vein drains into the

    a. inferior vena cava

    b. left internal iliac vein

    c. right internal iliac vein

    d. inferior mesenteric vein

    e. left renal vein

5. Which of the following is not contained within the spermatic cord?

    a. ductus deferens

    b. pampiniform plexus

    c. ejaculatory duct

    d. cremaster muscle

6. The peripheral zone is the largest zone of the glandular prostate.

    a. true

    b. false

7. The penis is composed of three cylindrical masses of tissue: two corpora spongiosa and a single corpus cavernosum.

    a. true

    b. false

8. Which of the following is not visualized during an ultrasound examination of normal scrotum?

    a. mediastinum testis

    b. head of the epididymis

    c. body of the epididymis

    d. spermatic cord

9. When scanning transrectally, the normal seminal vesicles will appear hyperechoic to the normal prostate gland.

    a. true

    b. false

10. The _____ zone is the only zone of the glandular prostate that can be individually differentiated on a transrectal ultrasound examination.

    a. peripheral

    b. central

    c. transition

    d. periurethral

11. When scanning transrectally in the transverse plane, the shape of the prostate will appear semilunar near the base and more rounded at the apex.

    a. true

    b. false

12. The cavernosal arteries are located within the corpus spongiosum of the penis.

    a. true

    b. false

13. Penile ultrasonography is most frequently used for the detection of fibrosis, tumors, and periurethral diseases.

    a. true

    b. false

14. Which of the following structures is the most echogenic on transrectal ultrasound?

    a. head of the epididymis

    b. testis

    c. mediastinum testis

    d. seminal vesicles

15. Which of the following structures is the most echolucent (hypoechoic) on transrectal ultrasound?

    a. corpus spongiosum

    b. lumen of the deep arteries

    c. corpus cavernosum

    d. septum penis

Identify the structures indicated in the following illustrations. These figures duplicate those found in *Sonography: Introduction to Normal Structure and Function.* Refer to the textbook if you need help.

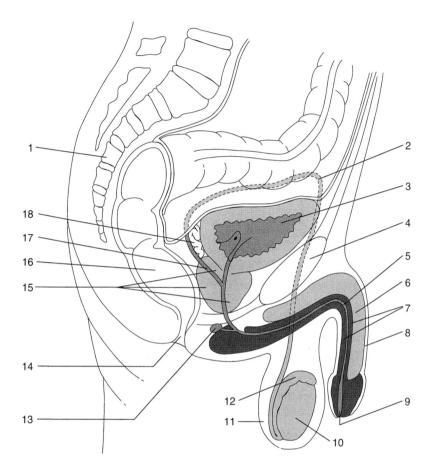

1 _____   10 _____

2 _____   11 _____

3 _____   12 _____

4 _____   13 _____

5 _____   14 _____

6 _____   15 _____

7 _____   16 _____

8 _____   17 _____

9 _____   18 _____

Figure 15-1 Male pelvis, sagittal section.

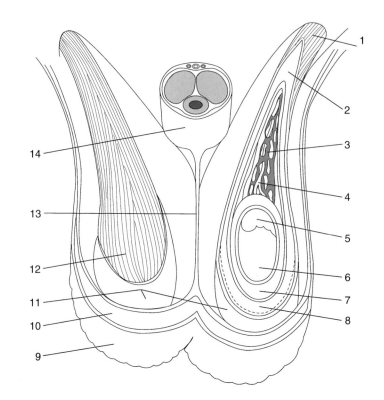

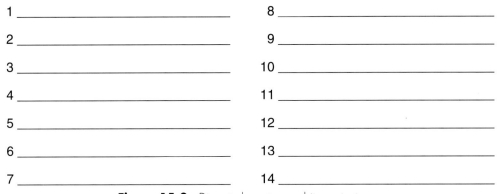

1 _____

2 _____

3 _____

4 _____

5 _____

6 _____

7 _____

8 _____

9 _____

10 _____

11 _____

12 _____

13 _____

14 _____

Figure 15-2 Dissected scrotum and its contents.

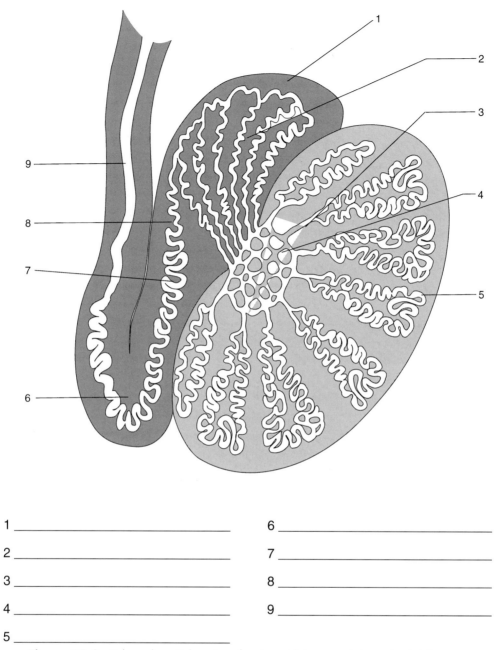

1 _____   6 _____

2 _____   7 _____

3 _____   8 _____

4 _____   9 _____

5 _____

Figure 15-3 Enlarged sagittal section of testis, epididymis, and ductus (vas) deferens.

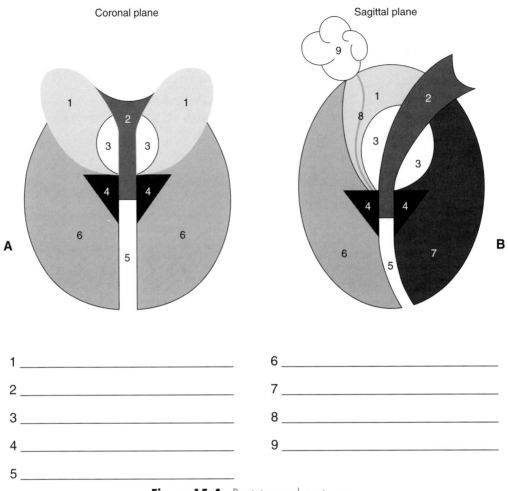

Coronal plane   Sagittal plane

A   B

1 _____   6 _____

2 _____   7 _____

3 _____   8 _____

4 _____   9 _____

5 _____

Figure 15-4 Prostate zonal anatomy.

1 _____

2 _____

3 _____

4 _____

5 _____

6 _____

7 _____

8 _____

9 _____

1 _____

2 _____

3 _____

4 _____

5 _____

6 _____

7 _____

8 _____

9 _____

10 _____

11 _____

12 _____

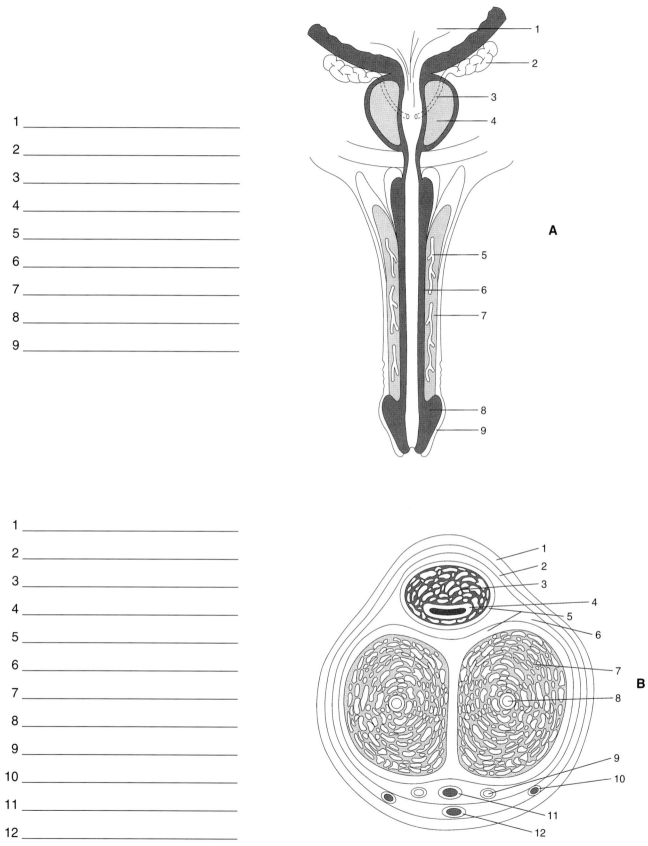

Figure 15-5 A, Penis anatomy, coronal plane. B, Penis anatomy, transverse plane.

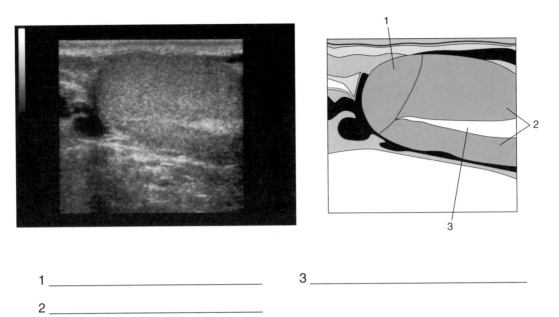

1 _____   3 _____

2 _____

Figure 15-6 Testis, sagittal section.

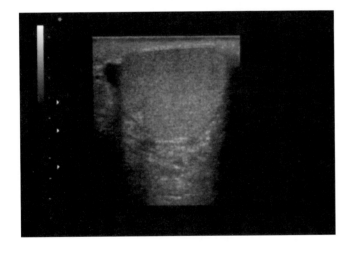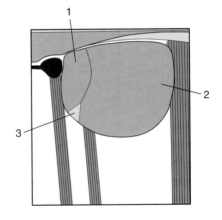

1 _____   3 _____

2 _____

Figure 15-7 Scrotum, transverse section.

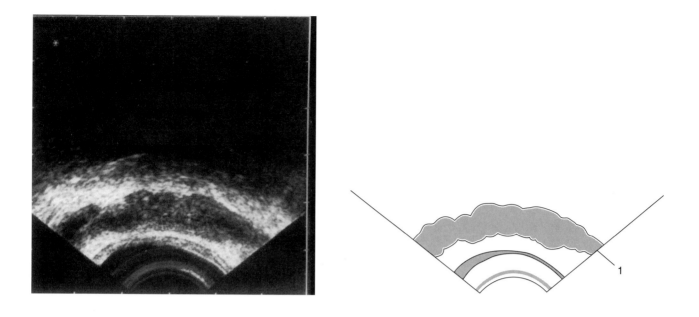

1 _____

Figure 15-8 Seminal vesicle, transverse section.

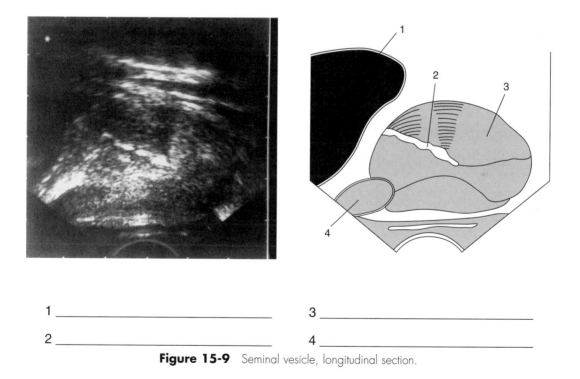

1 _____   3 _____

2 _____   4 _____

Figure 15-9 Seminal vesicle, longitudinal section.

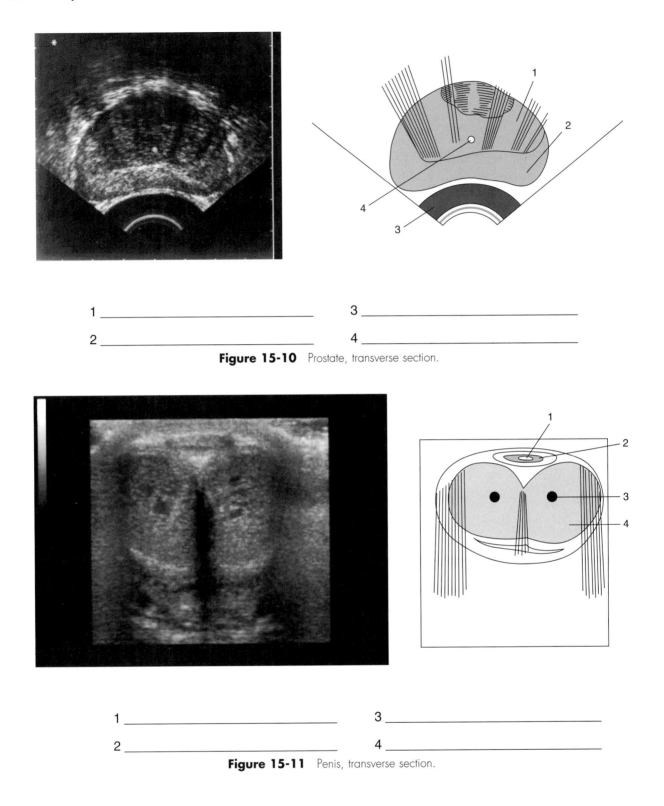

1 _____   3 _____

2 _____   4 _____

Figure 15-10 Prostate, transverse section.

1 _____   3 _____

2 _____   4 _____

Figure 15-11 Penis, transverse section.

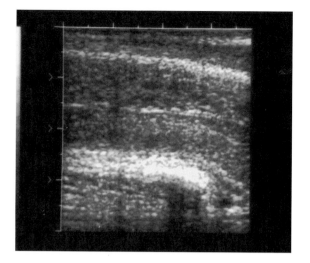 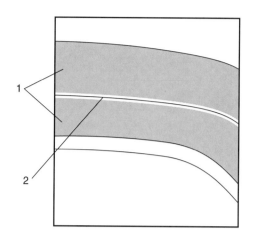

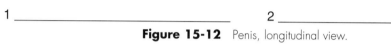

Figure 15-12 Penis, longitudinal view.

CHAPTER 16

The Female Pelvis

REVIEW QUESTIONS

1. Which of the following statements most accurately describes the anatomic relationships among the ovary, the ureter, and the internal iliac vessels?

    a. the ureter is posterior to the ovary, whereas the internal iliac vessels are anterior to the ovary

    b. the ureter is anterior to the ovary, whereas the internal iliac vessels are posterior to the ovary

    c. the ureter and internal iliac vessels both lie posterior to the ovary

    d. the ureter and internal iliac vessels both lie anterior to the ovary

2. Which of the following is used to divide the pelvic cavity into the pelvis major (false pelvis) and the pelvis minor (true pelvis)?

    a. pubic symphysis

    b. linea alba

    c. linea terminalis

    d. iliac crests

3. Which of the following muscles *do not* lie within the true pelvis?

    a. iliacus muscles

    b. piriformis muscles

    c. levator ani muscles

    d. obturator internus muscles

4. In which structure(s) are the hormones estrogen and progesterone produced in the female body?

    a. anterior pituitary gland

    b. ovarian medulla

    c. ovarian follicles

    d. uterine endometrium

5. The fibrous tissue mass remaining in the ovarian cortex following ovulation and the regression of the corpus luteum is called

    a. corpus albicans

    b. graafian follicle

    c. linea alba

    d. granulosa luteal cells

6. The arteries within the uterus that penetrate the myometrium are the

    a. spiral arteries

    b. arcuate arteries

    c. straight arteries

    d. radial arteries

7. The region of the uterus where the fallopian tube passes through the uterine wall and communicates with the uterine cavity is called the

    a. corpus

    b. cornu

    c. fundus

    d. infundibulum

8. Which of the following is the *outermost* layer of the ovary?

    a. tunica externa

    b. tunica albuginea

    c. visceral peritoneum

    d. germinal epithelium

9. Which of the following support structures anchors the ovary loosely to the uterine cornu?
   a. mesovarium
   b. ovarian ligament
   c. round ligament
   d. cardinal ligament
   e. infundibulopelvic ligament

10. Which of the following support structures extends from the uterine cornu, passes over the pelvic brim, through the inguinal canal, and is secured at the labia majora?
    a. round ligament
    b. broad ligament
    c. cardinal ligament
    d. uterosacral ligament

11. The most echogenic layer of the vagina is the
    a. vaginal mucosa
    b. muscular wall
    c. vaginal canal
    d. vaginal serosa

12. Bicornuate uterus is a congenital malformation caused by incomplete fusion of which structures during embryogenesis?
    a. wolffian ducts
    b. müllerian ducts
    c. urogenital sinuses
    d. mesonephros

13. On ultrasound, the skeletal muscles of the abdomen and pelvis appear _____ compared with their surrounding structures.
    a. hyperechoic
    b. hypoechoic
    c. isoechoic
    d. anechoic

14. The space between the pubic symphysis and the anterior wall of the urinary bladder is called the
    a. anterior cul de sac
    b. vesicouterine pouch
    c. uterovesical junction
    d. space of Retzius

15. Name the gonadotropin responsible for maintaining the corpus luteum.
    a. follicle stimulating hormone (FSH)
    b. estrogen
    c. progesterone
    d. luteinizing hormone (LH)

16. When the uterine body and fundus are tilted posteriorly, uterine position is described as
    a. anteflexed
    b. retroflexed
    c. retroverted
    d. anteverted

17. When the uterine body and fundus are situated posterior to the cervix, uterine position is described as
    a. anteflexed
    b. retroflexed
    c. retroverted
    d. anteverted

18. When the urinary bladder is empty, uterine position is described as
    a. anteflexed
    b. retroflexed
    c. retroverted
    d. anteverted

19. When the urinary bladder is fully distended, uterine position is described as
    a. anteflexed
    b. retroflexed
    c. retroverted
    d. anteverted

20. The portions of the large intestine contained within the true pelvis are the
    a. ascending colon and rectum
    b. transverse colon and rectum
    c. ascending and descending colon
    d. sigmoid colon and rectum

21. The vagina can be identified in the _____ portion of the pelvis between the _____ (anteriorly) and _____ (posteriorly).
    a. posterior/urinary bladder/rectum
    b. anterior/anterior cul de sac/urinary bladder
    c. inferior/urinary bladder/rectum
    d. superior/urinary bladder/posterior cul de sac

22. The thin, reflective, endometrial stripe describes the sonographic appearance of the
    a. endometrial canal
    b. basal layer of the endometrium
    c. inner layer of the myometrium
    d. functional zone of the endometrium

23. Anechoic areas seen between the outer and intermediate layers of the myometrium represent
    a. spiral arteries
    b. arcuate vessels
    c. areas of placental abruption
    d. the "sonographic halo"

24. The _____ phase is the best time to observe blood flow within the ovary.
    a. luteal
    b. proliferative
    c. secretory
    d. follicular

25. The muscles of the pelvic diaphragm and any fluid in the posterior cul de sac are visualized
    a. abutting the anterior cul de sac
    b. posterior to the vagina
    c. abutting the posterior bladder wall
    d. posterior to the rectum

Number in order from the most posterior to anterior pelvic layers. Label anatomy.
(See chapter opening figure.)

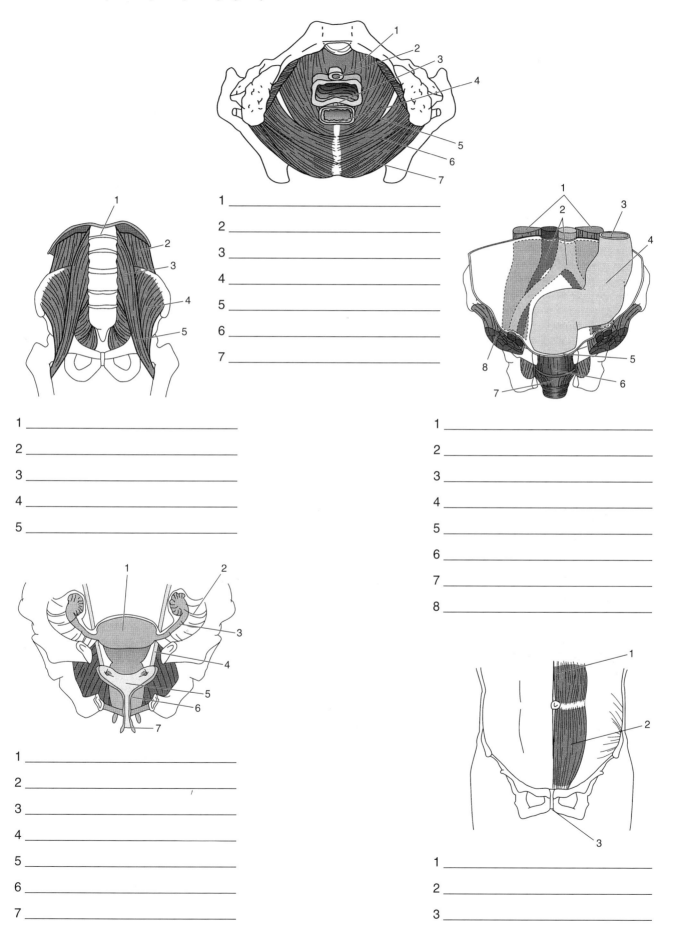

1 _____

2 _____

3 _____

4 _____

5 _____

6 _____

7 _____

1 _____

2 _____

3 _____

4 _____

5 _____

1 _____

2 _____

3 _____

4 _____

5 _____

6 _____

7 _____

8 _____

1 _____

2 _____

3 _____

4 _____

5 _____

6 _____

7 _____

1 _____

2 _____

3 _____

Identify the structures indicated in the following illustrations. These figures duplicate those found in *Sonography: Introduction to Normal Structure and Function.* Refer to the textbook if you need help.

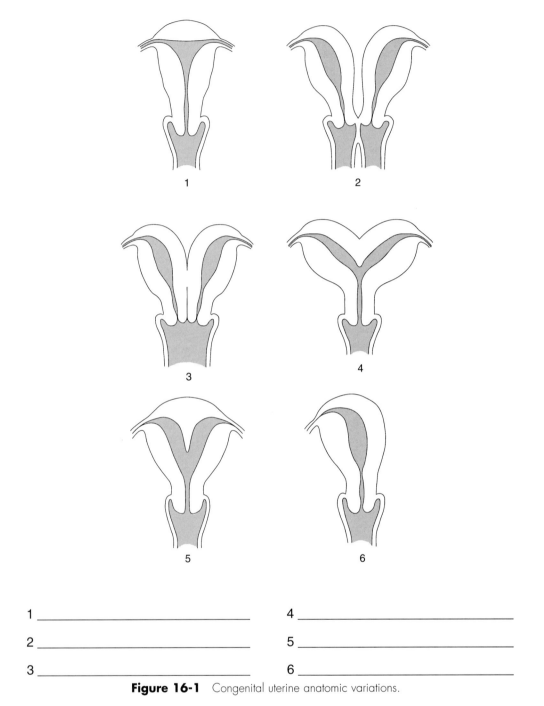

1 _____   4 _____

2 _____   5 _____

3 _____   6 _____

Figure 16-1 Congenital uterine anatomic variations.

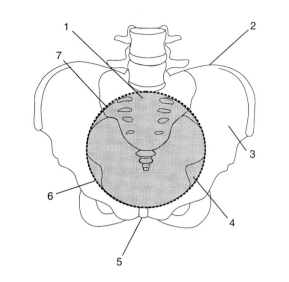

1 _____   5 _____

2 _____   6 _____

3 _____   7 _____

4 _____

Figure 16-3 The true and false pelves.

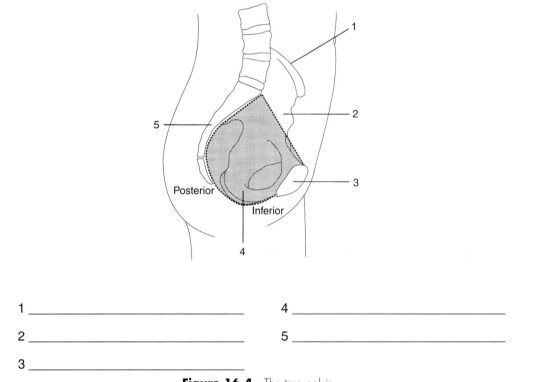

1 _____   4 _____

2 _____   5 _____

3 _____

Figure 16-4 The true pelvis.

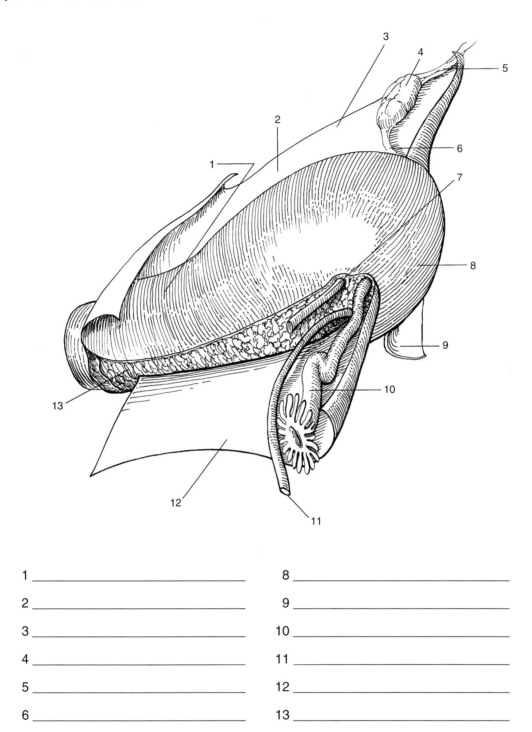

1 _____   8 _____

2 _____   9 _____

3 _____   10 _____

4 _____   11 _____

5 _____   12 _____

6 _____   13 _____

7 _____

Figure 16-5 Broad ligaments and surrounding structures.

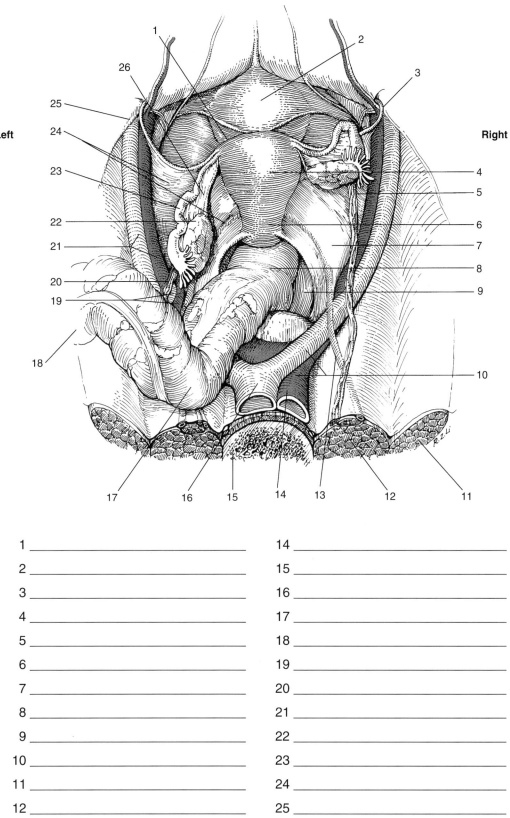

Left

Right

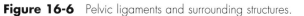

Figure 16-6 Pelvic ligaments and surrounding structures.

1 _____
2 _____
3 _____
4 _____
5 _____
6 _____
7 _____
8 _____
9 _____
10 _____
11 _____
12 _____
13 _____

14 _____
15 _____
16 _____
17 _____
18 _____
19 _____
20 _____
21 _____
22 _____
23 _____
24 _____
25 _____
26 _____

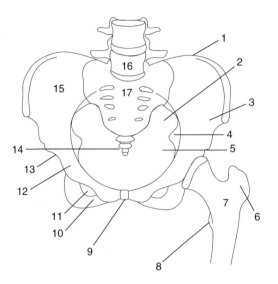

1 _____   10 _____

2 _____   11 _____

3 _____   12 _____

4 _____   13 _____

5 _____   14 _____

6 _____   15 _____

7 _____   16 _____

8 _____   17 _____

9 _____

Figure 16-7 The pelvic skeleton.

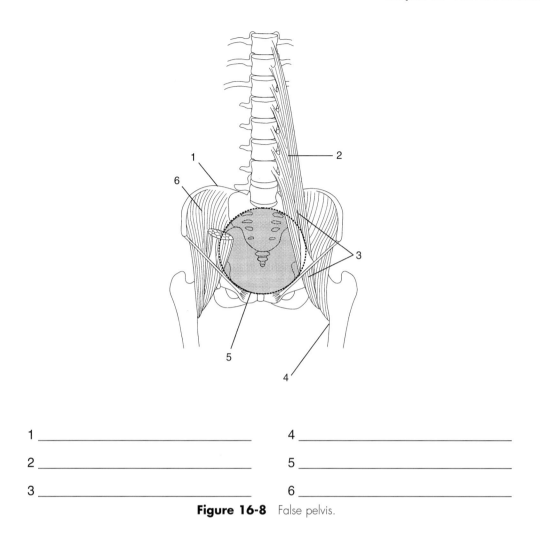

1 _____   4 _____

2 _____   5 _____

3 _____   6 _____

Figure 16-8 False pelvis.

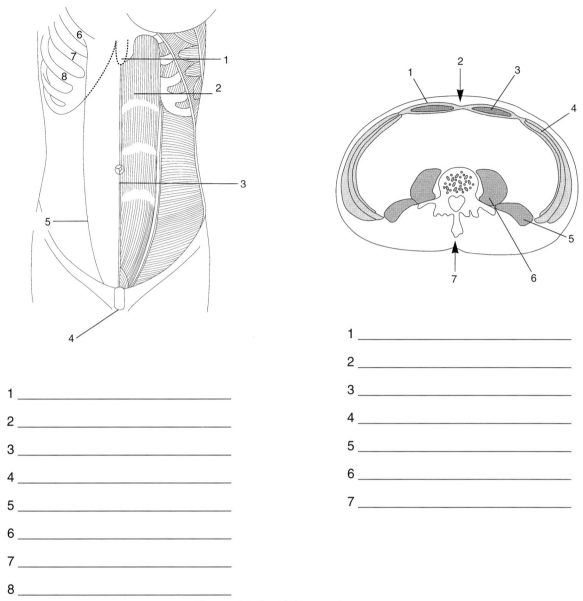

1 _____

2 _____

3 _____

4 _____

5 _____

6 _____

7 _____

8 _____

1 _____

2 _____

3 _____

4 _____

5 _____

6 _____

7 _____

Figure 16-9 Abdominopelvic cavity.

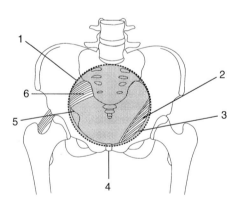

1 _____ 4 _____

2 _____ 5 _____

3 _____ 6 _____

Figure 16-10 True pelvis.

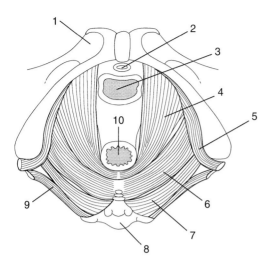

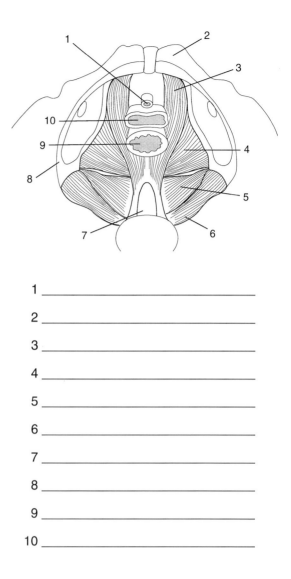

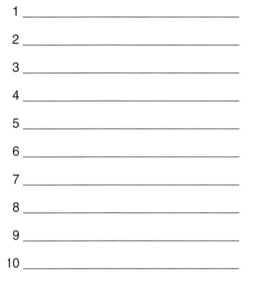

1 _____

2 _____

3 _____

4 _____

5 _____

6 _____

7 _____

8 _____

9 _____

10 _____

1 _____

2 _____

3 _____

4 _____

5 _____

6 _____

7 _____

8 _____

9 _____

10 _____

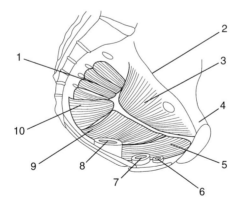

1 _____   6 _____

2 _____   7 _____

3 _____   8 _____

4 _____   9 _____

5 _____   10 _____

Figure 16-11

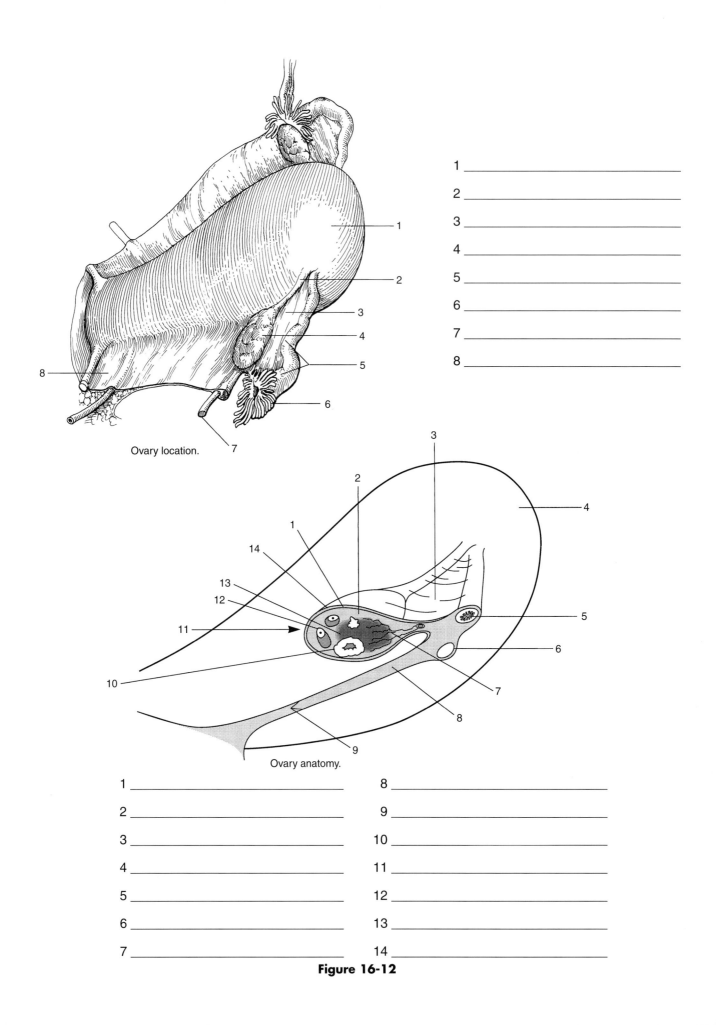

Ovary location.

1 _____
2 _____
3 _____
4 _____
5 _____
6 _____
7 _____
8 _____

Ovary anatomy.

1 _____   8 _____
2 _____   9 _____
3 _____   10 _____
4 _____   11 _____
5 _____   12 _____
6 _____   13 _____
7 _____   14 _____

Figure 16-12

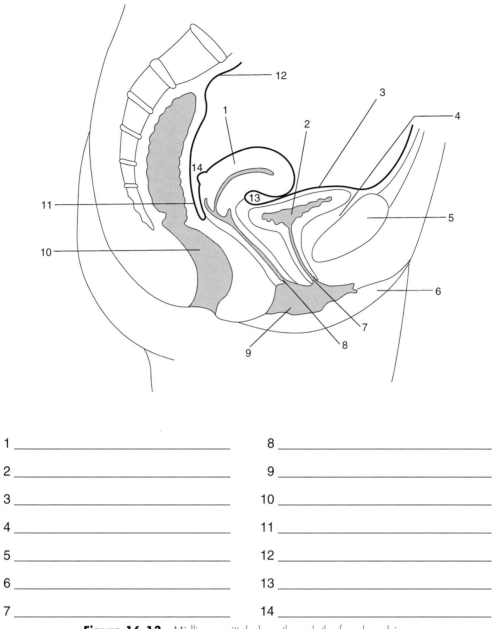

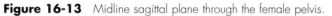

1 _____	8 _____
2 _____	9 _____
3 _____	10 _____
4 _____	11 _____
5 _____	12 _____
6 _____	13 _____
7 _____	14 _____

Figure 16-13 Midline sagittal plane through the female pelvis.

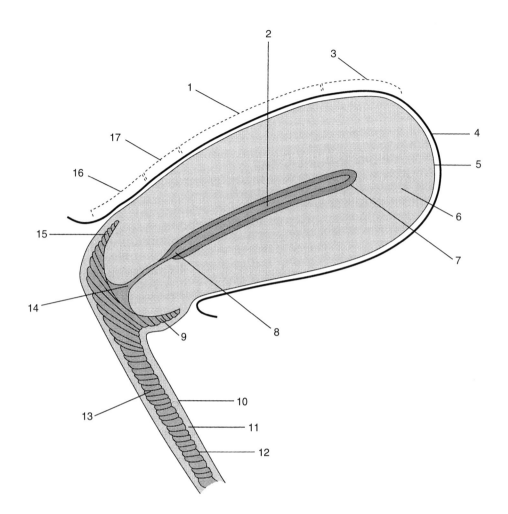

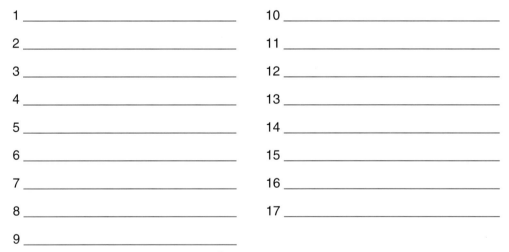

1 _____   10 _____

2 _____   11 _____

3 _____   12 _____

4 _____   13 _____

5 _____   14 _____

6 _____   15 _____

7 _____   16 _____

8 _____   17 _____

9 _____

Figure 16-14

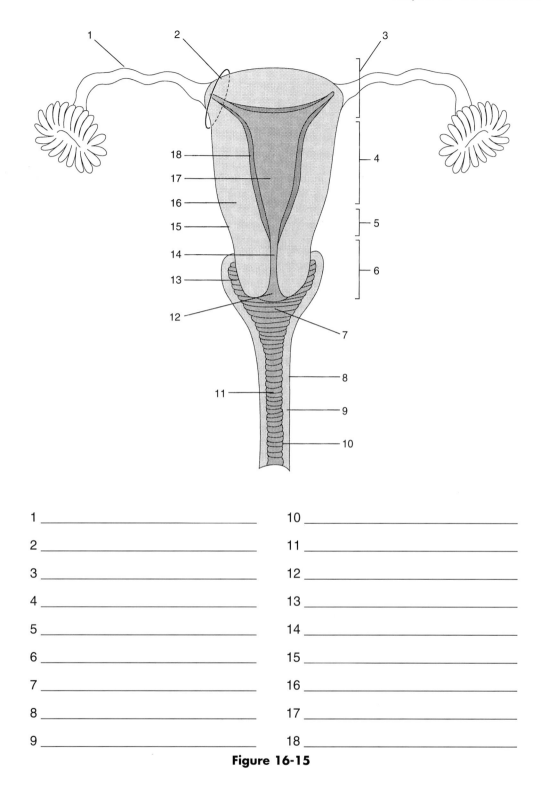

Figure 16-15

1 _____   10 _____

2 _____   11 _____

3 _____   12 _____

4 _____   13 _____

5 _____   14 _____

6 _____   15 _____

7 _____   16 _____

8 _____   17 _____

9 _____   18 _____

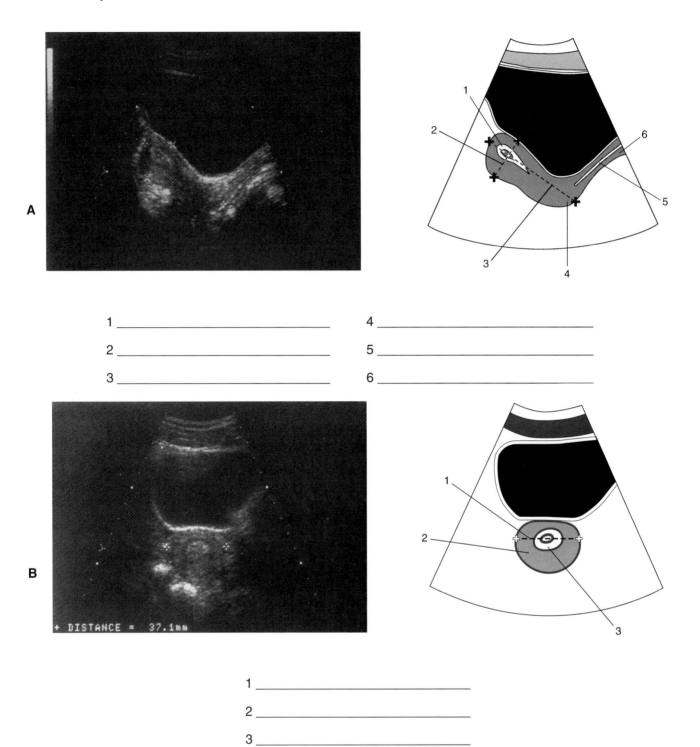

A

1 _____   4 _____

2 _____   5 _____

3 _____   6 _____

B

1 _____

2 _____

3 _____

Figure 16-16 A, Long axis uterine section. B, Short axis uterine section.

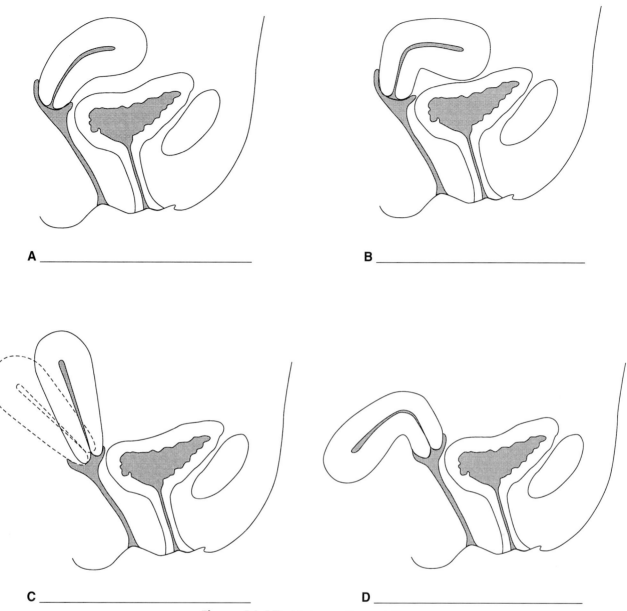

A _____

B _____

C _____

D _____

Figure 16-17 Uterine position variations.

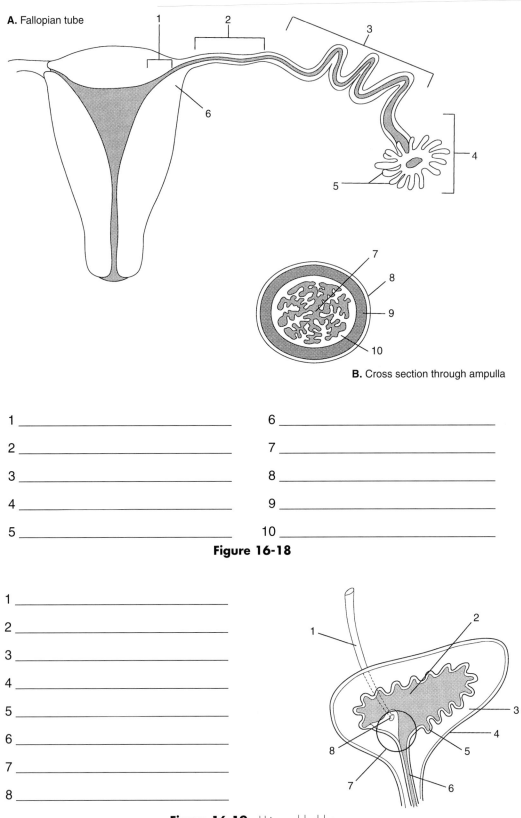

A. Fallopian tube

B. Cross section through ampulla

1 _____	6 _____
2 _____	7 _____
3 _____	8 _____
4 _____	9 _____
5 _____	10 _____

Figure 16-18

1 _____

2 _____

3 _____

4 _____

5 _____

6 _____

7 _____

8 _____

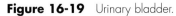

Figure 16-19 Urinary bladder.

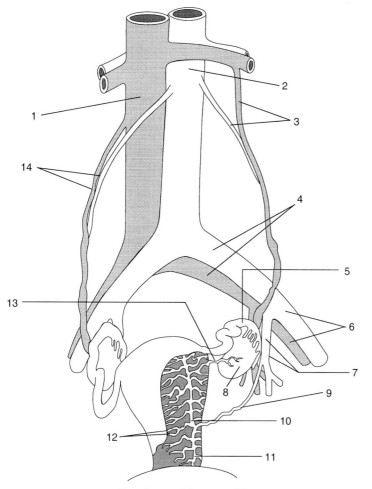

Vasculature of the true pelvis.

1	_____
2	_____
3	_____
4	_____
5	_____
6	_____
7	_____
8	_____
9	_____
10	_____
11	_____
12	_____
13	_____
14	_____

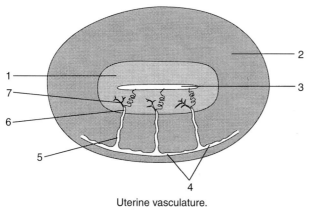

Uterine vasculature.

1	_____
2	_____
3	_____
4	_____
5	_____
6	_____
7	_____

Figure 16-20

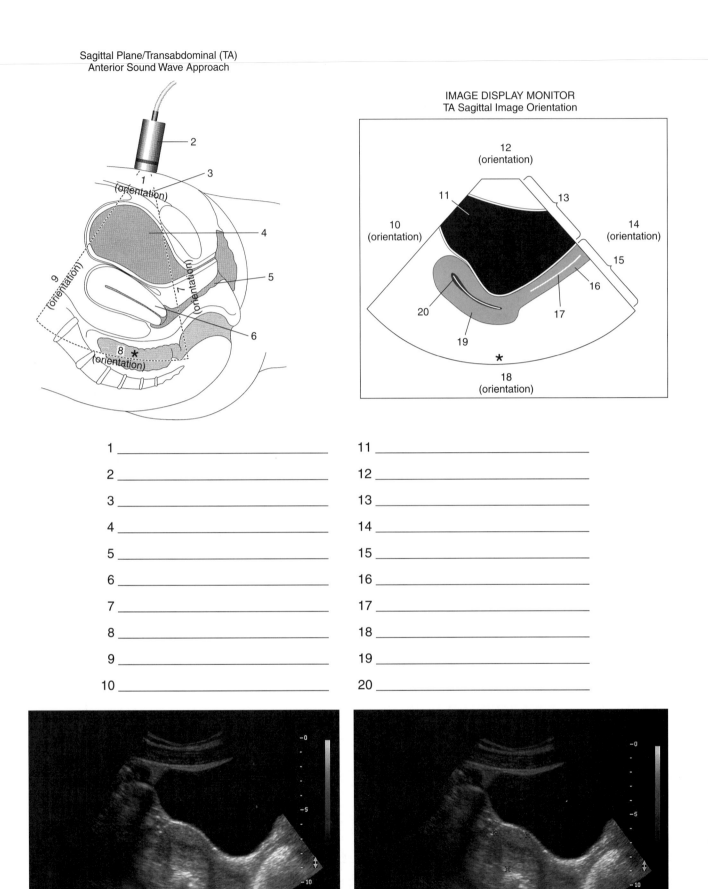

IMAGE DISPLAY MONITOR
TA Sagittal Image Orientation

1 _____

2 _____

3 _____

4 _____

5 _____

6 _____

7 _____

8 _____

9 _____

10 _____

11 _____

12 _____

13 _____

14 _____

15 _____

16 _____

17 _____

18 _____

19 _____

20 _____

Figure 16-23 TA, pelvic, sagittal plane view.

Transverse Plane/Transabdominal (TA)
Anterior Sound Wave Approach

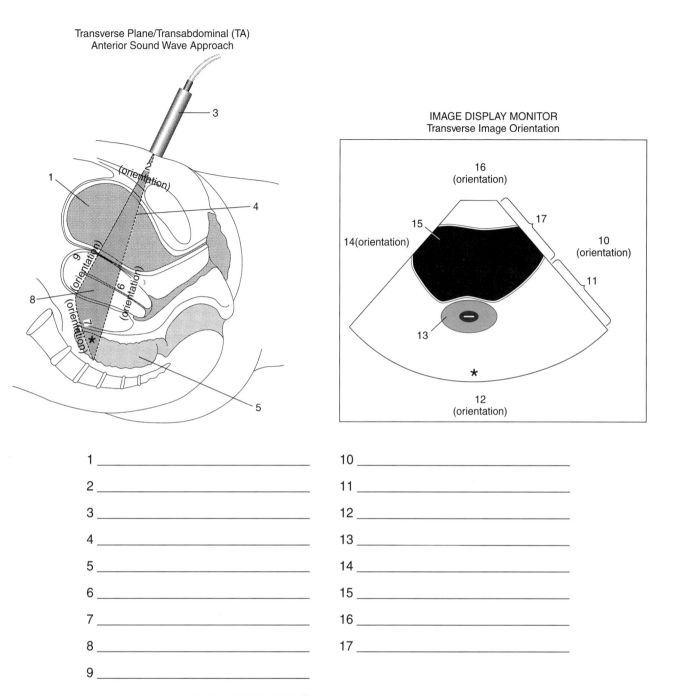

IMAGE DISPLAY MONITOR
Transverse Image Orientation

1 _____
2 _____
3 _____
4 _____
5 _____
6 _____
7 _____
8 _____
9 _____

10 _____
11 _____
12 _____
13 _____
14 _____
15 _____
16 _____
17 _____

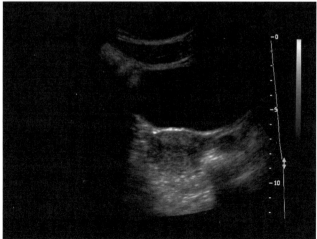

Figure 16-24 TA, pelvic, transverse plane view.

Transvaginal (TV) Sagittal Plane/Inferior Sound Wave Approach

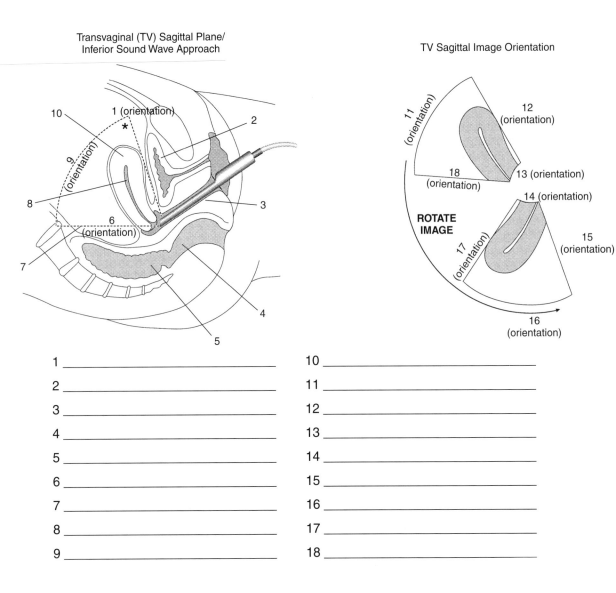

TV Sagittal Image Orientation

1 _____	10 _____
2 _____	11 _____
3 _____	12 _____
4 _____	13 _____
5 _____	14 _____
6 _____	15 _____
7 _____	16 _____
8 _____	17 _____
9 _____	18 _____

IMAGE DISPLAY MONITOR

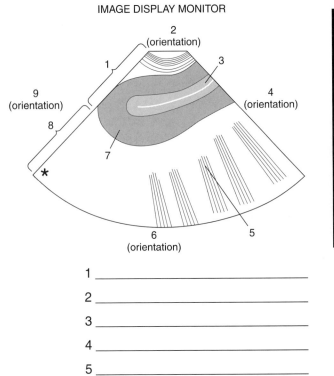

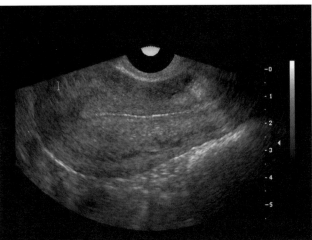

1 _____	6 _____
2 _____	7 _____
3 _____	8 _____
4 _____	9 _____
5 _____	

Figure 16-25 TV, pelvic, sagittal plane view.

Coronal Plane/Transvaginal (TV)
Inferior Sound Wave Approach

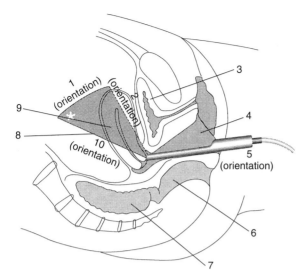

TV Coronal Image Orientation

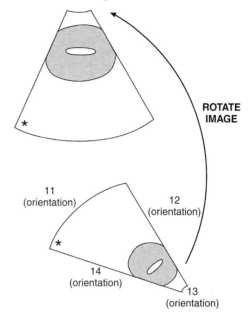

ROTATE IMAGE

1 _____   8 _____

2 _____   9 _____

3 _____   10 _____

4 _____   11 _____

5 _____   12 _____

6 _____   13 _____

7 _____   14 _____

IMAGE DISPLAY MONITOR

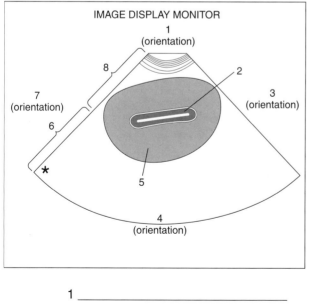

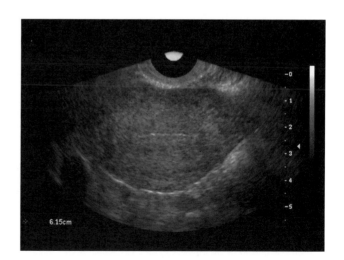

1 _____   5 _____

2 _____   6 _____

3 _____   7 _____

4 _____   8 _____

Figure 16-26 TV, pelvic, coronal plane view.

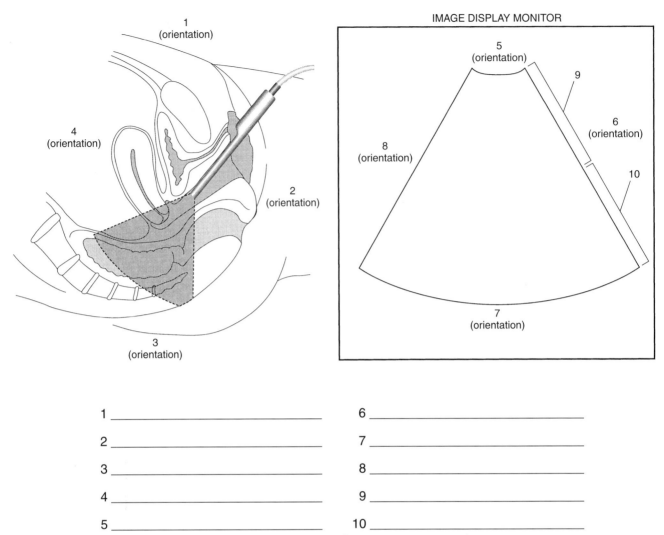

IMAGE DISPLAY MONITOR

1 _____	6 _____
2 _____	7 _____
3 _____	8 _____
4 _____	9 _____
5 _____	10 _____

Figure 16-27 TV imaging from an anterior approach.

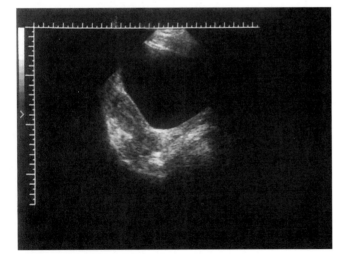

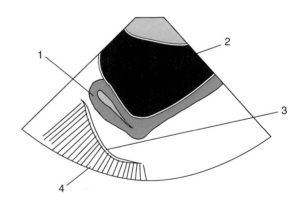

| 1 _____ | 3 _____ |
| 2 _____ | 4 _____ |

Figure 16-28 TA, sagittal pelvis view.

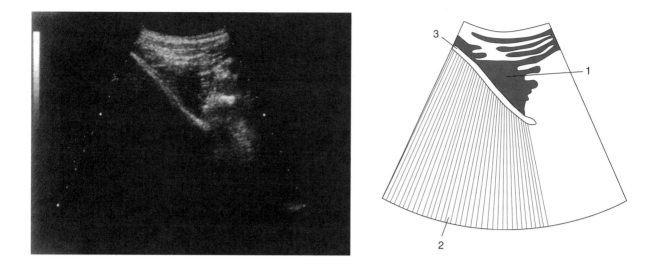

1 _____

2 _____

3 _____

Figure 16-29 TA, transverse pelvis view.

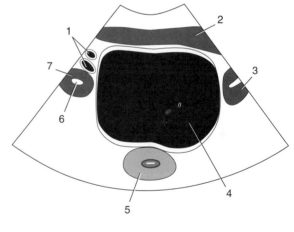
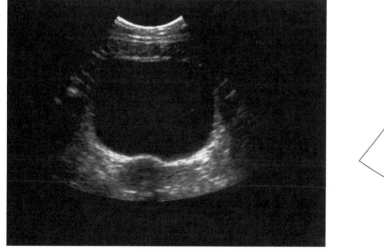

1 _____   5 _____

2 _____   6 _____

3 _____   7 _____

4 _____

Figure 16-30 TA, transverse pelvis view.

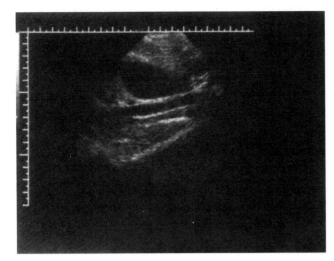
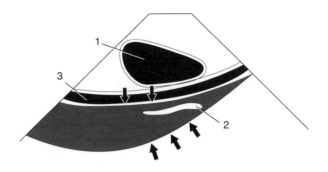

1 _____

2 _____

3 _____

4 Define the anatomic area indicated by

the arrows _____

Figure 16-31 TA, right parasagittal pelvis view.

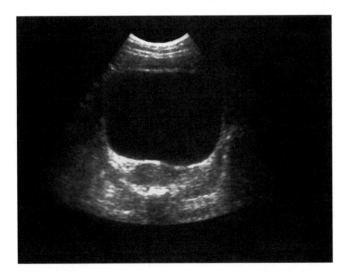
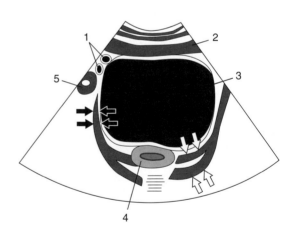

1 _____   5 _____

2 _____   6 Define the anatomic area indicated by

3 _____   the arrows _____

4 _____

Figure 16-32 TA, transverse pelvis view.

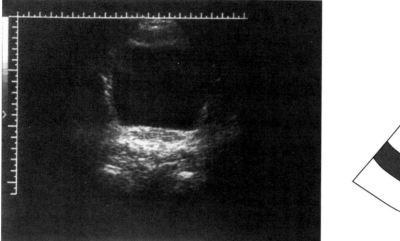

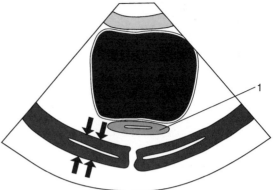

1 _____

2 Define the anatomic area indicated by

the arrows _____

Figure 16-33 TA, transverse pelvis view.

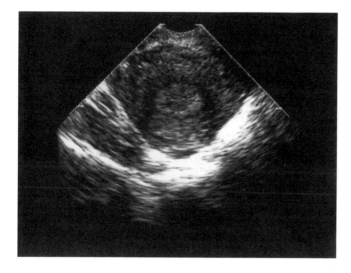

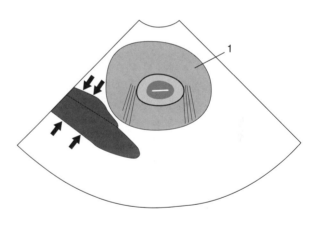

1 _____

2 Define the anatomic area indicated by

the arrows _____

Figure 16-34 TV, coronal view.

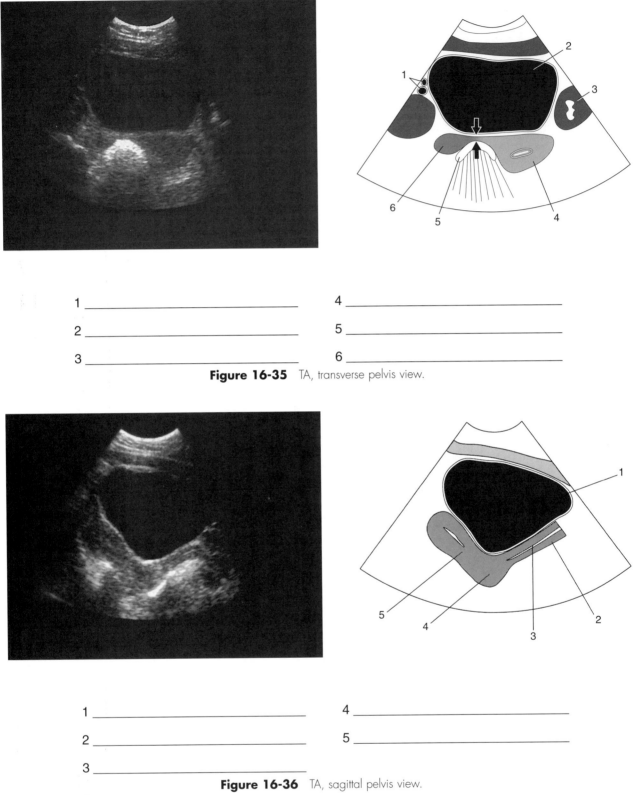

1 _____   4 _____

2 _____   5 _____

3 _____   6 _____

Figure 16-35 TA, transverse pelvis view.

1 _____   4 _____

2 _____   5 _____

3 _____

Figure 16-36 TA, sagittal pelvis view.

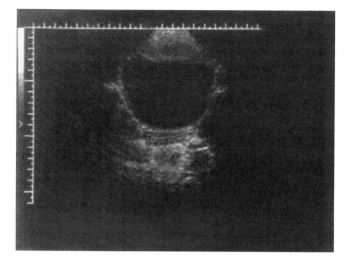
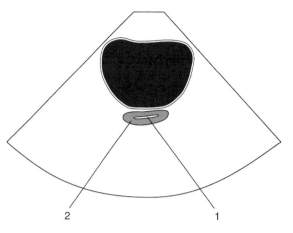

1 _____

2 _____

Figure 16-37 TA, transverse pelvis view.

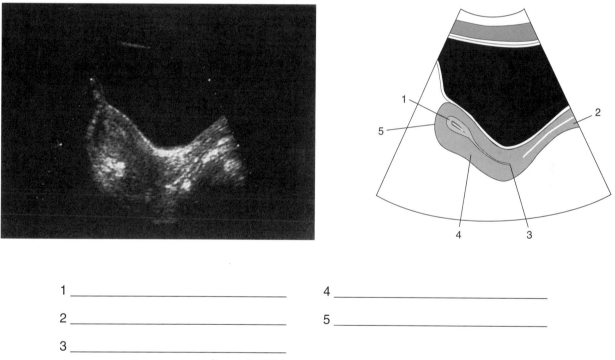

1 _____   4 _____

2 _____   5 _____

3 _____

Figure 16-38 TA, sagittal pelvis view.

A

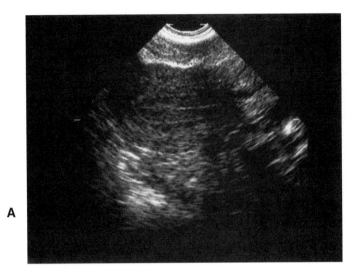
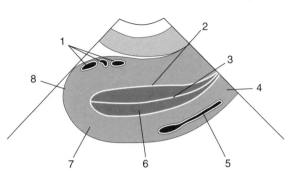

1 _____   5 _____

2 _____   6 _____

3 _____   7 _____

4 _____   8 _____

B

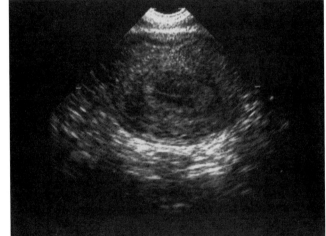
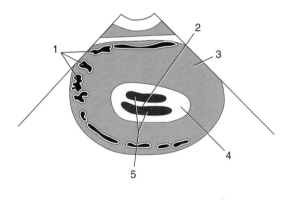

1 _____   4 _____

2 _____   5 _____

3 _____

Figure 16-40 A, TV, sagittal view. B, TV, coronal view.

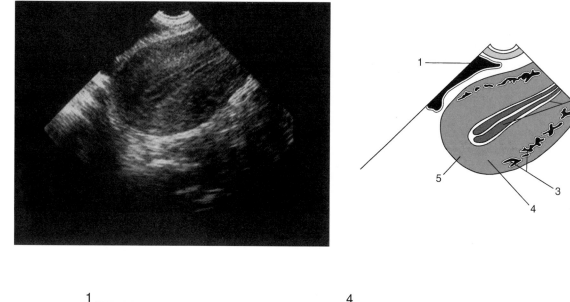

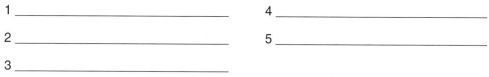

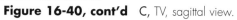

1 _____   4 _____

2 _____   5 _____

3 _____

Figure 16-40, cont'd C, TV, sagittal view.

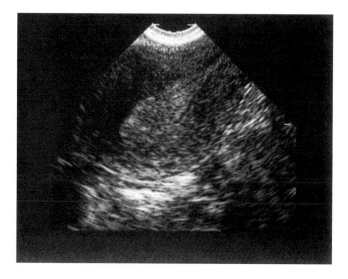

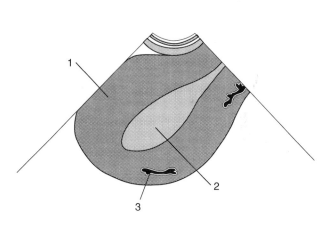

1 _____

2 _____

3 _____

Figure 16-41 TV, sagittal view.

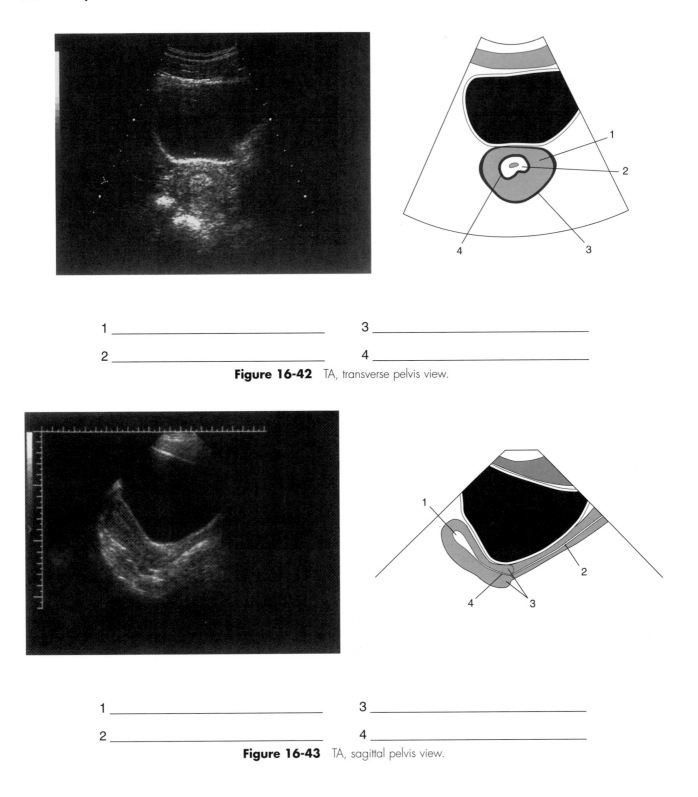

1 _____   3 _____

2 _____   4 _____

Figure 16-42 TA, transverse pelvis view.

1 _____   3 _____

2 _____   4 _____

Figure 16-43 TA, sagittal pelvis view.

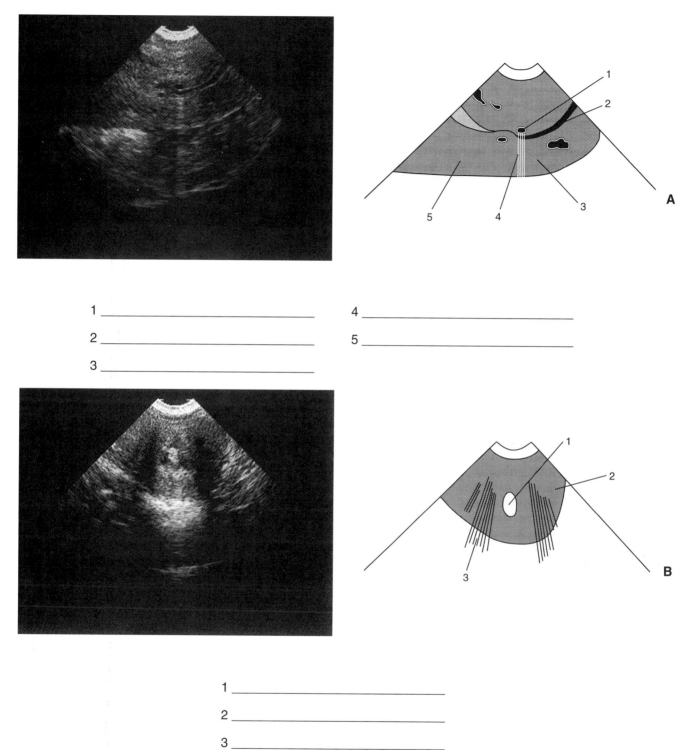

1 _____   4 _____

2 _____   5 _____

3 _____

1 _____

2 _____

3 _____

Figure 16-44 A, TV, sagittal view. B, TV, coronal view.   *continued*

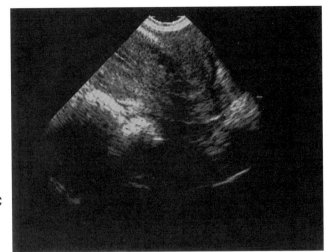

C

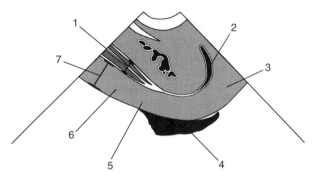

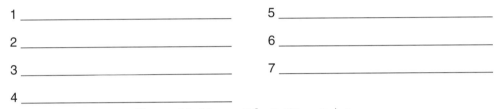

1 _____   5 _____

2 _____   6 _____

3 _____   7 _____

4 _____

Figure 16-44, cont'd C, TV, sagittal view.

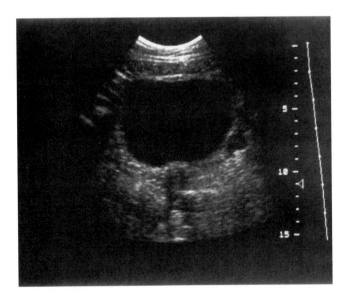

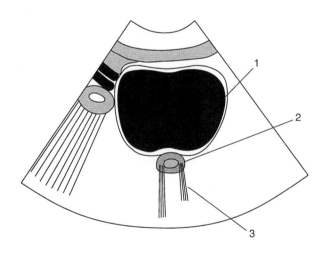

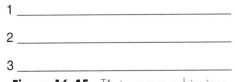

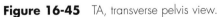

1 _____

2 _____

3 _____

Figure 16-45 TA, transverse pelvis view.

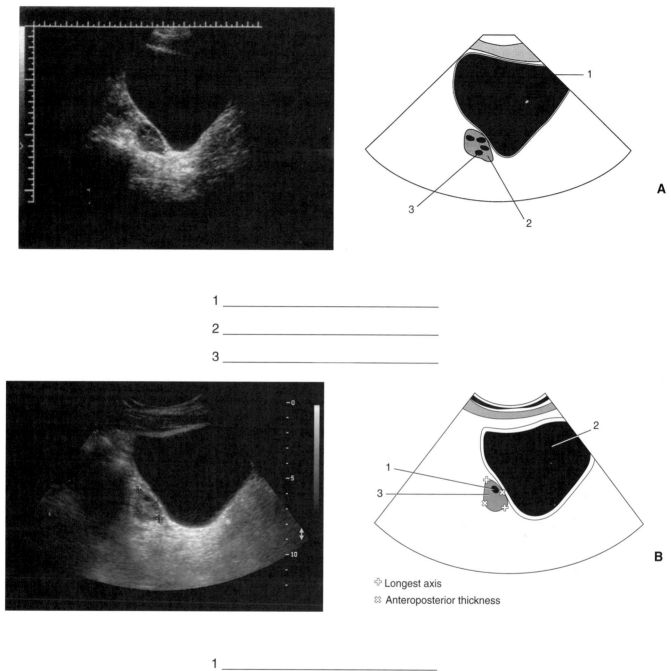

A

1 _____

2 _____

3 _____

⊕ Longest axis
⊗ Anteroposterior thickness

B

1 _____

2 _____

3 _____

Figure 16-46 A, TA, right parasagittal pelvis view. B, TA, sagittal view. *continued*

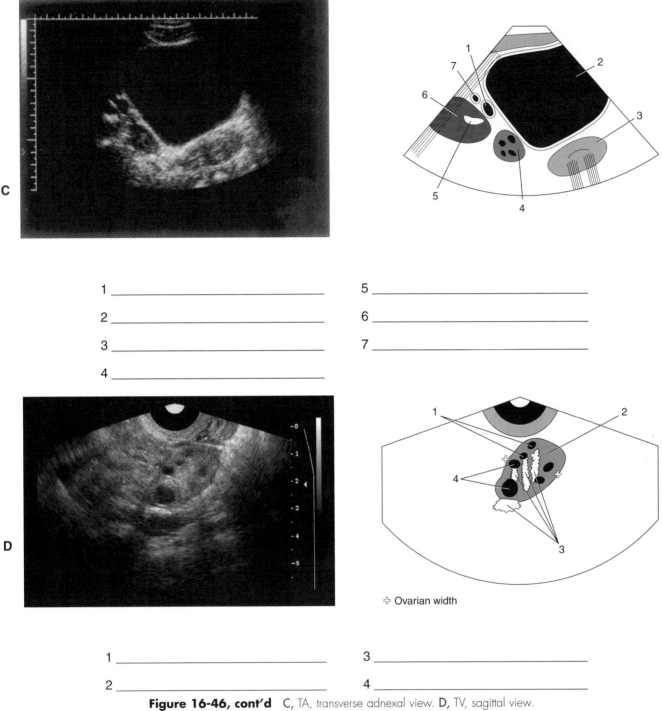

1 _____   5 _____

2 _____   6 _____

3 _____   7 _____

4 _____

1 _____   3 _____

2 _____   4 _____

Figure 16-46, cont'd   C, TA, transverse adnexal view. D, TV, sagittal view.

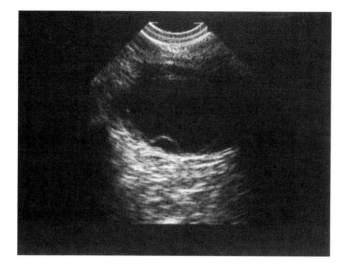
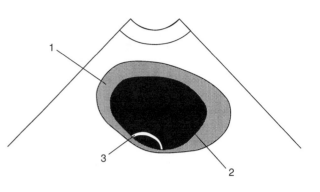

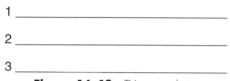

1 _____

2 _____

3 _____

Figure 16-48 TV, coronal view.

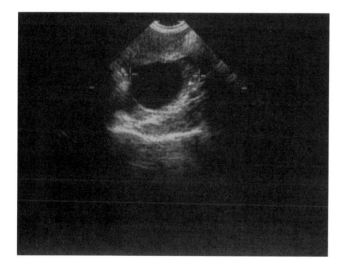
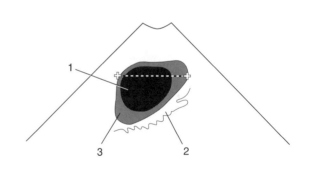

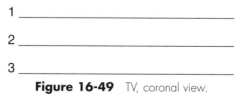

1 _____

2 _____

3 _____

Figure 16-49 TV, coronal view.

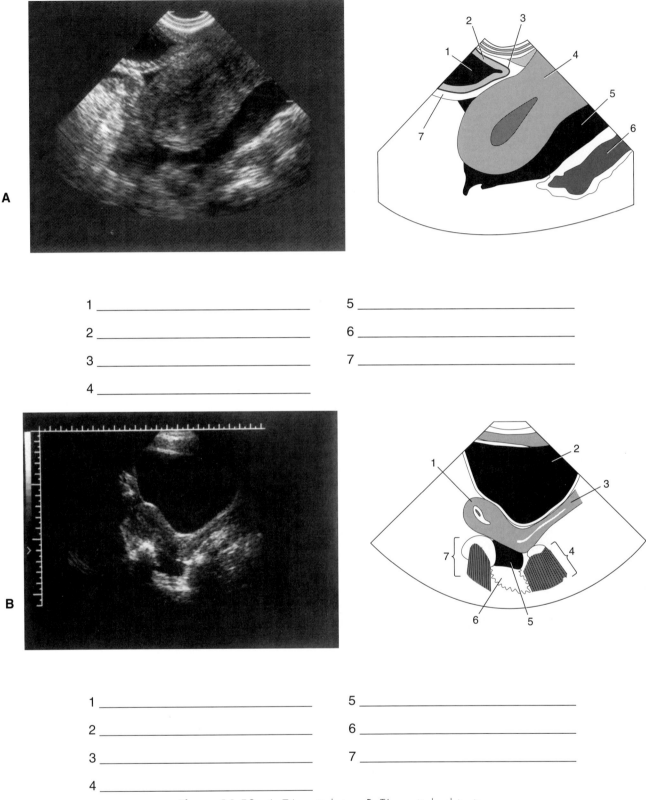

1 _____   5 _____

2 _____   6 _____

3 _____   7 _____

4 _____

B

1 _____   5 _____

2 _____   6 _____

3 _____   7 _____

4 _____

Figure 16-50 A, TV, sagittal view. B, TA, sagittal pelvis view.

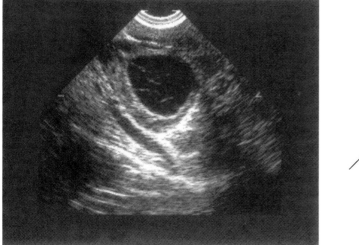

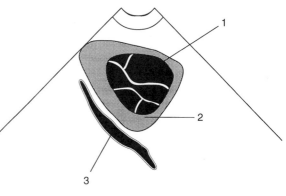

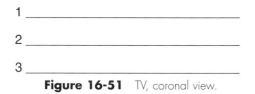

1 _____

2 _____

3 _____

Figure 16-51 TV, coronal view.

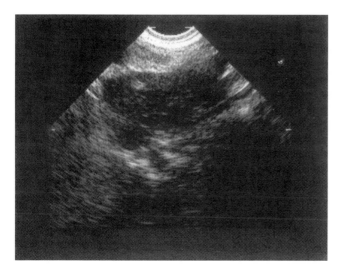

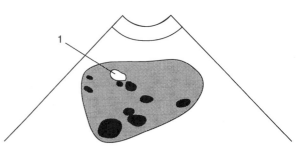

1 _____

Figure 16-52 TV, sagittal view.

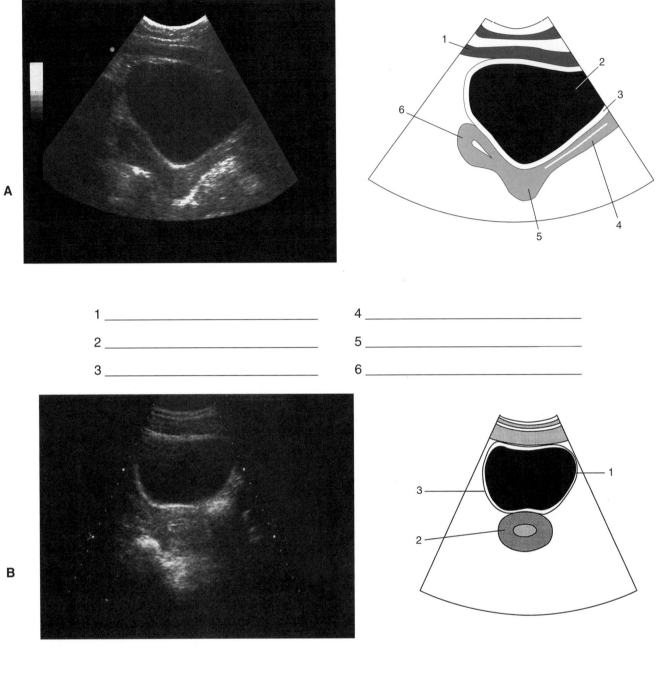

1 _____   4 _____

2 _____   5 _____

3 _____   6 _____

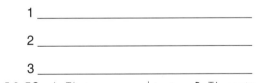

1 _____

2 _____

3 _____

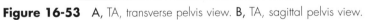

Figure 16-53 A, TA, transverse pelvis view. B, TA, sagittal pelvis view.

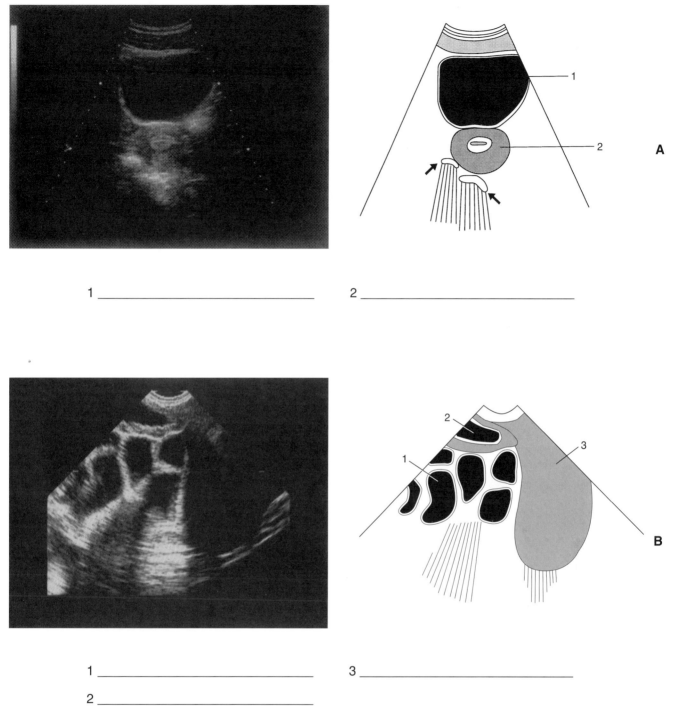

1 _____ 2 _____

A

1 _____ 3 _____

2 _____

B

Figure 16-55 A, TA, sagittal pelvis view. B, TA, transverse pelvis view.

1 _____

2 _____

3 _____

4 _____

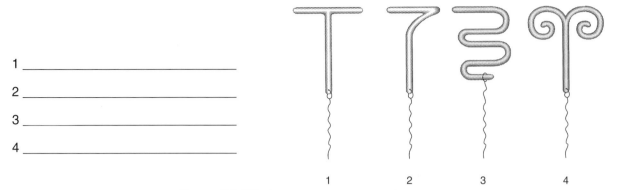

Figure 16-57 Intrauterine contraceptive devices.

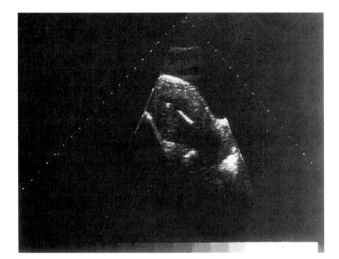

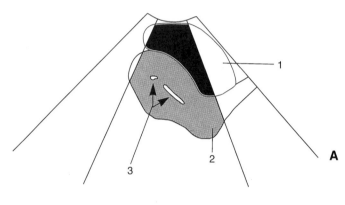

A

1 _____

2 _____

3 _____

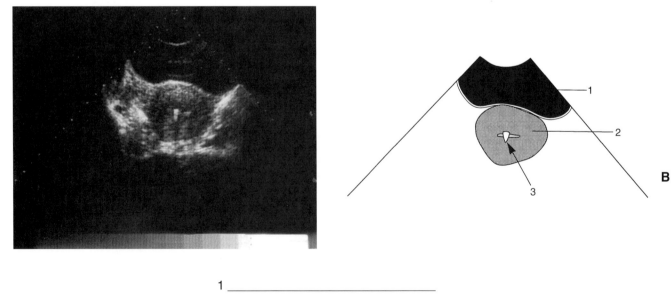

B

1 _____

2 _____

3 _____

Figure 16-58 A, TA, longitudinal uterine section. B, TA, short axis uterine section.

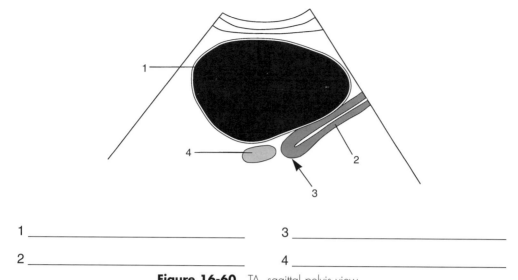

Figure 16-60 TA, sagittal pelvis view.

1 _____ 3 _____

2 _____ 4 _____

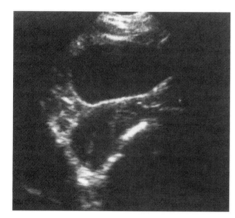
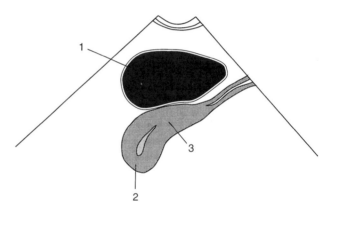

1 _____

2 _____

3 _____

Figure 16-61 TA, sagittal pelvis view.

CHAPTER 17

First Trimester Obstetrics (0 to 12 Weeks)

REVIEW QUESTIONS

1. Progesterone is produced by the
   a. uterus
   b. pituitary gland
   c. corpus luteum
   d. none of the above
   e. all of the above

2. Human chorionic gonadotropin (HCG) is found in
   a. urine
   b. blood
   c. amniotic fluid
   d. a and b
   e. b and c

3. Lacunae are structures within the
   a. ovary
   b. fetal brain
   c. amnion
   d. placenta
   e. none of the above

4. The most accurate method of dating a gestation is the
   a. sac size
   b. crown-rump length (CRL)
   c. biparietal diameter
   d. femur length
   e. yolk sac size

5. The yolk sac is
   a. outside both chorion and amnion
   b. inside both chorion and amnion
   c. outside the amnion but inside the chorion
   d. outside the chorion but inside the amnion

6. Fetal heart activity should usually be detected as early as the last menstrual period dating of
   a. 3 weeks
   b. 5 weeks
   c. 7 weeks
   d. 10 weeks
   e. 12 weeks

7. Separation of chorion and amnion membranes at 14 weeks is
   a. a sign of fetal death
   b. a sign of twins
   c. due to a large yolk sac
   d. normal
   e. none of the above

8. Which of the following is not a common indication for a first trimester ultrasound examination?
   a. vaginal bleeding
   b. size bigger than dates
   c. size smaller than dates
   d. pain
   e. no sensation of fetal movement

9. The secondary yolk sac can
  a. be bigger than the embryo
  b. be cystic in appearance
  c. be visualized before the embryo
  d. disappear before the end of the first trimester
  e. all of the above

10. A retroverted uterus
  a. prevents pregnancy
  b. is due to infection
  c. may make the ultrasound examination more difficult
  d. none of the above
  e. is extremely rare

11. The term "gestational sac" describes the
  a. endometrial cavity
  b. pseudo sac
  c. yolk sac
  d. chorionic cavity
  e. blastocyst

12. Amniotic fluid volume (AFV) is normally reduced by
  a. fetal regurgitation
  b. maternal urination
  c. fetal swallowing
  d. maternal fluid retention
  e. fetal urination

13. What uterine position causes the fundus to appear "echo free"?
  a. anteflexed
  b. anteverted and anteflexed
  c. retroverted and anteflexed
  d. retroflexed
  e. none of the above

14. What is the first structure identified within the gestational sac?
  a. amniotic membrane
  b. yolk sac
  c. double bleb sign
  d. embryo
  e. synechia

15. The embryo is sonographically visible with transvaginal scanning
  a. as early as 3 to 4 weeks' gestational age (GA)
  b. when it retreats from the amnion
  c. at 5 to 6 weeks' gestational age (GA)
  d. following obliteration of the chorionic cavity
  e. at 5 to 6 mm in length

16. The embryo's sonographic appearance is
  a. echogenic and hyperechoic to adjacent structures
  b. homogeneous
  c. heterogeneous
  d. low-level echoes and hypoechoic to adjacent structures
  e. complex

17. When viewed in short axis, the umbilical cord presents as
  a. one large, round, anechoic vessel flanked by two small, round, anechoic vessels encircled by thick, bright walls
  b. one small, round, anechoic vessel interposed between two large, round, hypoechoic vessels
  c. two linear, anechoic vessels with bright walls that join the fetal portal vein and one linear, anechoic vessel with hyperechoic walls that joins the urinary bladder
  d. one large, anechoic vessel flanked by two linear, anechoic vessels
  e. Three small, round, anechoic vessels enclosed by thin, bright walls

18. Embryonic gut herniation
  a. is into the small bowel
  b. occurs at 5 to 6 weeks' gestational age (GA)
  c. is into the base of the umbilical cord
  d. occurs at 10 to 10.5 weeks' gestational age (GA)
  e. is into the amnion

19. An anechoic area identified sonographically within the embryonic skull at 8 weeks is
  a. abnormal
  b. the vitelline duct
  c. the hindbrain
  d. the midbrain
  e. enlarged ventricles

20. A sonographic marker of the chorionic cavity is

    a. echogenic fluid

    b. triple membranes

    c. anechoic fluid

    d. oligohydramnios

    e. polyhdramnios

21. Gestational sac size is determined by

    a. two right angle measurements in a longitudinal section

    b. the mean sac diameter (MSD)

    c. adding the number 30 to the sac depth

    d. the 6th gestational week

    e. adding the number 30 to the crown-rump length (CRL)

22. Gestational age (GA) in days is calculated by

    a. dividing the mean sac diameter by 30

    b. dividing the largest sac dimension by 30

    c. volume measurement of the gestational sac

    d. adding the number 30 to the length of the embryo

    e. adding 30 to the mean sac diameter (MSD)

23. The most accurate assessment of gestational age (GA) is considered to be

    a. gestational sac size

    b. gestational sac size when the yolk sac is visualized

    c. when the embryo measures 1 to 2 mm in length

    d. embryo neck-rump length

    e. embryo crown-rump length (CRL)

24. When the amnion and chorion completely fuse between 12 and 16 weeks' gestational age (GA)

    a. the chorionic membrane is no longer visible sonographically

    b. the amniotic membrane is no longer visible sonographically

    c. the double bleb becomes smaller

    d. neck-rump and crown-rump measurements begin

    e. the double sac sign is easier to differentiate sonographically

25. Crown-rump length (CRL) (in mm) determines gestational age (GA) by

    a. length × 2 = gestational age

    b. length + 30 = gestational age

    c. MSD + CRL = gestational age

    d. applying the length to methodology tables that have already correlated lengths and ages

    e. converting crown-rump length mm measurement to cm measurement

Identify the structures indicated in the following illustrations. These figures duplicate those found in *Sonography: Introduction to Normal Structure and Function.* Refer to the textbook if you need help.

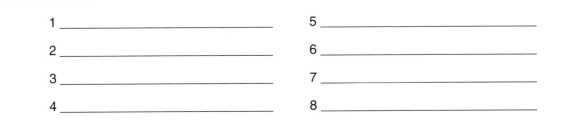

1 _____

2 _____

3 _____

4 _____

5 _____

6 _____

7 _____

8 _____

NORMAL EVENTS IN THE FIRST FOUR WEEKS OF GESTATION

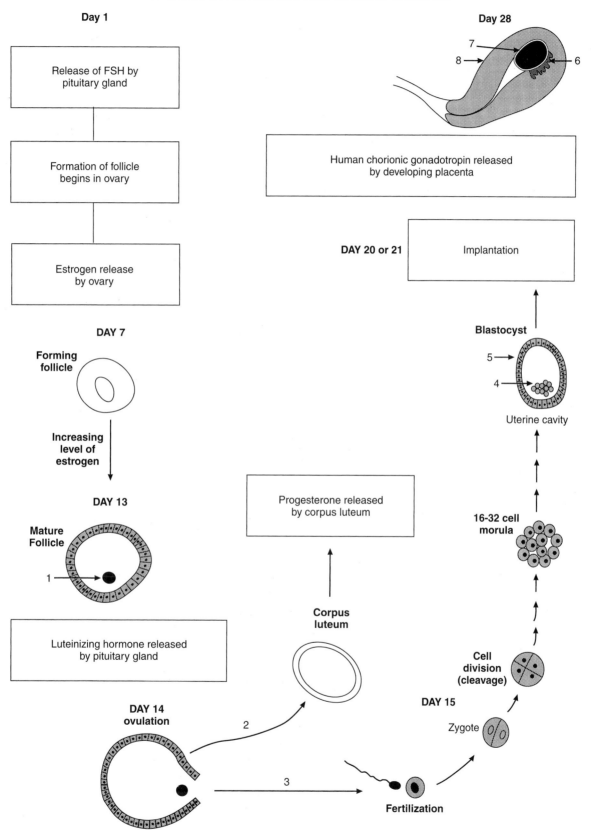

Figure 17-1

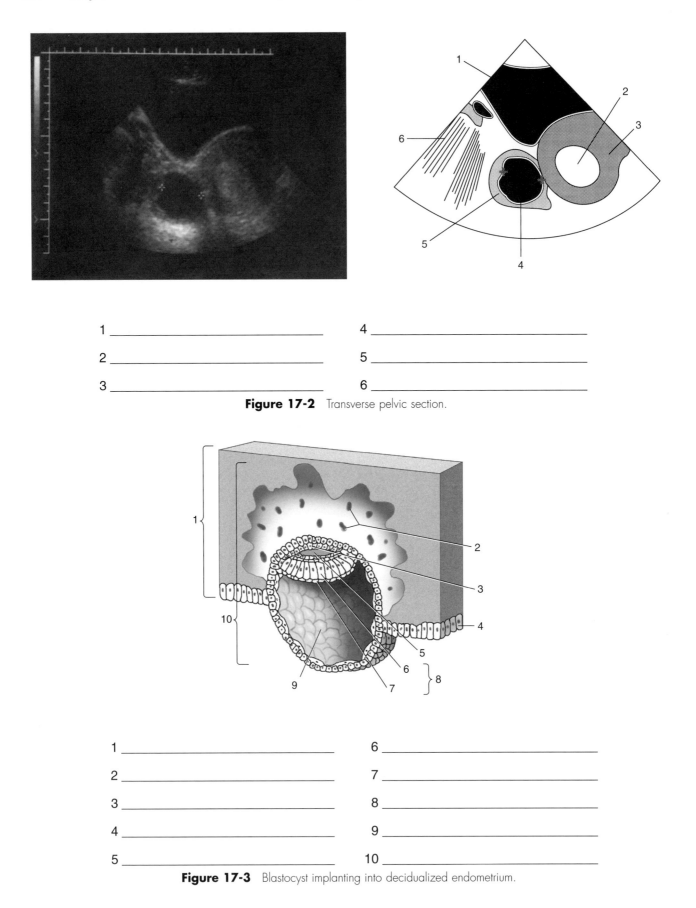

1 _____   4 _____

2 _____   5 _____

3 _____   6 _____

Figure 17-2 Transverse pelvic section.

1 _____   6 _____

2 _____   7 _____

3 _____   8 _____

4 _____   9 _____

5 _____   10 _____

Figure 17-3 Blastocyst implanting into decidualized endometrium.

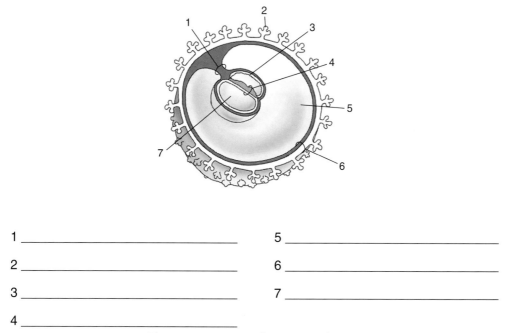

1 _____	5 _____
2 _____	6 _____
3 _____	7 _____
4 _____	

Figure 17-4   5 weeks' gestational age.

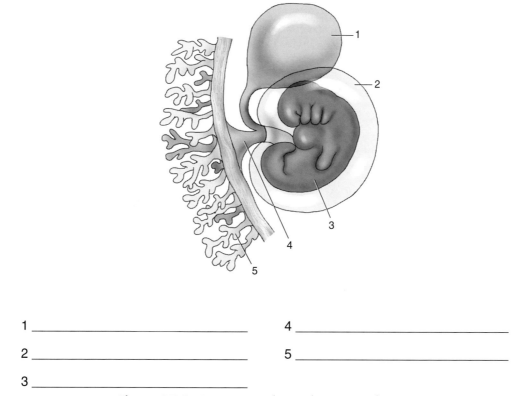

1 _____	4 _____
2 _____	5 _____
3 _____	

Figure 17-5   Between 7 and 8 weeks' gestational age.

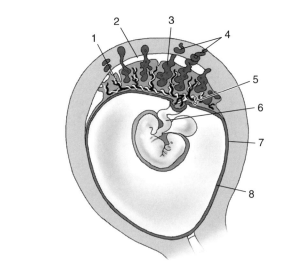

1 _____	5 _____
2 _____	6 _____
3 _____	7 _____
4 _____	8 _____

Figure 17-6 Embryo-maternal circulation.

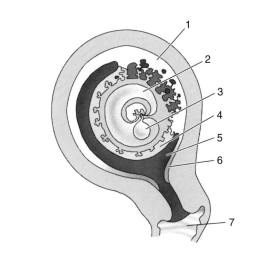

1 _____	5 _____
2 _____	6 _____
3 _____	7 _____
4 _____	

Figure 17-7 7 weeks' gestational age.

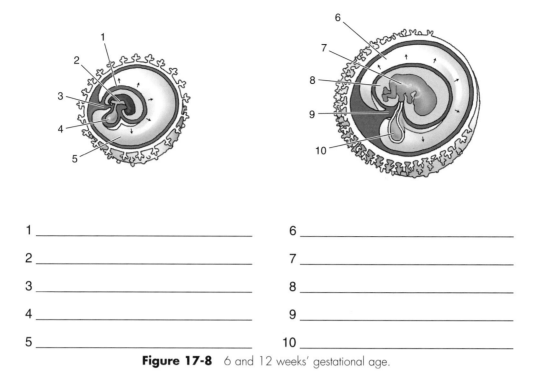

1 _____   6 _____

2 _____   7 _____

3 _____   8 _____

4 _____   9 _____

5 _____   10 _____

Figure 17-8 6 and 12 weeks' gestational age.

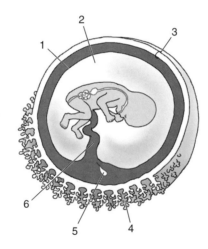

1 _____   4 _____

2 _____   5 _____

3 _____   6 _____

Figure 17-9 22 weeks' gestational age.

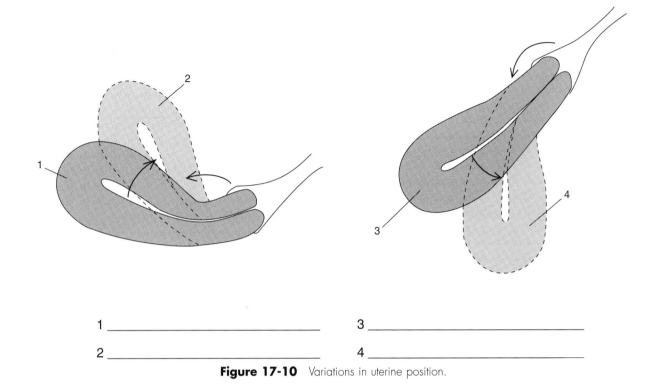

1 _____   3 _____

2 _____   4 _____

Figure 17-10 Variations in uterine position.

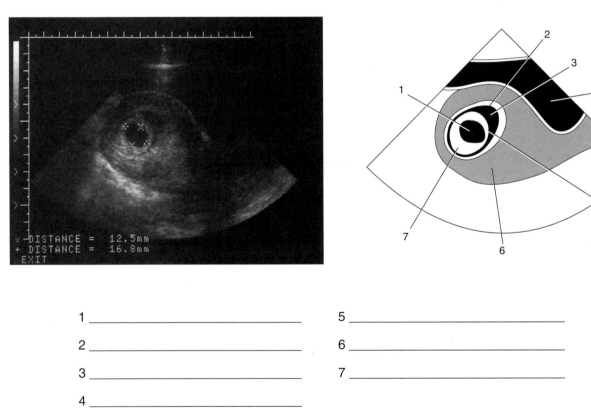

1 _____   5 _____

2 _____   6 _____

3 _____   7 _____

4 _____

Figure 17-11 Double sac sign.

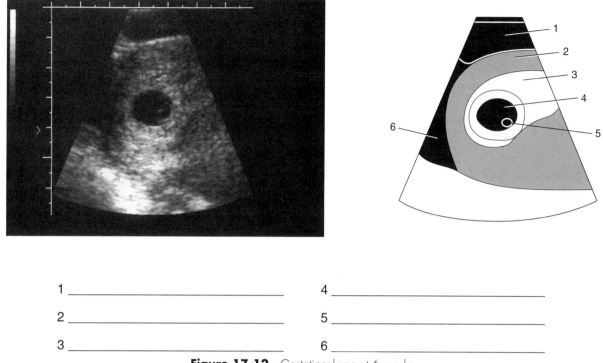

1 _____   4 _____

2 _____   5 _____

3 _____   6 _____

Figure 17-12 Gestational sac at 6 weeks.

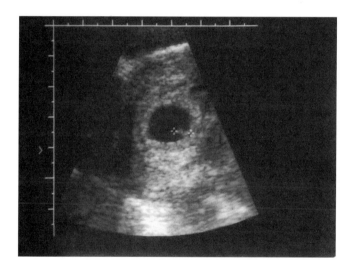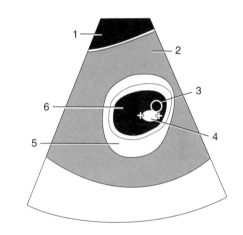

1 _____   4 _____

2 _____   5 _____

3 _____   6 _____

Figure 17-13 Gravid uterus.

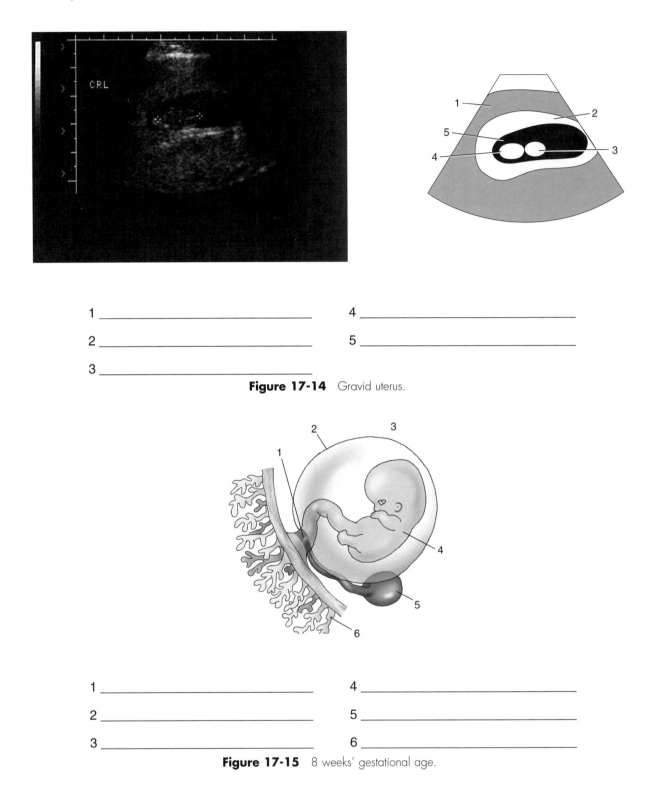

1 _____   4 _____

2 _____   5 _____

3 _____

Figure 17-14 Gravid uterus.

1 _____   4 _____

2 _____   5 _____

3 _____   6 _____

Figure 17-15 8 weeks' gestational age.

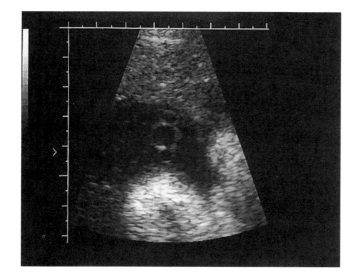
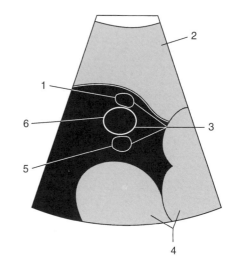

1 _____   4 _____

2 _____   5 _____

3 _____   6 _____

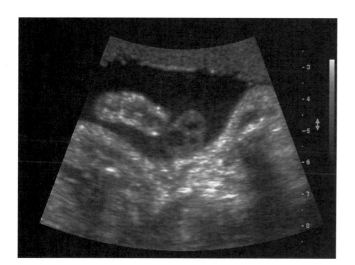
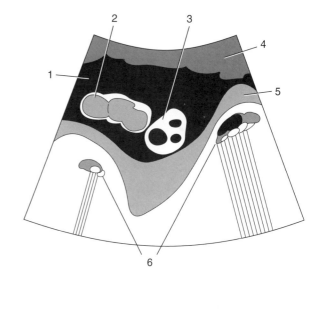

1 _____   4 _____

2 _____   5 _____

3 _____   6 _____

Figure 17-16 Short axis umbilical cord. (Bottom half-tone image courtesy University of Virginia Health System, Department of Radiology, Division of Ultrasound, Charlottesville, Virginia.)

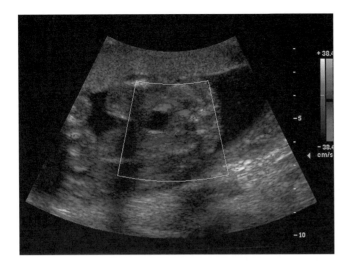
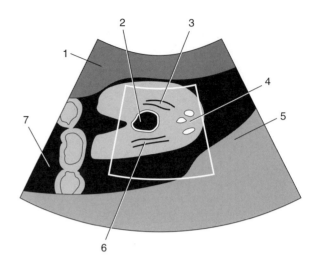

1 _____ 5 _____

2 _____ 6 _____

3 _____ 7 _____

4 _____

Figure 17-17 Longitudinal section of fetal abdominopelvic area. (Half-tone image courtesy University of Virginia Health System, Department of Radiology, Division of Ultrasound, Charlottesville, Virginia.)

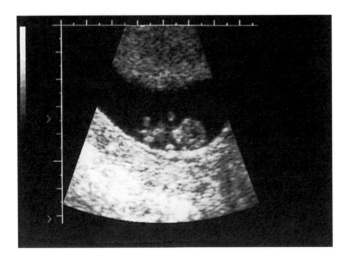
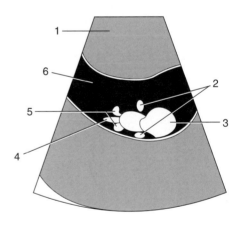

1 _____ 4 _____

2 _____ 5 _____

3 _____ 6 _____

Figure 17-18 9.5 weeks' gestational age.

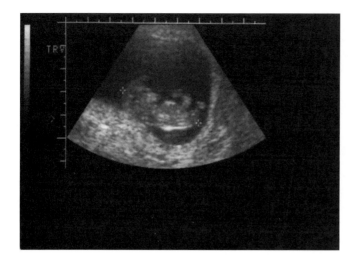
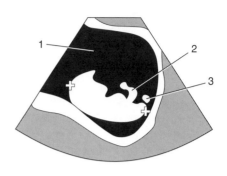
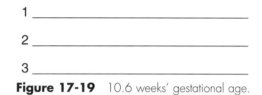

1 _____

2 _____

3 _____

Figure 17-19 10.6 weeks' gestational age.

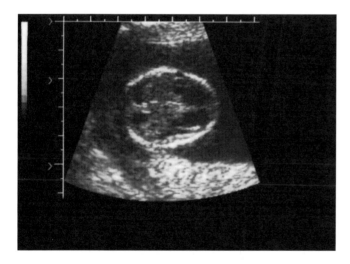
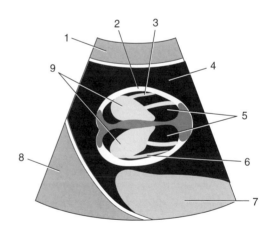

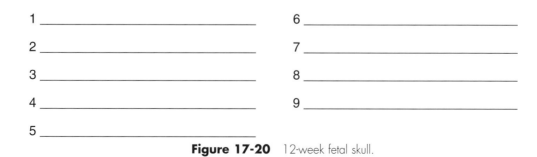

1 _____   6 _____

2 _____   7 _____

3 _____   8 _____

4 _____   9 _____

5 _____

Figure 17-20 12-week fetal skull.

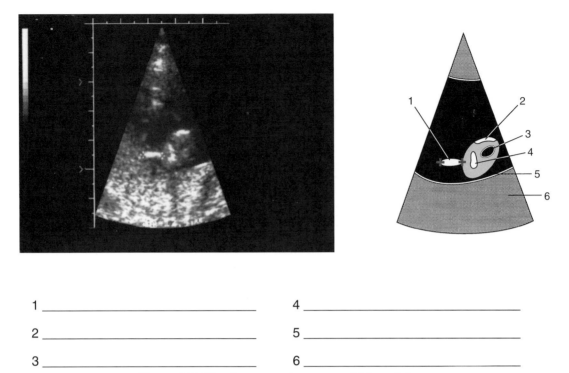

1 _____   4 _____

2 _____   5 _____

3 _____   6 _____

Figure 17-21 Short axis pelvis section of 12-week fetus.

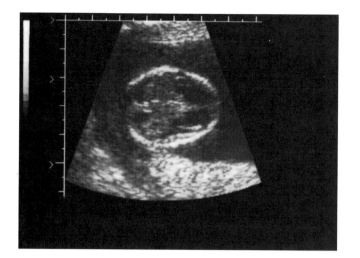
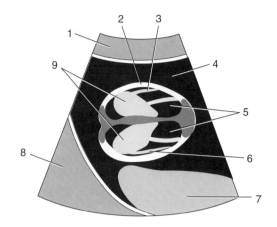

1 _____   6 _____

2 _____   7 _____

3 _____   8 _____

4 _____   9 _____

5 _____

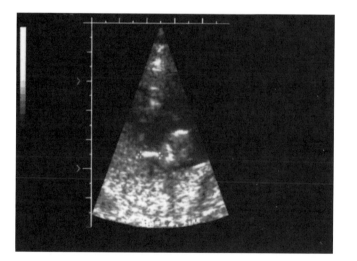
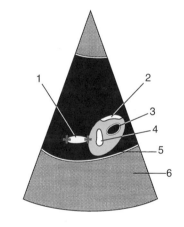

1 _____   4 _____

2 _____   5 _____

3 _____   6 _____

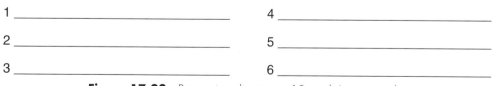

Figure 17-22 Bone mineralization at 12 weeks' gestational age.

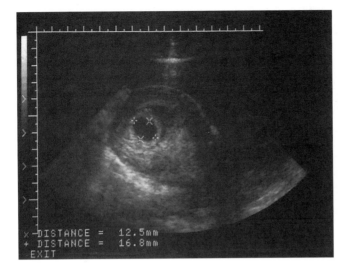
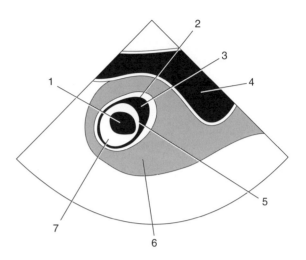

1 _____   5 _____

2 _____   6 _____

3 _____   7 _____

4 _____

Figure 17-23 Gravid endometrium.

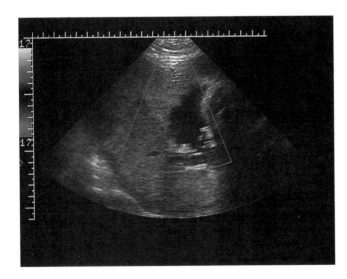
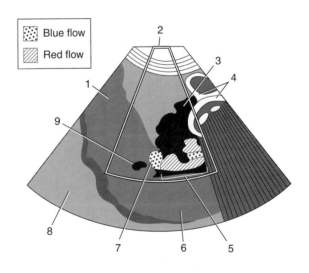

1 _____   6 _____

2 _____   7 _____

3 _____   8 _____

4 _____   9 _____

5 _____

Figure 17-24 Umbilical cord insertion.

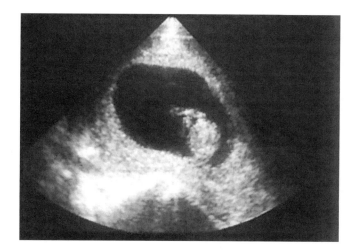
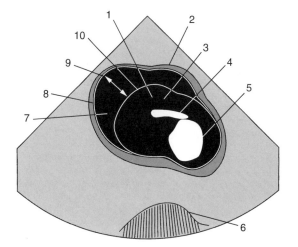

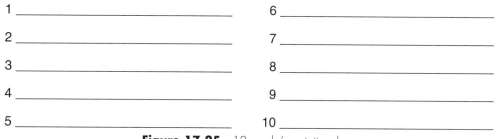

1 _____	6 _____
2 _____	7 _____
3 _____	8 _____
4 _____	9 _____
5 _____	10 _____

Figure 17-25 12 weeks' gestational age.

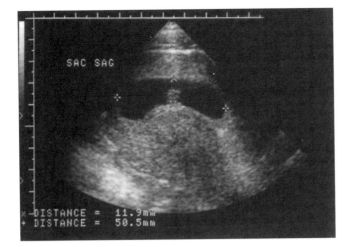
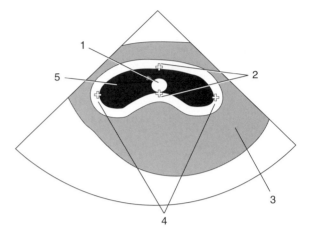

1 _____   4 _____

2 _____   5 _____

3 _____

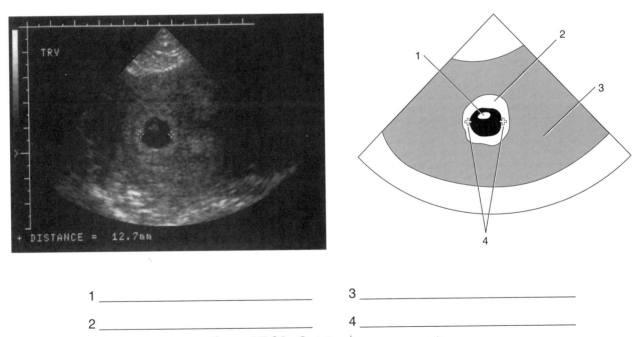

1 _____   3 _____

2 _____   4 _____

Figure 17-26 Gestational sac measurements.

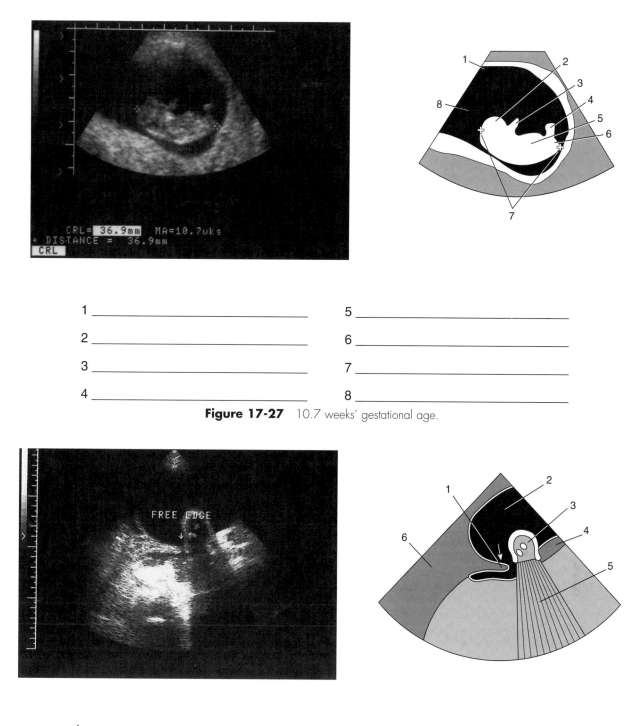

1 _____	5 _____
2 _____	6 _____
3 _____	7 _____
4 _____	8 _____

Figure 17-27 10.7 weeks' gestational age.

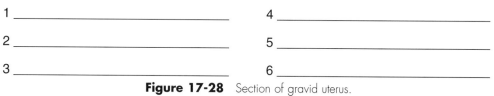

1 _____	4 _____
2 _____	5 _____
3 _____	6 _____

Figure 17-28 Section of gravid uterus.

CHAPTER 18

Second and Third Trimester Obstetrics (13 to 42 Weeks)

REVIEW QUESTIONS

1. The fetal spine closes
   a. from head to rump
   b. uniformly, all at once
   c. from ends to middle
   d. from middle to ends
   e. from rump to head

2. Cerebrospinal fluid is produced in the fetus by the
   a. cerebellum
   b. pons
   c. choroid plexus
   d. spine and brain
   e. meninges

3. The fetal lungs can function as early as
   a. 15 weeks
   b. 20 weeks
   c. 25 weeks
   d. 35 weeks
   e. none of the above

4. The umbilical cord has
   a. one vessel
   b. two vessels
   c. three vessels
   d. four vessels
   e. six vessels

5. A grade III placenta may have
   a. cystic areas
   b. calcification
   c. segments
   d. calcified base plate
   e. all of the above

6. A grade I placenta may have
   a. cystic areas
   b. calcification
   c. segments
   d. calcified base plate
   e. none of the above

7. What vessels comprise the umbilical cord?
   a. portal vein and umbilical artery
   b. two umbilical arteries and one umbilical vein
   c. one umbilical artery and two umbilical veins
   d. umbilical artery and right and left portal veins
   e. umbilical vein and right and left portal veins

8. Anechoic tubular structures on the uterine surface of the placenta are
   a. lacunae
   b. maternal marginal veins
   c. fetal marginal veins
   d. venous lakes
   e. placental abruption

9. Placenta previa occurs
    a. from accelerated calcifications
    b. with a grade III placenta
    c. when a portion of the placenta covers the internal os of the cervix
    d. when a portion of the placenta covers a portion of the external os of the cervix
    e. with a fetal breech position

10. An accurate biparietal diameter (BPD) measurement can be obtained through any plane of section that intersects the
    a. thalami, third ventricle, and cavum septum pellucidum
    b. thalami and cavum septum pellucidum
    c. thalami, cavum septum pellucidum, and cerebellum
    d. thalami and third ventricle
    e. thalami, third ventricle, cavum septum pellucidum, and cerebellum

11. The cisterna magna is a(n)
    a. moderately echogenic portion of the brain stem
    b. anechoic medullary pyramid
    c. anechoic subarachnoid space
    d. highly reflective brain fissure
    e. remnant that becomes the highly reflective ligamentum teres

12. The atrial septal opening is the
    a. ductus venosus
    b. mitral valve
    c. foramen ovale
    d. ductus arteriosus
    e. tricuspid valve

13. The thalami are
    a. centrally located in the brain and appear anechoic
    b. centrally located in the brain and appear homogeneous and mid gray
    c. the highly echogenic lines seen dividing the cerebrum
    d. the bright, drumstick-shaped portions of the lateral ventricles
    e. the cartilaginous end of the femurs

14. Collapsed, the fetal colon typically
    a. appears hyperechoic compared with adjacent structures
    b. presents with anechoic, thick walls and hyperechoic lumen
    c. appears hypoechoic compared with adjacent structures
    d. is never seen sonographically
    e. indicates a gastrointestinal abnormality

15. Sonographic identification of the fetal _____ is necessary to establish renal function.
    a. urinary bladder
    b. kidneys
    c. renal sinus
    d. urine-filled medullary pyramids
    e. ureters

16. The fetal adrenal glands appear _____ to the liver, spleen, and renal cortex.
    a. hyperechoic
    b. hypoechoic
    c. anechoic
    d. posteroinferior
    e. anterolateral

17. The _____ of bone(s) _____ sound waves.
    a. mineralization/determines width of
    b. density/causes posterior enhancement of
    c. type/determines the degree of posterior enhancement
    d. attenuation/passes
    e. density/attenuates

18. Muscles usually appear _____ compared with adjacent structures.
    a. hyperechoic
    b. dense
    c. hypoechoic
    d. echodense
    e. highly reflective

19. Head circumference (HC) is best obtained through (a) _____ plane(s) of section perpendicular to the _____.

a. single/thalami, cavum septum pellucidum, and tentorium

b. multiple/thalami, cavum septum pellucidum, and tentorium

c. single/thalami, third ventricle, cavum septum pellucidum, and tentorium

d. multiple/thalami, third ventricle, cavum septum pellucidum, and tentorium

e. multiple/thalami and cavum septum pellucidum

20. Abdominal circumference (AC) is measured through (a) _____ plane(s) of section where the _____ are continuous with one another.

a. single/right and left portal veins

b. multiple/right and left portal veins

c. single/right and left hepatic ducts

d. multiple/right and left hepatic ducts

e. single/umbilical vein and right hepatic vein

Identify the structures indicated in the following illustrations. These figures duplicate those found in *Sonography: Introduction to Normal Structure and Function*. Refer to the textbook if you need help.

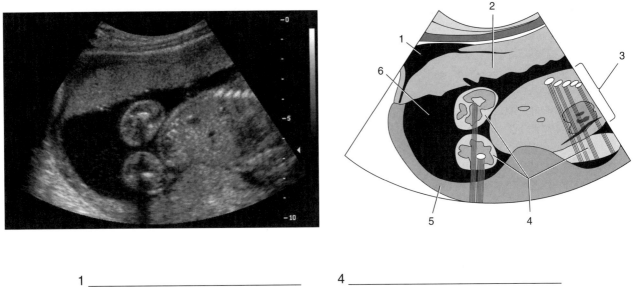

1 _____   4 _____

2 _____   5 _____

3 _____   6 _____

Figure 18-1 Amniotic sac/fetal section. (Half-tone image courtesy the University of Virginia Health System, Department of Radiology, Division of Ultrasound, Charlottesville, Virginia.)

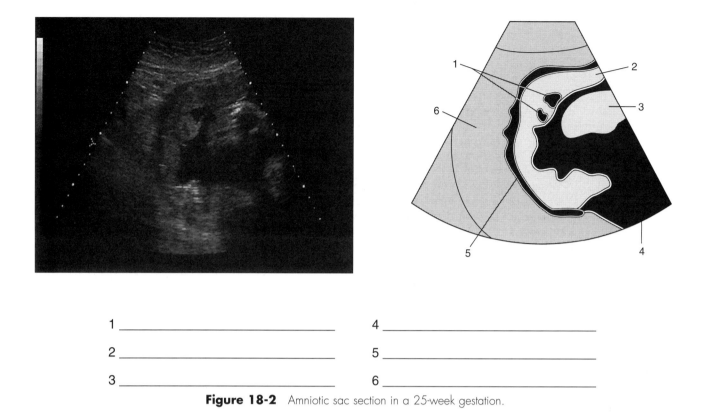

1 _____   4 _____

2 _____   5 _____

3 _____   6 _____

Figure 18-2 Amniotic sac section in a 25-week gestation.

A. PLACENTAL GRADING

Grade 0

Grade I

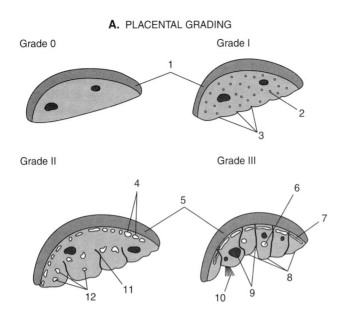

Grade II

Grade III

1 _____

2 _____

3 _____

4 _____

5 _____

6 _____

7 _____

8 _____

9 _____

10 _____

11 _____

12 _____

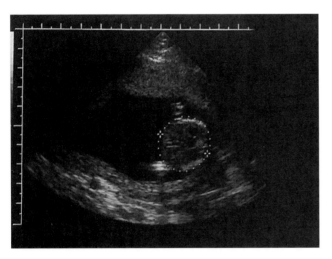

B. 13 _____

C. 14 _____

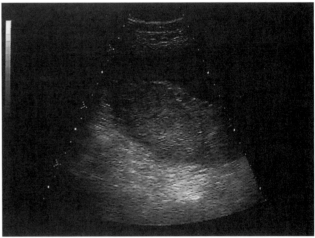

D. 15 _____

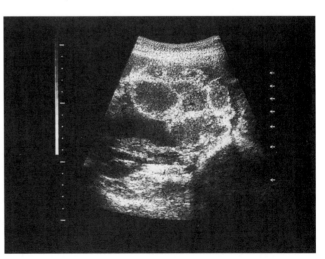

E. 16 _____

Figure 18-3 Placental grading.

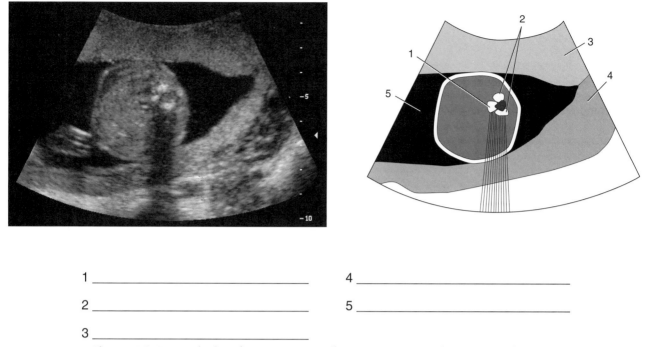

1 _____   4 _____

2 _____   5 _____

3 _____

Figure 18-4 Vertebral ossification center. (Half-tone image courtesy the University of Virginia Health System, Department of Radiology, Division of Ultrasound, Charlottesville, Virginia.)

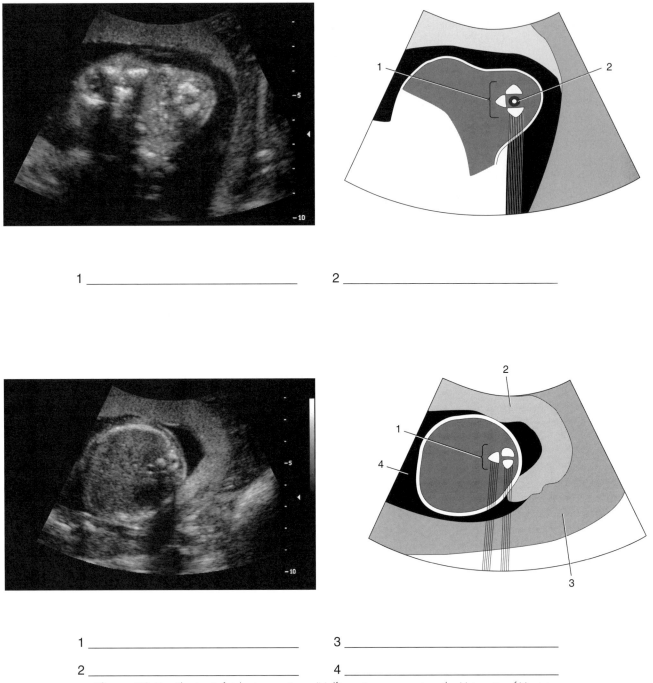

1 _____   2 _____

1 _____   3 _____

2 _____   4 _____

Figure 18-5 Short axis fetal spine sections. (Half-tone images courtesy the University of Virginia Health System, Department of Radiology, Division of Ultrasound, Charlottesville, Virginia.)

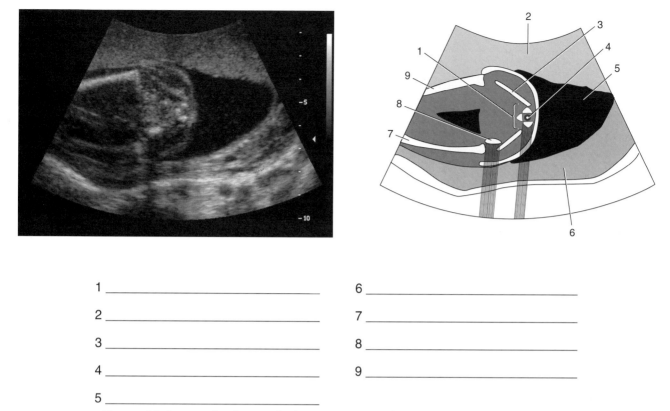

1 _____   6 _____

2 _____   7 _____

3 _____   8 _____

4 _____   9 _____

5 _____

Figure 18-5, cont'd   Short axis fetal spine sections. (Half-tone image courtesy the University of Virginia Health System, Department of Radiology, Division of Ultrasound, Charlottesville, Virginia.)

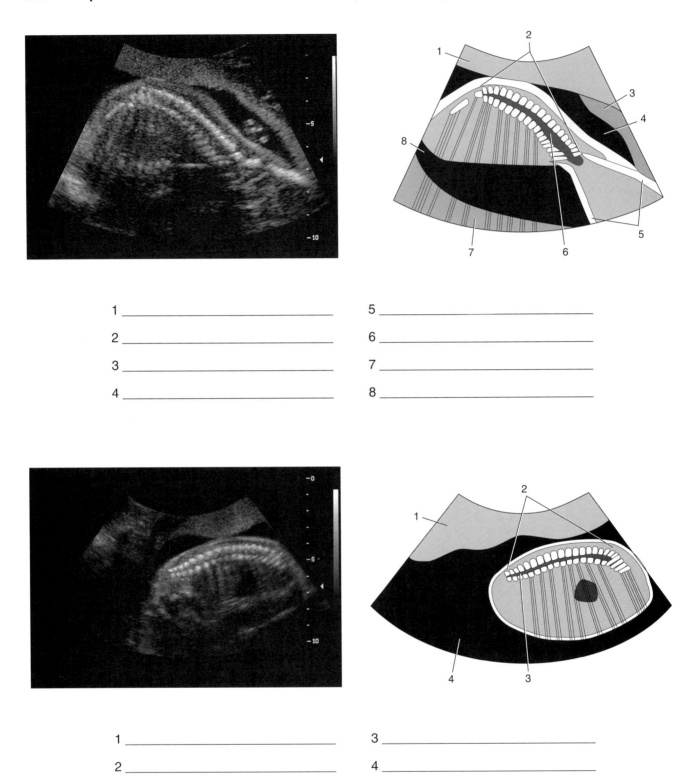

1 _____   5 _____

2 _____   6 _____

3 _____   7 _____

4 _____   8 _____

1 _____   3 _____

2 _____   4 _____

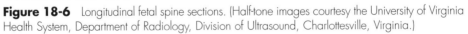

Figure 18-6 Longitudinal fetal spine sections. (Half-tone images courtesy the University of Virginia Health System, Department of Radiology, Division of Ultrasound, Charlottesville, Virginia.)

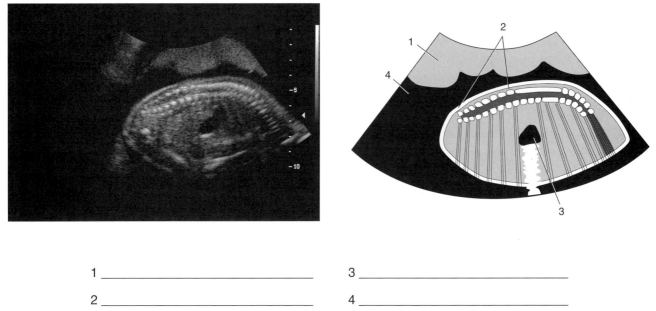

1 _____   3 _____

2 _____   4 _____

Figure 18-6, cont'd Longitudinal fetal spine sections. (Half-tone image courtesy the University of Virginia Health System, Department of Radiology, Division of Ultrasound, Charlottesville, Virginia.)

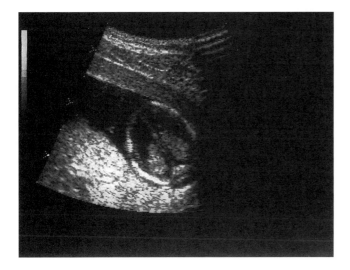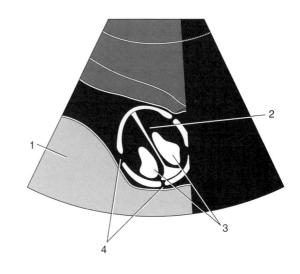

1 _____   3 _____

2 _____   4 _____

Figure 18-7 Fetal head.

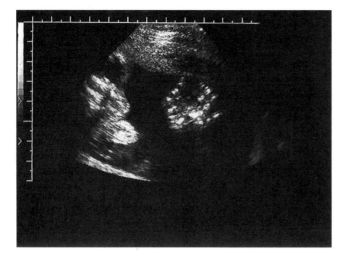
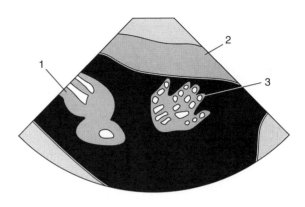

1 _____

2 _____

3 _____

Figure 18-8 Fetal hand.

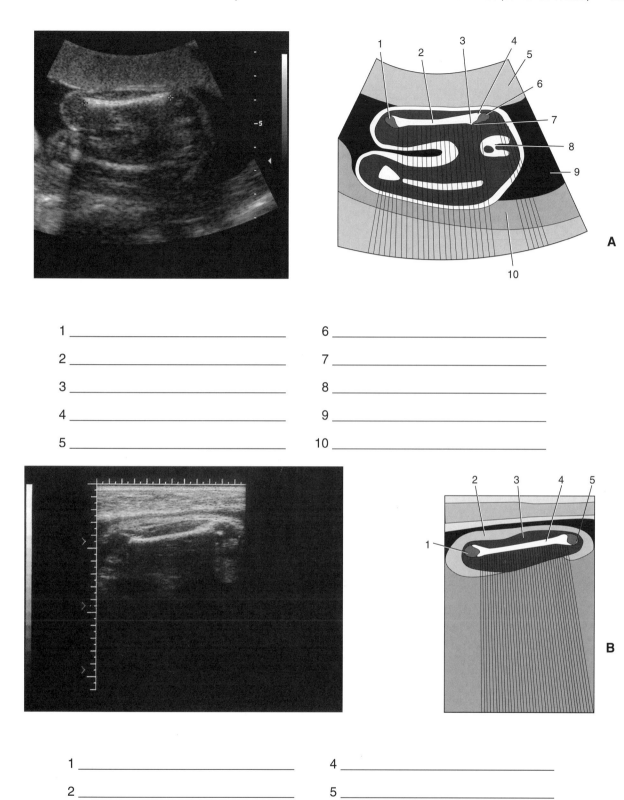

1 _____ 6 _____

2 _____ 7 _____

3 _____ 8 _____

4 _____ 9 _____

5 _____ 10 _____

1 _____ 4 _____

2 _____ 5 _____

3 _____

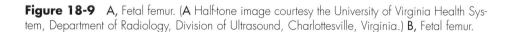

Figure 18-9 **A,** Fetal femur. (**A** Half-tone image courtesy the University of Virginia Health System, Department of Radiology, Division of Ultrasound, Charlottesville, Virginia.) **B,** Fetal femur.

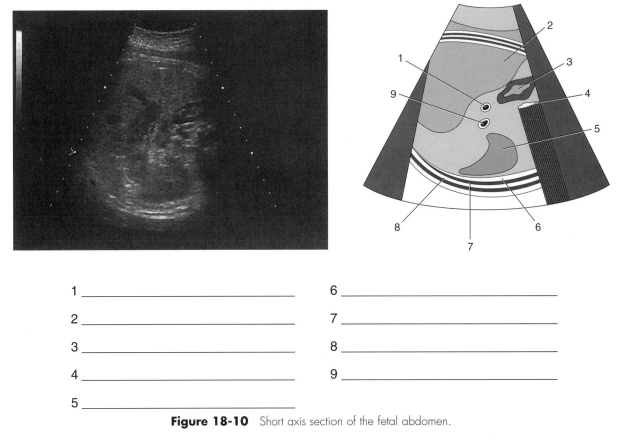

1 _____   6 _____

2 _____   7 _____

3 _____   8 _____

4 _____   9 _____

5 _____

Figure 18-10 Short axis section of the fetal abdomen.

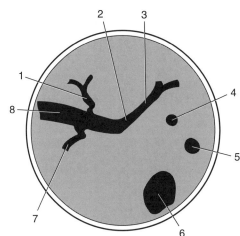

1 _____   5 _____

2 _____   6 _____

3 _____   7 _____

4 _____   8 _____

Figure 18-11 Fetal/left portal circulation.

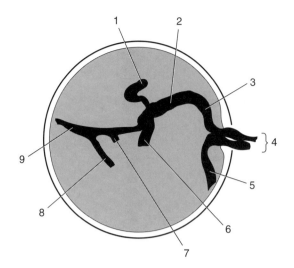

1 _____   6 _____

2 _____   7 _____

3 _____   8 _____

4 _____   9 _____

5 _____

Figure 18-12 Umbilical circulation.

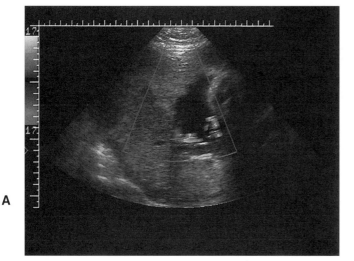
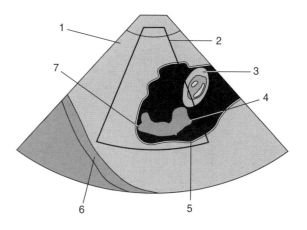

A

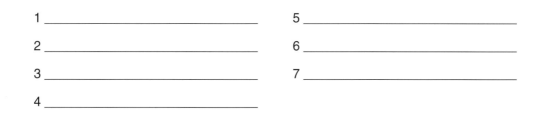

1 _____   5 _____

2 _____   6 _____

3 _____   7 _____

4 _____

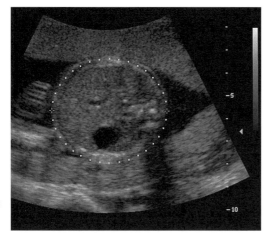
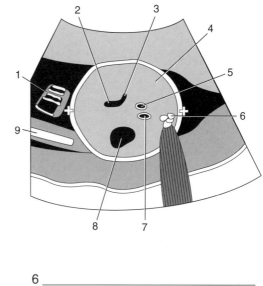

B

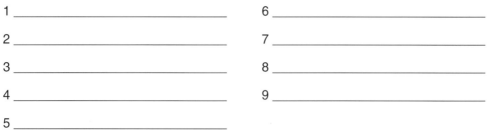

1 _____   6 _____

2 _____   7 _____

3 _____   8 _____

4 _____   9 _____

5 _____

Figure 18-13 A, Umbilical cord insertion sites. B, Umbilical cord insertion sites. (Half-tone images courtesy the University of Virginia Health System, Department of Radiology, Division of Ultrasound, Charlottesville, Virginia.)

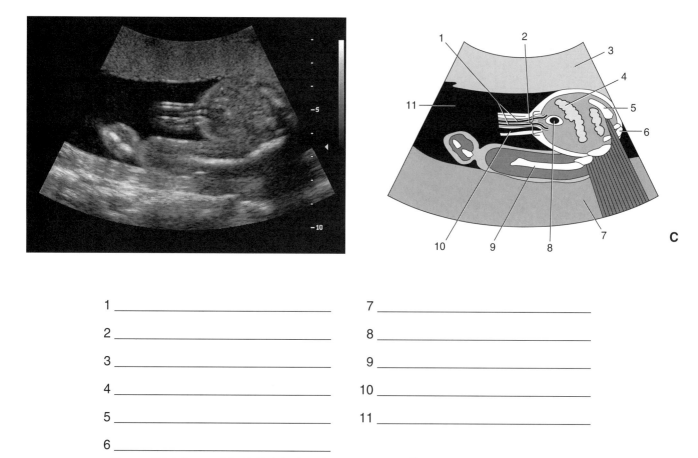

1 _____   7 _____

2 _____   8 _____

3 _____   9 _____

4 _____   10 _____

5 _____   11 _____

6 _____

Figure 18-13, cont'd C, Umbilical cord insertion sites. (Half-tone image courtesy the University of Virginia Health System, Department of Radiology, Division of Ultrasound, Charlottesville, Virginia.)

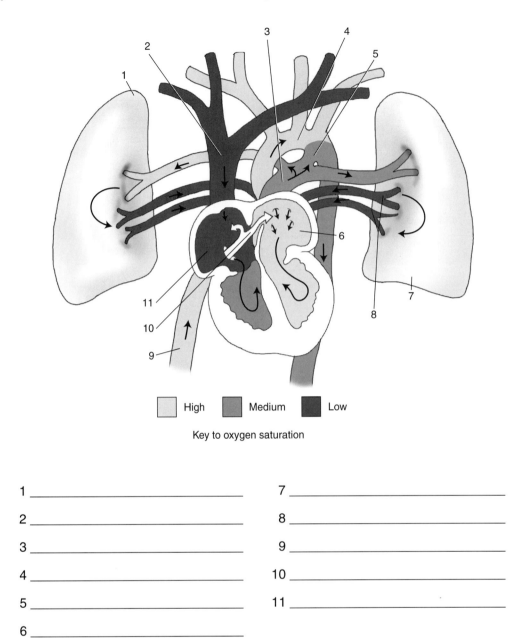

High   Medium   Low

Key to oxygen saturation

1 _____   7 _____

2 _____   8 _____

3 _____   9 _____

4 _____   10 _____

5 _____   11 _____

6 _____

Figure 18-14 Fetal circulation.

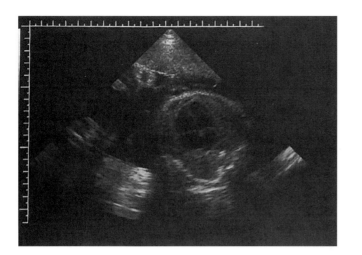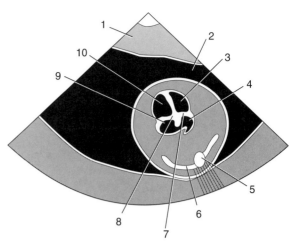

1 _____ 6 _____

2 _____ 7 _____

3 _____ 8 _____

4 _____ 9 _____

5 _____ 10 _____

Figure 18-15 Short axis section of the fetal thorax.

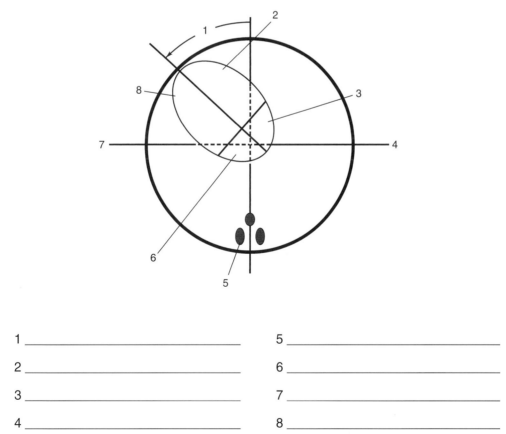

1 _____ 5 _____

2 _____ 6 _____

3 _____ 7 _____

4 _____ 8 _____

Figure 18-16 Illustrates the normal position of the fetal heart as viewed in a short axis section of the fetal thorax.

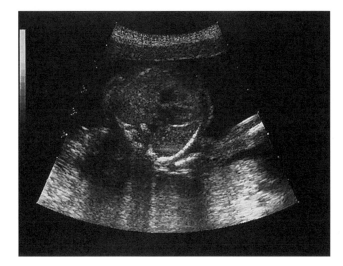
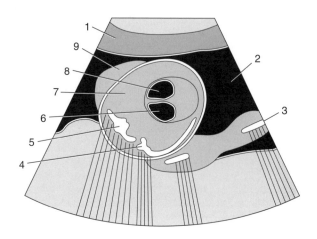

1 _____   6 _____
2 _____   7 _____
3 _____   8 _____
4 _____   9 _____
5 _____

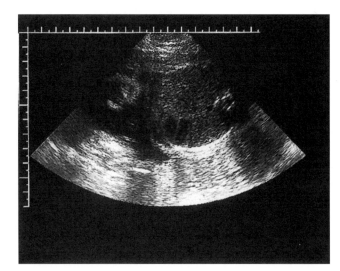
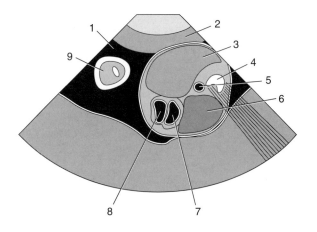

1 _____   6 _____
2 _____   7 _____
3 _____   8 _____
4 _____   9 _____
5 _____

Figure 18-17 Short axis sections of the fetal thorax.

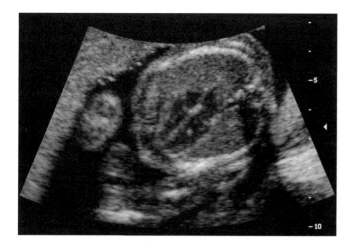

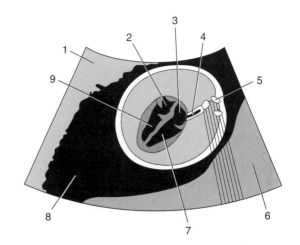

1 _____   6 _____

2 _____   7 _____

3 _____   8 _____

4 _____   9 _____

5 _____

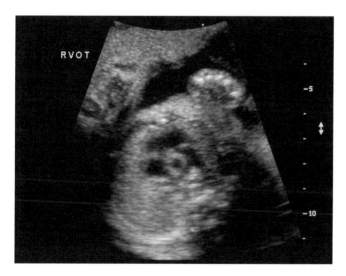

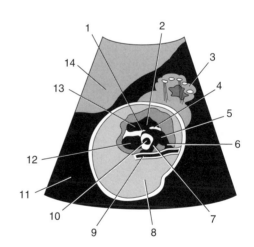

1 _____   8 _____

2 _____   9 _____

3 _____   10 _____

4 _____   11 _____

5 _____   12 _____

6 _____   13 _____

7 _____   14 _____

Figure 18-18 Fetal heart and great vessels. (Half-tone images courtesy the University of Virginia Health System, Department of Radiology, Division of Ultrasound, Charlottesville, Virginia.)

continued

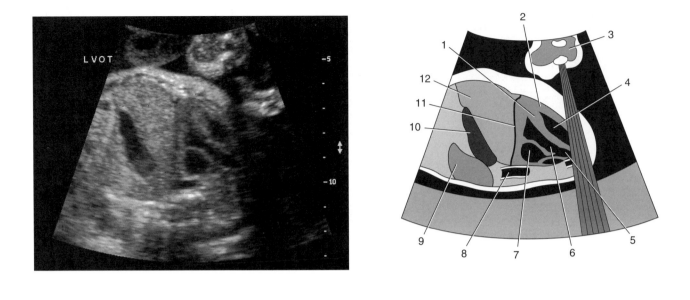

1 _____ 7 _____

2 _____ 8 _____

3 _____ 9 _____

4 _____ 10 _____

5 _____ 11 _____

6 _____ 12 _____

Figure 18-18, cont'd Fetal heart and great vessels. (Half-tone image courtesy the University of Virginia Health System, Department of Radiology, Division of Ultrasound, Charlottesville, Virginia.)

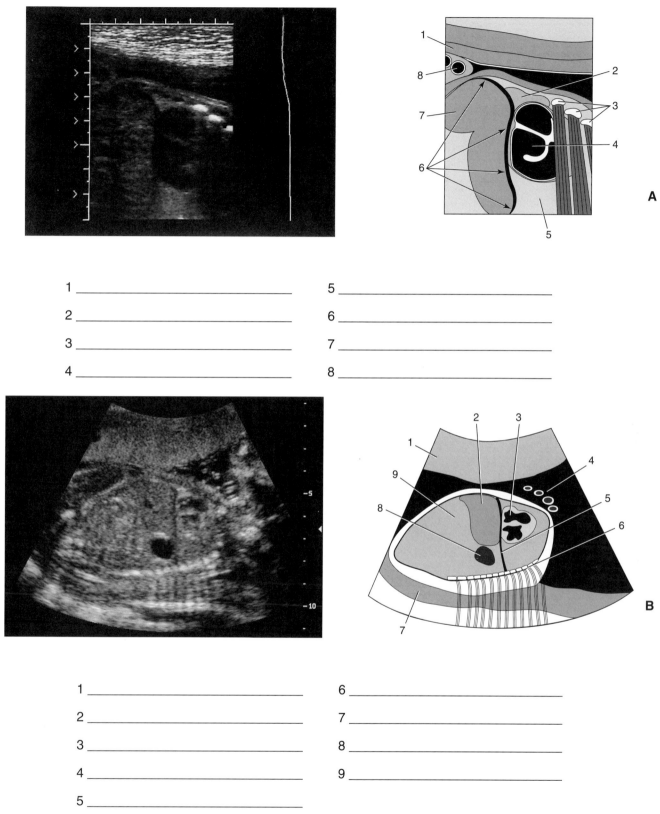

1 _____   5 _____

2 _____   6 _____

3 _____   7 _____

4 _____   8 _____

1 _____   6 _____

2 _____   7 _____

3 _____   8 _____

4 _____   9 _____

5 _____

Figure 18-19 A, Longitudinal sections of the fetal thorax and abdominal cavity. B, Longitudinal sections of the fetal thorax and abdominal cavity. (Half-tone images courtesy the University of Virginia Health System, Department of Radiology, Division of Ultrasound, Charlottesville, Virginia.)

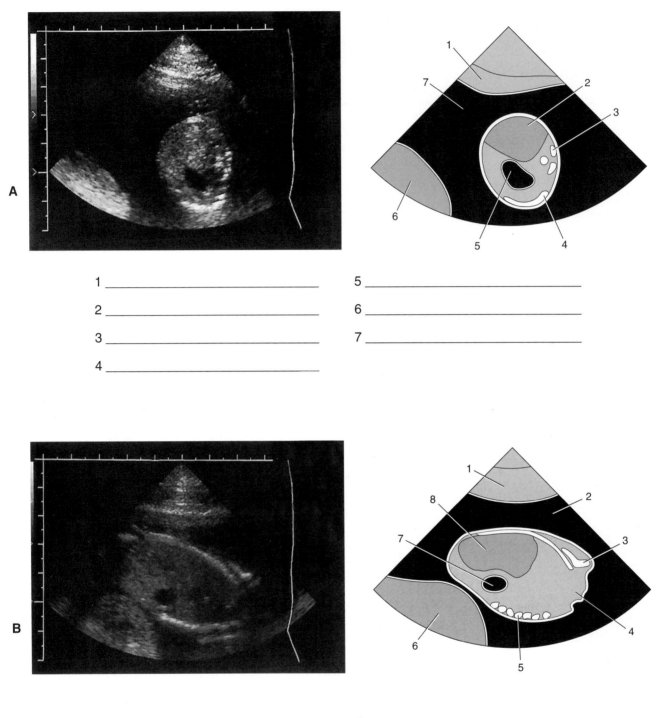

1 _____   5 _____

2 _____   6 _____

3 _____   7 _____

4 _____

1 _____   5 _____

2 _____   6 _____

3 _____   7 _____

4 _____   8 _____

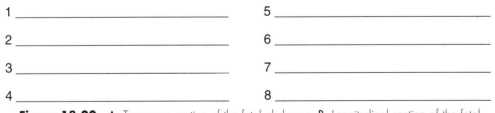

Figure 18-20 A, Transverse section of the fetal abdomen. B, Longitudinal section of the fetal abdomen.

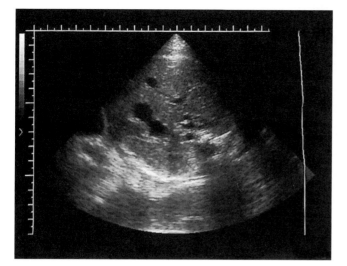
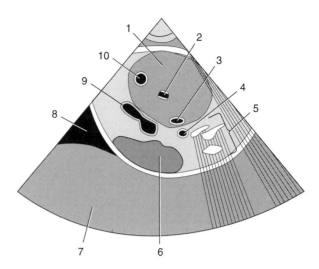

1 _____ 6 _____

2 _____ 7 _____

3 _____ 8 _____

4 _____ 9 _____

5 _____ 10 _____

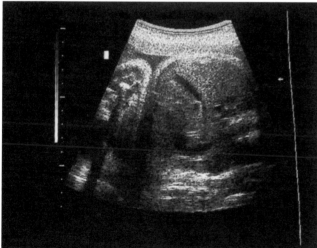
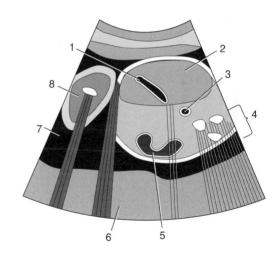

1 _____ 5 _____

2 _____ 6 _____

3 _____ 7 _____

4 _____ 8 _____

Figure 18-21 Short axis sections of the fetal abdomen.

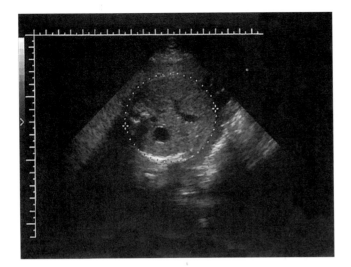

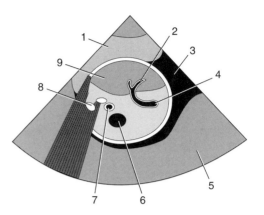

1 _____   6 _____

2 _____   7 _____

3 _____   8 _____

4 _____   9 _____

5 _____

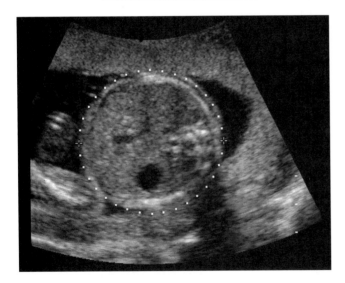

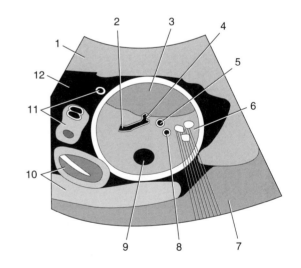

1 _____   7 _____

2 _____   8 _____

3 _____   9 _____

4 _____   10 _____

5 _____   11 _____

6 _____   12 _____

Figure 18-22 Short axis sections of the fetal abdomen. (Bottom half-tone image courtesy the University of Virginia Health System, Department of Radiology, Division of Ultrasound, Charlottesville, Virginia.)

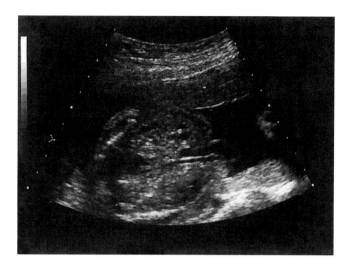
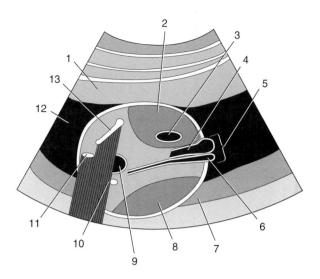

1	_____	8	_____
2	_____	9	_____
3	_____	10	_____
4	_____	11	_____
5	_____	12	_____
6	_____	13	_____
7	_____		

Figure 18-23 Short axis section of the fetal abdomen.

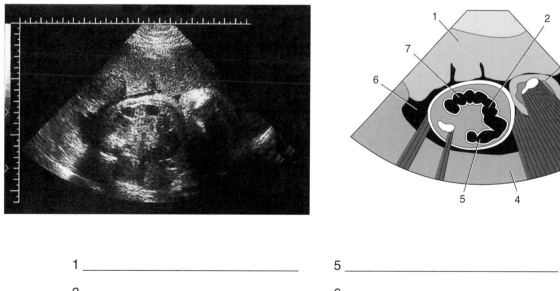

1	_____	5	_____
2	_____	6	_____
3	_____	7	_____
4	_____		

Figure 18-24 Short axis section of the abdominopelvic cavity.

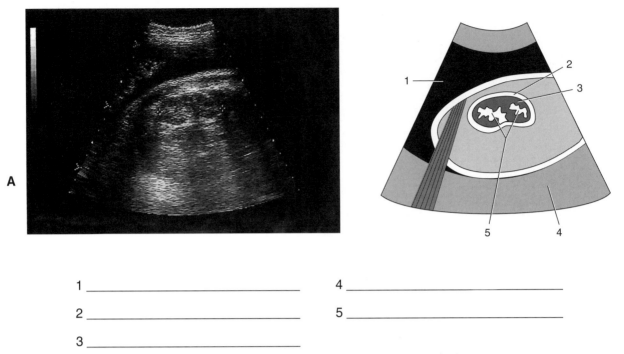

1 _____   4 _____

2 _____   5 _____

3 _____

Figure 18-25 A, Longitudinal section of the right side of the fetal abdomen.

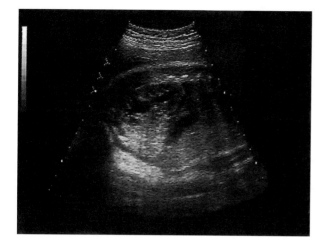
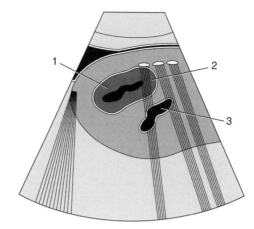

B

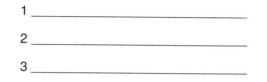

1 _____

2 _____

3 _____

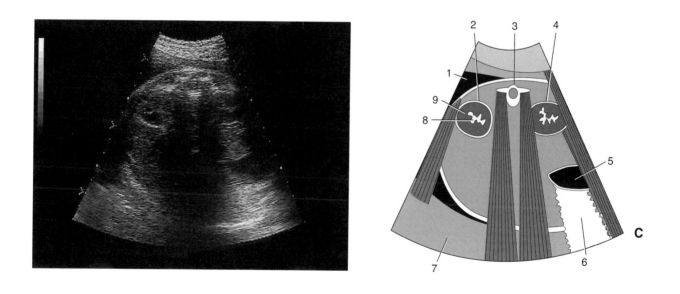

C

1 _____   6 _____

2 _____   7 _____

3 _____   8 _____

4 _____   9 _____

5 _____

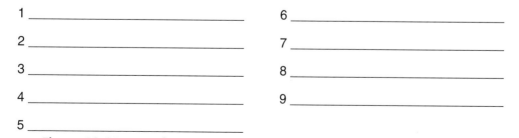

Figure 18-25, cont'd B, Longitudinal section of the left side of the fetal abdomen. C, Short axis section of the fetal abdomen.

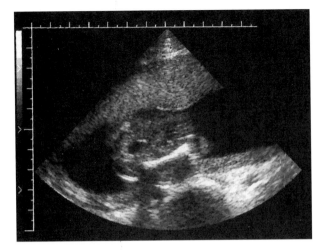

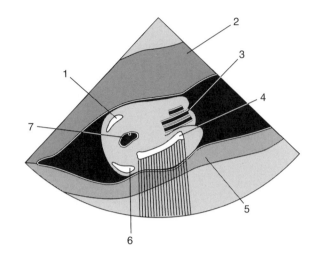

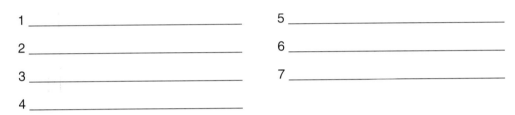

1 _____   5 _____

2 _____   6 _____

3 _____   7 _____

4 _____

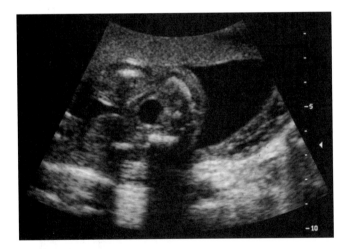

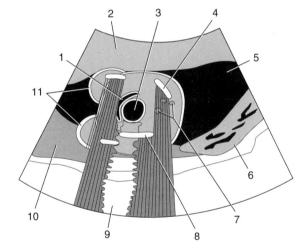

1 _____   7 _____

2 _____   8 _____

3 _____   9 _____

4 _____   10 _____

5 _____   11 _____

6 _____

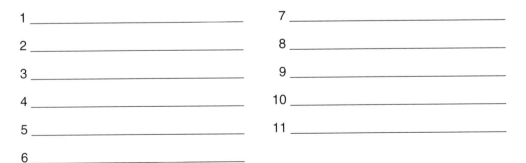

Figure 18-26 Short axis sections of the fetal pelvis. (Bottom half-tone image courtesy the University of Virginia Health System, Department of Radiology, Division of Ultrasound, Charlottesville, Virginia.)

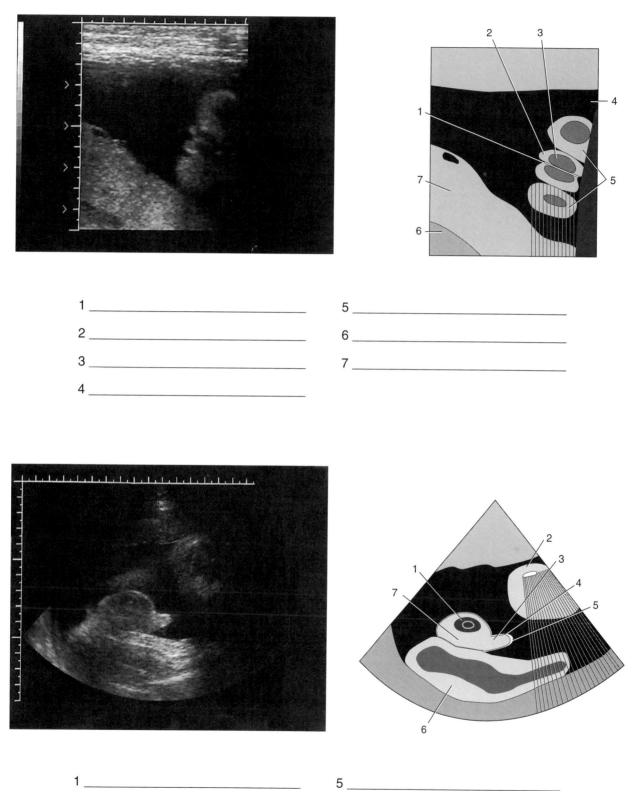

1 _____   5 _____

2 _____   6 _____

3 _____   7 _____

4 _____

1 _____   5 _____

2 _____   6 _____

3 _____   7 _____

4 _____

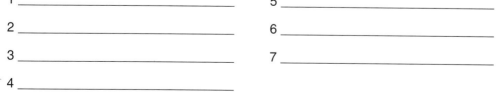

Figure 18-27 Fetal male and female genitalia.

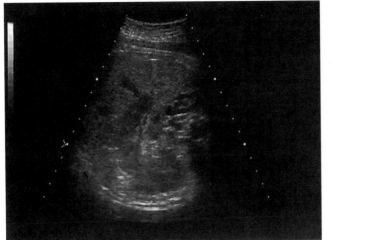
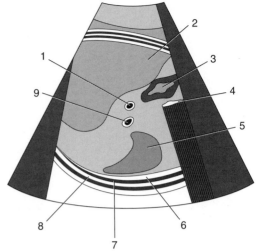

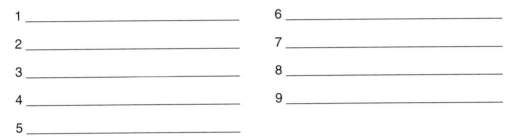

1 _____   6 _____

2 _____   7 _____

3 _____   8 _____

4 _____   9 _____

5 _____

Figure 18-28   Short axis section of the fetal abdomen.

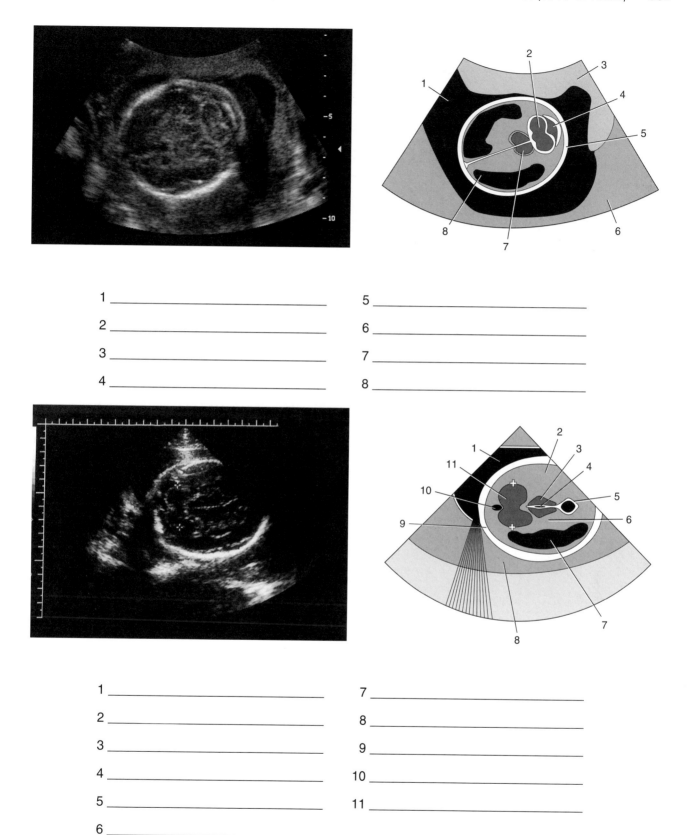

1 _____   5 _____

2 _____   6 _____

3 _____   7 _____

4 _____   8 _____

1 _____   7 _____

2 _____   8 _____

3 _____   9 _____

4 _____   10 _____

5 _____   11 _____

6 _____

Figure 18-29 Fetal brain sections. (Top half-tone image courtesy the University of Virginia Health System, Department of Radiology, Division of Ultrasound, Charlottesville, Virginia.)

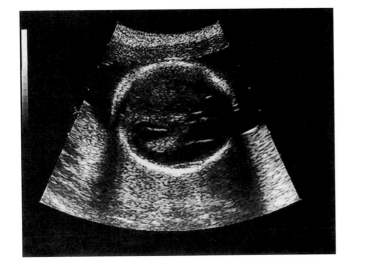
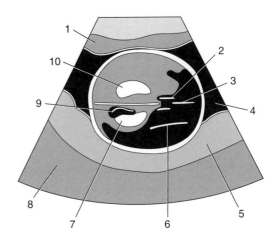

1 _____   6 _____

2 _____   7 _____

3 _____   8 _____

4 _____   9 _____

5 _____   10 _____

Figure 18-30 Fetal brain section.

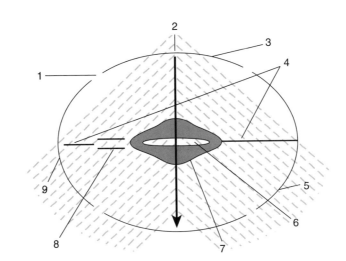

1 _____   6 _____

2 _____   7 _____

3 _____   8 _____

4 _____   9 _____

5 _____

Figure 18-31 Illustrates direction and plane for a fetal head measurement.

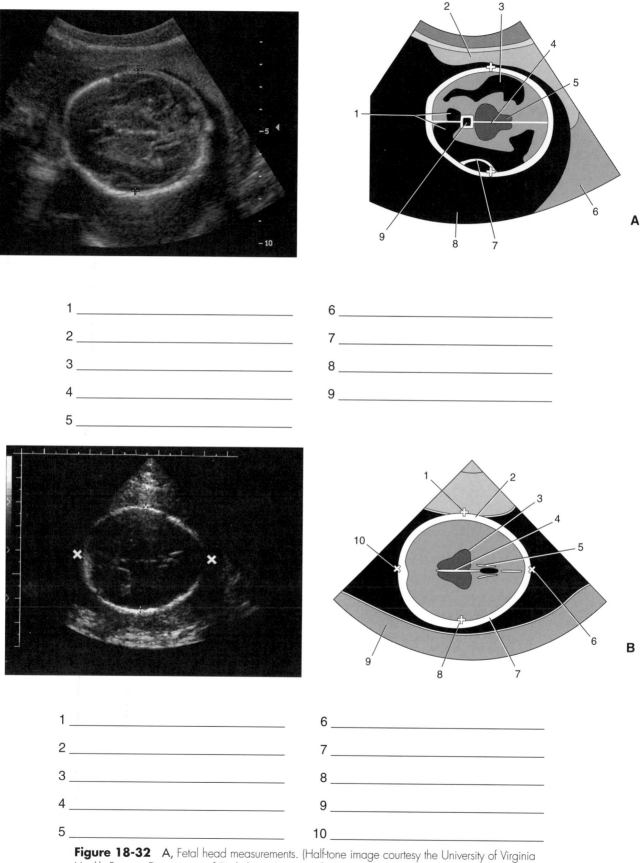

1 _____   6 _____

2 _____   7 _____

3 _____   8 _____

4 _____   9 _____

5 _____

1 _____   6 _____

2 _____   7 _____

3 _____   8 _____

4 _____   9 _____

5 _____   10 _____

Figure 18-32   **A,** Fetal head measurements. (Half-tone image courtesy the University of Virginia Health System, Department of Radiology, Division of Ultrasound, Charlottesville, Virginia.) **B,** Fetal head measurements.

continued

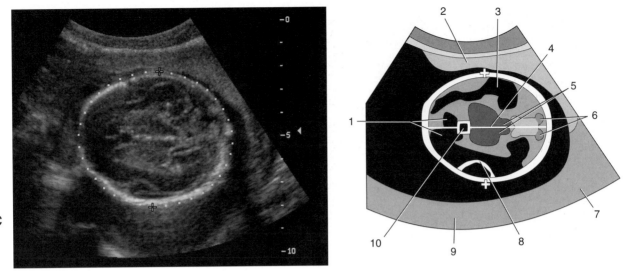

1 _____   6 _____

2 _____   7 _____

3 _____   8 _____

4 _____   9 _____

5 _____   10 _____

Figure 18-32, cont'd C, Fetal head measurements. (Half-tone image courtesy the University of Virginia Health System, Department of Radiology, Division of Ultrasound, Charlottesville, Virginia.)

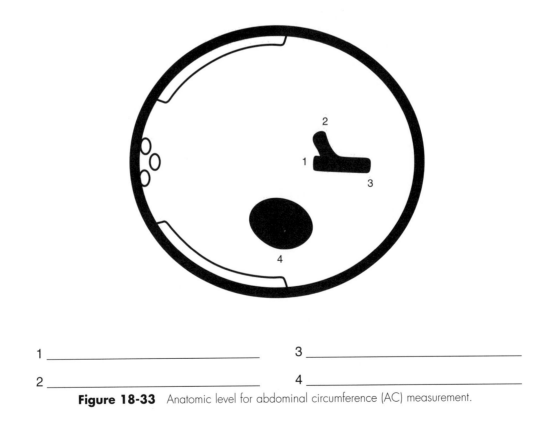

1 _____   3 _____

2 _____   4 _____

Figure 18-33 Anatomic level for abdominal circumference (AC) measurement.

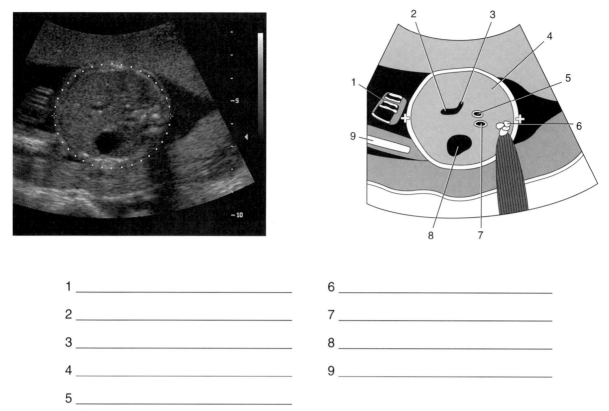

1 _____   6 _____

2 _____   7 _____

3 _____   8 _____

4 _____   9 _____

5 _____

Figure 18-34 Fetal abdominal measurement. (Half-tone image courtesy the University of Virginia Health System, Department of Radiology, Division of Ultrasound, Charlottesville, Virginia.)

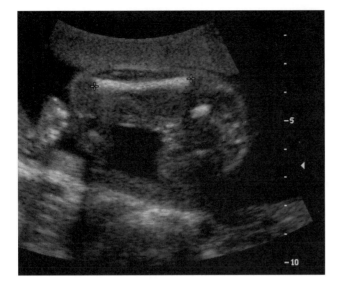
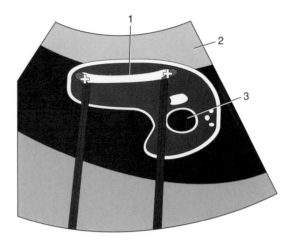

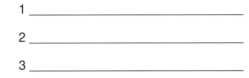

1 _____

2 _____

3 _____

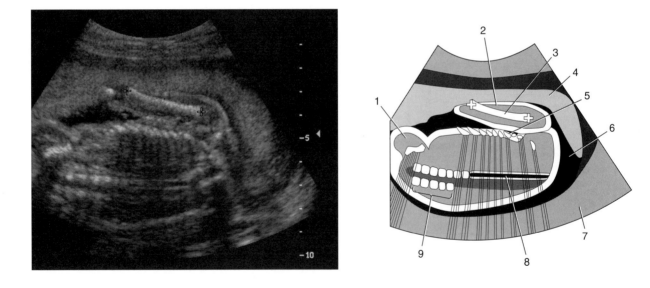

1 _____   6 _____

2 _____   7 _____

3 _____   8 _____

4 _____   9 _____

5 _____

Figure 18-35   Fetal long bones. (Half-tone images courtesy the University of Virginia Health System, Department of Radiology, Division of Ultrasound, Charlottesville, Virginia.)

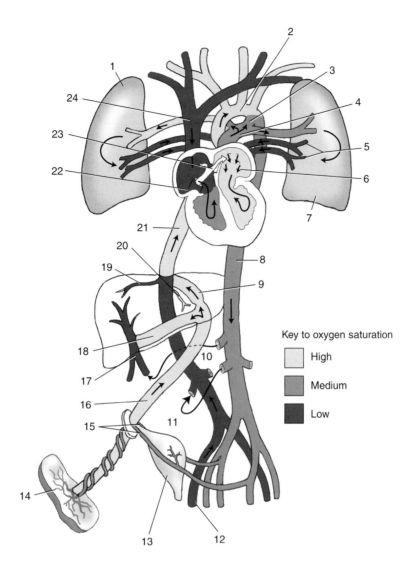

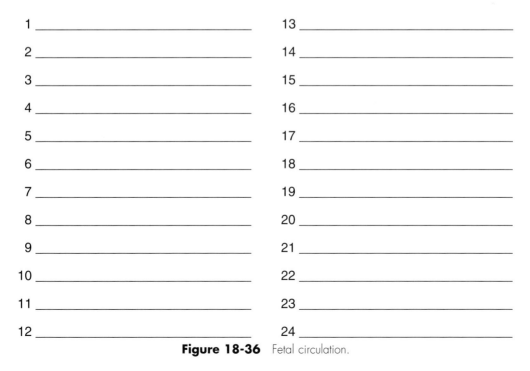

1 _____	13 _____
2 _____	14 _____
3 _____	15 _____
4 _____	16 _____
5 _____	17 _____
6 _____	18 _____
7 _____	19 _____
8 _____	20 _____
9 _____	21 _____
10 _____	22 _____
11 _____	23 _____
12 _____	24 _____

Figure 18-36 Fetal circulation.

CHAPTER 19

High-Risk Obstetric Sonography

REVIEW QUESTIONS

1. Fetal biophysical variables observed and scored to predict perinatal outcome include
   a. _____
   b. _____
   c. _____
   d. _____
   e. _____
   f. _____

2. Abnormal fetal aortic flow velocity waveforms have been associated with
   a. musculoskeletal abnormalities
   b. genitourinary dysfunctions
   c. neurologic dysfunctions
   d. cardiac dysfunctions
   e. liver abnormalities

3. The lecithin-sphingomyelin (L-S) ratio is used to
   a. determine whether abnormalities are present
   b. rule out infections
   c. determine cardiac activity
   d. determine lung maturity
   e. date the early pregnancy for chorionic villus sampling (CVS)

4. Which of the following procedures is done earliest in a pregnancy?
   a. CVS
   b. amniocentesis for L-S ratio
   c. amniocentesis for genetic analysis
   d. cord Doppler
   e. cord transfusions

5. Amniocentesis is associated with which of the following risks?
   a. infection
   b. needle injury
   c. premature delivery
   d. a and b
   e. a, b, and c

6. Which component of amniotic fluid increases beyond normal limits when certain defects are present?
   a. hCG (human chorionic gonadotropin)
   b. AFP (alpha-fetoprotein)
   c. LH (luteinizing hormone)
   d. estrogen
   e. progesterone

7. What ultrasound studies are utilized for high-risk pregnancies?

8. How is the amniotic fluid index (AFI) determined?

9. What are the indications for prenatal ultrasound studies in high-risk pregnancies?

10. Scores lower than 8 on a biophysical profile are
    a. usually followed up with additional testing or induced labor
    b. considered normal
    c. followed up with a fetal intravascular transfusion
    d. considered questionable and followed up with another profile in 6 weeks
    e. associated with good perinatal outcome

11. In a twin gestation, division of the zygote prior to day 4 postfertilization results in
    a. a monochorionic-monoamniotic gestation
    b. a monochorionic-diamniotic gestation
    c. a dichorionic-monoamniotic gestation
    d. the demise of one twin
    e. a dichorionic-diamniotic gestation

12. If division occurs to the embryonic disk more than 13 days postfertilization, the result is
    a. the demise of one twin
    b. a monochorionic-monoamniotic gestation
    c. conjoined twins
    d. congenital anomalies such as anencephaly (absence of the head)
    e. a dichorionic-diamniotic gestation

13. In multifetal gestations, identifying chorionicity (placentae) is most accurate
    a. from the 6th through 10th gestational weeks
    b. from the 14th through the 16th gestational weeks
    c. during the last trimester
    d. at exactly 12 gestational weeks
    e. when the gestation is triplets

14. If twin fetuses are of opposite gender, they are always
    a. monochorionic and monoamniotic
    b. monochorionic and diamniotic
    c. dichorionic and monoamniotic
    d. identical
    e. dichorionic and diamniotic

15. The interfetal membrane
    a. is a congenital malformation found with multifetal gestations
    b. is identifiable in a diamniotic twin gestation
    c. is only associated with same gender, twin gestations
    d. is predominantly part of the cord
    e. is only associated with opposite gender, twin gestations

Identify the structures indicated in the following illustration. This figure duplicates that found in *Sonography: Introduction to Normal Structure and Function.* Refer to the textbook if you need help.

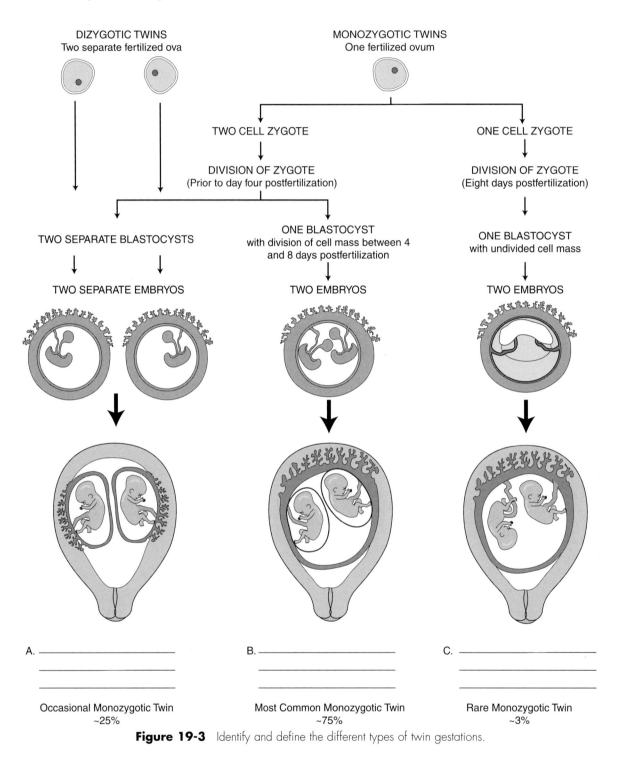

A. _____

B. _____

C. _____

Occasional Monozygotic Twin
~25%

Most Common Monozygotic Twin
~75%

Rare Monozygotic Twin
~3%

Figure 19-3 Identify and define the different types of twin gestations.

CHAPTER 20

The Thyroid and Parathyroid Glands

REVIEW QUESTIONS

1. The thyroid is an endocrine gland that secretes three hormones, which are
   a. triiodothyronine (T_4), thyroxine (T_5), and calcitonin
   b. triiodothyronine (T_3), thyroxine (T_4), and calcitonin
   c. triiodothyronine (T_3), thyroxine (T_4), and iron
   d. triiodothyronine (T_3), thyroxine (T_7), and iron

2. Each of the following statements regarding the thyroid gland is true *except*
   a. it lies anterior to the trachea
   b. it is composed of right and left lobes
   c. a pyramidal lobe is present in approximately 15% to 30% of the population
   d. it is an exocrine gland

3. The average weight of the thyroid gland is approximately
   a. 2 to 15 g
   b. 30 to 40 g
   c. 25 to 35 g
   d. 10 to 15 g

4. Which one of the following statements is *not* true regarding the thyroid gland?
   a. measures approximately 4 to 6 cm in length, 2.0 to 3.0 cm in anteroposterior (AP) diameter, and 1.5 to 2 cm in width
   b. in cross-section is outlined laterally by the common carotid artery and the internal jugular vein
   c. the isthmus measures approximately 1 to 2 mm in AP diameter
   d. plays a major role in growth and development, and regulates basal metabolism by the synthesis, storage, and secretion of thyroid hormones

5. Neck muscles located anterolateral to the thyroid gland include all of the following *except*
   a. the sternothyroid (ST) and sternohyoid (SH)
   b. the longus colli (LCM)
   c. the sternocleidomastoid
   d. the omohyoid and thyrohyoid

6. The sonographic appearance of the normal thyroid gland is uniformly
   a. hypoechoic with scattered hyperechoic regions
   b. echogenic with medium-level echoes similar to the liver and testes
   c. hyperechoic with high-level echoes
   d. hypoechoic with medium-level echoes

7. The following statements are true regarding the sonographic appearance of neck muscles and the esophagus *except*
   a. the esophagus appears hypoechoic with an echogenic center representing mucosa
   b. the longus colli muscle (LCM) is hyperechoic compared with the thyroid gland
   c. the sternocleidomastoid muscle is hypoechoic compared with the thyroid gland
   d. the infrahyoid muscles are hypoechoic relative to the thyroid gland

8. The secretion of triiodothyronine (T_3), thyroxine (T_4), and calcitonin is regulated by the
   a. liver and pituitary gland
   b. hypothalamus and the pituitary gland
   c. hypothalamus only
   d. parafollicular cells (C cells)

9. The thyroid gland is composed of follicles filled with a substance called
   a. thyrotropin
   b. colloid
   c. calcitonin
   d. none of the above

10. Each of the following statements regarding parathyroid glands is true *except*
    a. most people (about 80% to 85%) have four parathyroid glands located in a symmetric position (two upper and two lower)
    b. parathyroid glands are situated posterior to the thyroid gland
    c. parathyroid glands may be intrathyroidal
    d. ectopic parathyroid glands represent approximately 5% of the total

11. Parathyroid glands develop from the
    a. first and second pharyngeal pouches
    b. third and fifth pharyngeal pouches
    c. third and fourth pharyngeal pouches
    d. none of the above

12. Which of the following statements is *not* true regarding parathyroid glands?
    a. ectopic parathyroid glands represent approximately 15% to 20% of the total
    b. ectopic locations include the carotid bulb, retroesophageal, thymus, and intrathyroidal
    c. normal parathyroid glands measure approximately 5 to 7 mm in length, 3 to 4 mm in width, and 1 to 2 mm in thickness
    d. the shape of parathyroid glands varies; they are generally elongated

13. The sonographic appearance of parathyroid glands is
    a. always hyperechoic compared with the thyroid gland
    b. hypoechoic to anechoic without through transmission
    c. anechoic with through transmission
    d. none of the above

14. Each of the following statements regarding parathyroid glands is true *except*
    a. normal parathyroid glands are usually not seen by sonography
    b. parathyroid glands are situated posterior to the thyroid gland and anterior to the longus colli muscle (LCM)
    c. a prominent longus colli muscle (LCM) may be mistaken for a parathyroid adenoma
    d. the minor neurovascular bundle is never mistaken for a parathyroid adenoma

15. Each of the following statements regarding parathyroid gland physiology is true *except*
    a. parathyroid glands secrete parathyroid hormone, also called PTH or parathormone
    b. parathyroid glands maintain homeostasis of blood calcium by promoting calcium absorption into the blood and preventing hypocalcemia
    c. when serum calcium levels are low, the parathyroid hormone lowers serum calcium by releasing calcium from the bone
    d. hypercalcemia (calcium levels greater than 10.2 mg/dl in adults and 10.7 mg/dl in children) is an indication for localizing abnormal parathyroid glands

16. When ultrasound fails to identify abnormal parathyroid glands preoperatively and postoperatively, which of the following tests is used?
    a. computed tomography, radionuclide scanning, or magnetic resonance imaging
    b. arteriography and magnetic resonance imaging
    c. computed tomography and spine radiography
    d. none of the above

17. High resolution sonography recommended for the evaluation of parathyroid adenomas is between
    a. 3.5 and 5.0 MHz
    b. 5.0 MHz only
    c. 7.5 and 10.0 MHz
    d. 2.5 MHz only

18. Superior and inferior parathyroid glands are supplied
    a. by superior thyroid arteries only
    b. by both superior and inferior thyroid arteries
    c. by the venous plexus only
    d. by all of the above

19. Which statement is true regarding the thyroid gland?
    a. exocrine gland that secretes; triiodothyronine (T_4), thyroxine (T_5), and calcitonin
    b. endocrine gland that secretes; triiodothyronine (T_3), thyroxine (T_4), and calcitonin
    c. exocrine gland that secretes; triiodothyronine (T_3), thyroxine (T_4), and iron
    d. endocrine gland that secretes; triiodothyronine (T_3), thyroxine (T_4), and iron

20. Each of the following statements regarding the thyroid gland is true *except*
    a. it lies inferior to the trachea
    b. it is composed of right and left lobes
    c. in cross-section is outlined posterolaterally by the common carotid artery (CCA) and internal jugular vein (IJV), and posteriorly by the LCM, esophagus, and major neurovascular branch
    d. connected across the midline by the isthmus

21. Each of the following statements regarding the size and shape of the thyroid gland is true *except*
    a. tall, thin individuals have short lateral lobes measuring 5 cm in length
    b. short, obese patients tend to exhibit oval lateral lobes measuring less than 5 cm in length
    c. tall, thin patients have elongated lateral lobes that can measure up to 7 to 8 cm in the longitudinal plane
    d. thyroid gland measurements have a wide range of variability

22. Which one of the following statements is *not* true regarding the adult thyroid gland?
    a. measures approximately 4 to 6 cm in length, 1.3 to 8 cm in AP diameter, and 1.5 to 2 cm in width
    b. in cross-section, is outlined posterolaterally by the CCA and the IJV
    c. the isthmus measures approximately 2 to 6 mm in AP diameter
    d. plays a major role in growth and development, and regulates basal metabolism by the synthesis, storage, and secretion of thyroid hormones

23. Neck muscles located anterolateral to the thyroid gland include all of the following *except*
    a. the sternothyroid (ST) and sternohyoid (SH)
    b. the omohyoid (OH) and thyrohyoid
    c. the sternocleidomastoid
    d. the longus colli muscle (LCM)

24. The following statements are true regarding the sonographic appearance of the normal thyroid gland *except*
    a. more uniformly hypoechoic than that of contiguous muscles and vascular structures
    b. uniformly echogenic with medium-level echoes similar to the liver and testes
    c. 1- to 2-mm anechoic tubular structures representing thyroid arteries and veins
    d. more echogenic than that of contiguous muscles and vascular structures

25. Each of the following statements regarding parathyroid glands is true *except*
    a. the most common indication for parathyroid imaging is hypercalcemia (greater than 10.5 mg/dl)
    b. primary hyperparathyroidism is caused by a solitary parathyroid adenoma in 80% to 90% of cases
    c. most people (about 80% to 85%) have four parathyroid glands located in a symmetric position, posterior to the thyroid lobe and anterior to the LCM
    d. the typical sonographic appearance of a parathyroid adenoma is an oval or bean-shaped hyperechoic to anechoic structure without through transmission

26. Which of the following statements is *not* true regarding parathyroid glands and parathyroid adenomas?
    a. ectopic parathyroid glands account for approximately 15% of the total
    b. the carotid bulb, thymus, retroesophageal, and intrathyroidal regions represent ectopic locations
    c. normal parathyroid glands are never detected by sonography
    d. normal cervical structures such as the longus colli muscle (LCM), esophagus, and small extrathyroidal arteries and veins can mimic parathyroid adenomas

27. Which of the following statements is *not* true regarding parathyroid imaging?

    a. high-resolution (7.5 to 15 MHz) linear transducers are routinely used to image abnormal parathyroid glands

    b. patients with thick necks may require 5 MHz to enhance acoustic visualization

    c. sonography is routinely performed on patients with normal calcium levels

    d. use the swallow maneuver to best locate inferior parathyroid adenomas

28. Which of the following statements is *not* true regarding parathyroid adenomas?

    a. measure between 0.8 and 1.5 cm in length

    b. homogeneous and hypoechoic, various shapes, with enlargement inhomogeneity and cystic degeneration

    c. hypervascular

    d. never coexist with thyroid nodules

Identify the structures indicated in the following illustrations. These figures duplicate those found in *Sonography: Introduction to Normal Structure and Function.* Refer to the textbook if you need help.

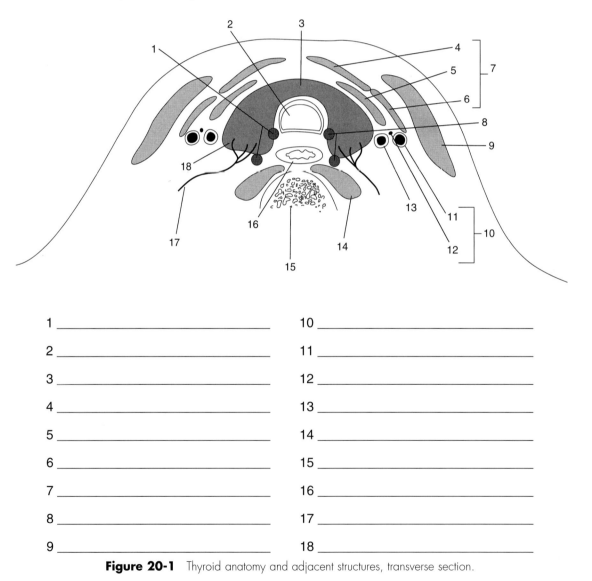

1 _____	10 _____
2 _____	11 _____
3 _____	12 _____
4 _____	13 _____
5 _____	14 _____
6 _____	15 _____
7 _____	16 _____
8 _____	17 _____
9 _____	18 _____

Figure 20-1 Thyroid anatomy and adjacent structures, transverse section.

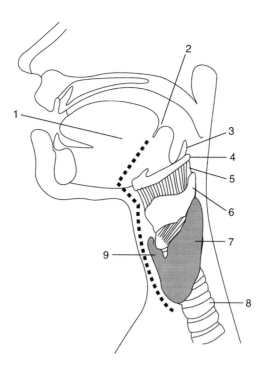

1 _____   6 _____

2 _____   7 _____

3 _____   8 _____

4 _____   9 _____

5 _____

Figure 20-2 Embryonic migration of the thyroid gland. Broken line indicates path of migration.

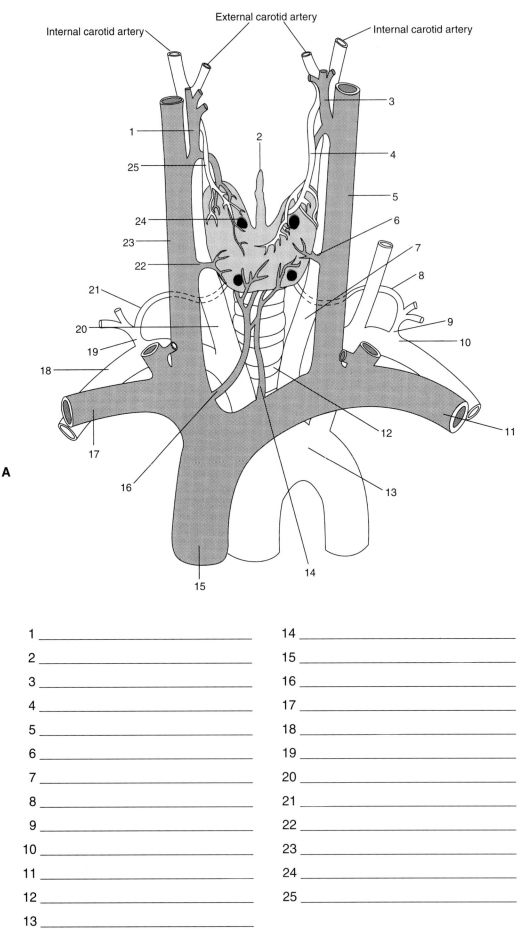

Internal carotid artery
External carotid artery
Internal carotid artery

1
2
3
4
5
6
7
8
9
10
11
12
13
14
15
16
17
18
19
20
21
22
23
24
25

A

1 _____   14 _____
2 _____   15 _____
3 _____   16 _____
4 _____   17 _____
5 _____   18 _____
6 _____   19 _____
7 _____   20 _____
8 _____   21 _____
9 _____   22 _____
10 _____   23 _____
11 _____   24 _____
12 _____   25 _____
13 _____

Figure 20-3 A, Illustration of frontal view of thyroid and parathyroid regions.

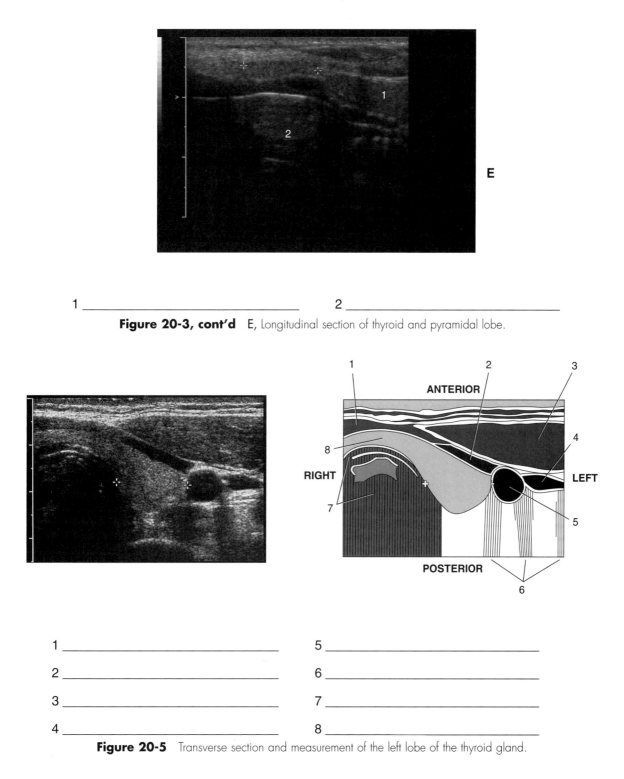

1 _____   2 _____

Figure 20-3, cont'd E, Longitudinal section of thyroid and pyramidal lobe.

1 _____   5 _____

2 _____   6 _____

3 _____   7 _____

4 _____   8 _____

Figure 20-5 Transverse section and measurement of the left lobe of the thyroid gland.

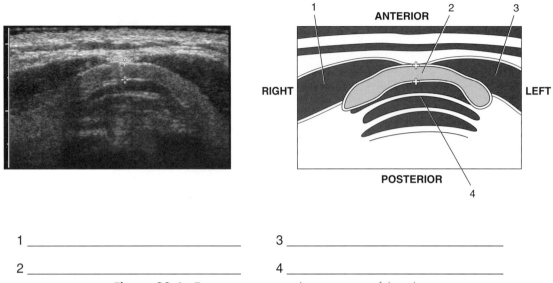

1 _____   3 _____

2 _____   4 _____

Figure 20-6 Transverse section and measurement of the isthmus.

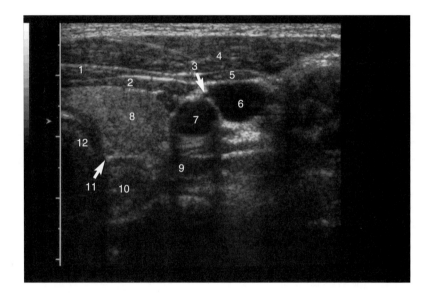

1 _____   7 _____

2 _____   8 _____

3 _____   9 _____

4 _____   10 _____

5 _____   11 _____

6 _____   12 _____

Figure 20-8 Transverse section of thyroid gland and adjacent structures.

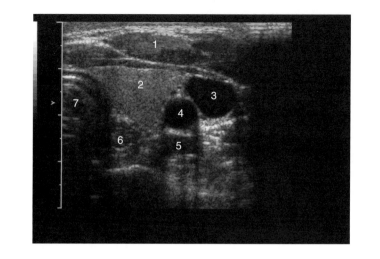

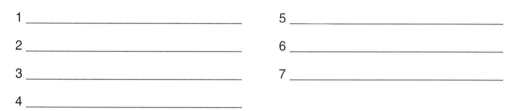

1 _____   5 _____

2 _____   6 _____

3 _____   7 _____

4 _____

Figure 20-9 Transverse section of thyroid gland and adjacent structures.

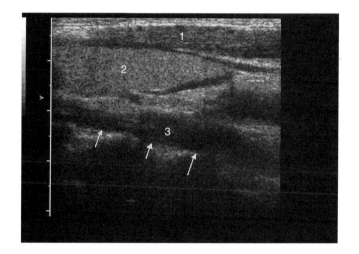

1 _____

2 _____

3 _____

Figure 20-10 Longitudinal section of strap muscle and longus colli muscle (LCM).

1 _____

2 _____

3 _____

4 _____

5 _____

6 _____

7 _____

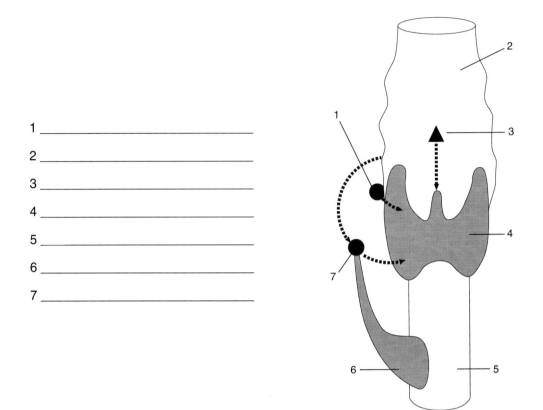

Figure 20-11 Migration of the thymus and parathyroid glands.

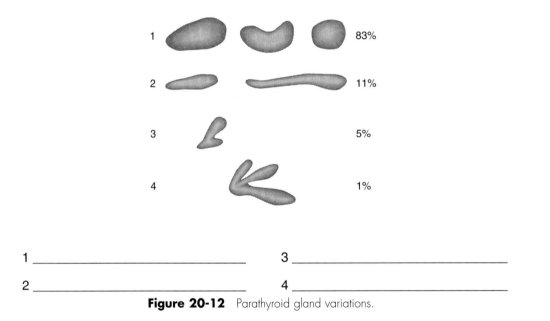

1 _____   3 _____

2 _____   4 _____

Figure 20-12 Parathyroid gland variations.

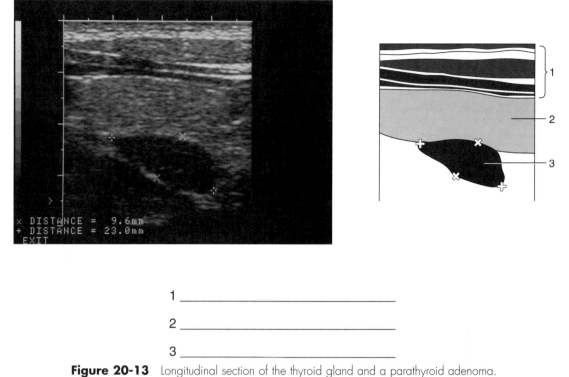

1 _____

2 _____

3 _____

Figure 20-13 Longitudinal section of the thyroid gland and a parathyroid adenoma.

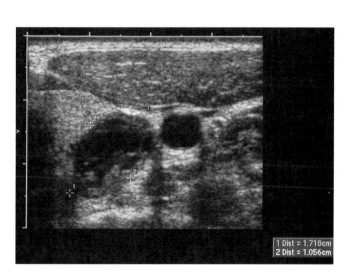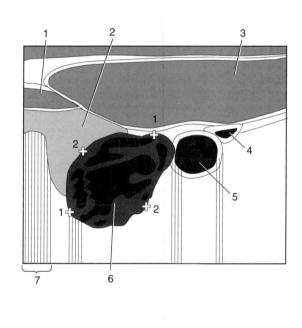

1 _____   5 _____

2 _____   6 _____

3 _____   7 _____

4 _____

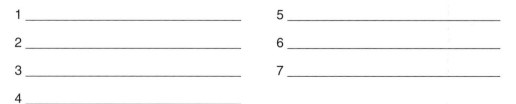

Figure 20-14 Transverse section through the mid left lobe of the thyroid gland and a parathyroid adenoma.

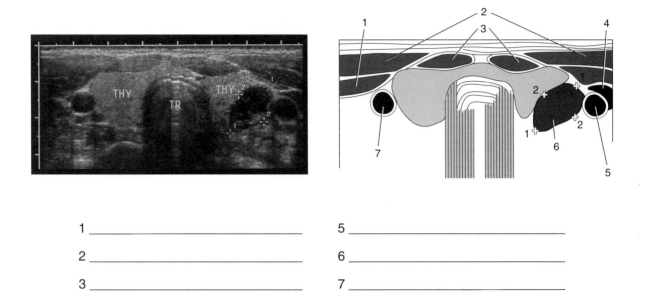

1 _____   5 _____

2 _____   6 _____

3 _____   7 _____

4 _____

Figure 20-15 Transverse section of the thyroid gland showing a left parathyroid adenoma.

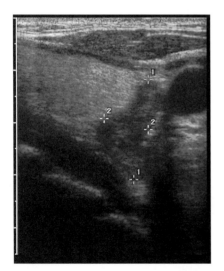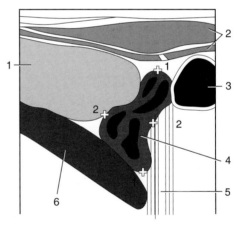

1 _____   4 _____

2 _____   5 _____

3 _____   6 _____

Figure 20-16 Longitudinal section of the right lower lobe of the thyroid gland showing a lobulated parathyroid adenoma.

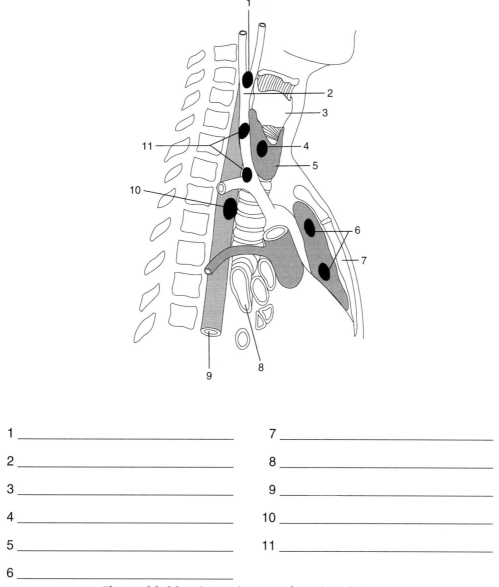

1 _____

2 _____

3 _____

4 _____

5 _____

6 _____

7 _____

8 _____

9 _____

10 _____

11 _____

Figure 20-23   Aberrant locations of parathyroid glands.

CHAPTER 21

Breast Sonography

REVIEW QUESTIONS

1. Which of the following hormones does *not* affect the breast?

    a. prolactin

    b. progesterone

    c. alkaline phosphatase

    d. estrogen

2. Which of the following best describes the image shown?

    a. normal breast tissue

    b. fatty breast tissue

    c. fibrocystic breast changes

    d. breast mass

    e. breast cyst

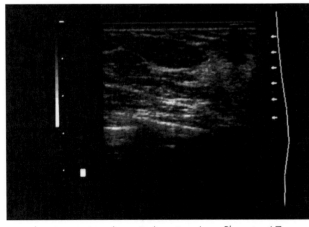

Image courtesy Acoustic Imaging, Inc., Phoenix, AZ.

3. Which of the following best describes the image shown?

    a. normal breast tissue

    b. fatty breast tissue

    c. fibrocystic breast changes

    d. breast mass

    e. breast cyst

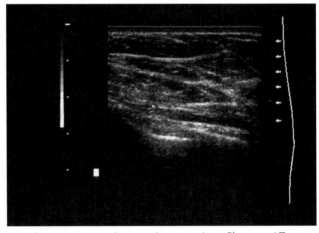

Image courtesy Acoustic Imaging, Inc., Phoenix, AZ.

4. Which of the following best describes the image shown?

    a. normal breast tissue

    b. fatty breast tissue

    c. fibrocystic breast changes

    d. breast mass

    e. breast cyst

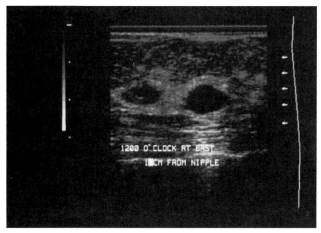

Image courtesy Acoustic Imaging, Inc., Phoenix, AZ.

5. The breast arises from which embryonic layer?

a. endoderm

b. mesoderm

c. mesenchyme

d. ectoderm

6. Which of the following best describes the image shown?

a. normal breast tissue

b. fatty breast tissue

c. fibrocystic breast changes

d. breast mass

e. breast cyst

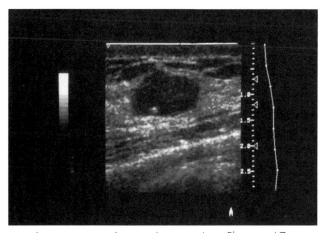

Image courtesy Acoustic Imaging, Inc., Phoenix, AZ.

7. Support of the breast parenchyma is provided by

a. lactiferous ducts

b. acini

c. Cooper's ligaments

d. the pectoralis major muscle

8. Which of the following statements best describes the anatomic location of the breast?

a. anterior to the pectoralis major muscle, bordered inferiorly by the fifth and sixth costal cartilages

b. anterior to the pectoralis major muscle, bordered superiorly by the second and third ribs

c. medial to the sternum, anterior to the second rib

d. anterior to the serratus muscle, lateral to the margin of the axilla

9. Most lymph drainage from the breast occurs in which manner?

a. subcutaneously

b. through the thoracic lymph nodes

c. through the acini

d. through the axillary lymph nodes

10. Which of the following statements is (are) true?

a. mammary glands are modified sweat glands

b. mammary glands are endocrine glands

c. mammary glands arise from the ectoderm

d. all of the above are true

11. The mammary glands are endocrine organs whose main function is lactation during pregnancy.

a. true

b. false

12. The breast is located anteriorly to the pectoralis minor, serratus, and internal oblique muscles and the sixth rib.

a. true

b. false

13. The normal breast is composed of 15 to 20 lobes, which are separated by adipose tissue, which then divide into lobules.

a. true

b. false

14. The suspensory ligaments of Cooper support the breast tissue and run between each two lobules from the deep muscle fascia to the skin surface.

a. true

b. false

15. The sonographic appearance of the fat components of the breast appears more echogenic than surrounding parenchymal breast tissue.

a. true

b. false

16. The glandular tissue of the breast appears homogeneous in texture, with medium-level to low-level echogenicity.

a. true

b. false

17. The fibrocystic breast is a very common normal variant on ultrasound in women of childbearing age.

a. true

b. false

18. It should be noted that breasts appear more fatty after menopause because the fat components become more prominent as the mammary ducts begin to atrophy.

a. true

b. false

19. Oxytocin is a hormone produced and stored by the ovaries that causes duct contraction and allows for the flow of milk during nursing.

a. true

b. false

20. Arterial blood supply to the breast is via the internal thoracic or the internal mammary artery.

a. true

b. false

Identify the structures indicated in the following illustrations. These figures duplicate those found in *Sonography: Introduction to Normal Structure and Function.* Refer to the textbook if you need help.

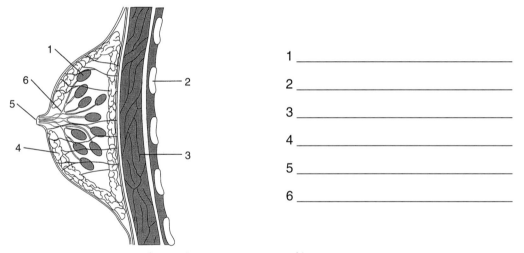

1 _____

2 _____

3 _____

4 _____

5 _____

6 _____

Figure 21-1   Cross-section of breast anatomy.

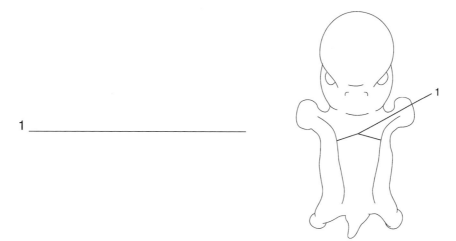

1 _____

Figure 21-2 Prenatal development of fetus.

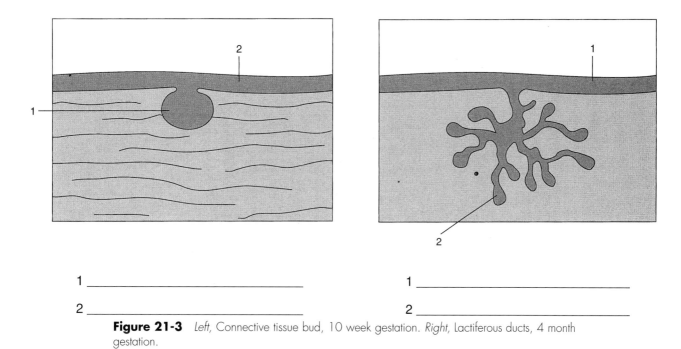

1 _____

2 _____

1 _____

2 _____

Figure 21-3 *Left,* Connective tissue bud, 10 week gestation. *Right,* Lactiferous ducts, 4 month gestation.

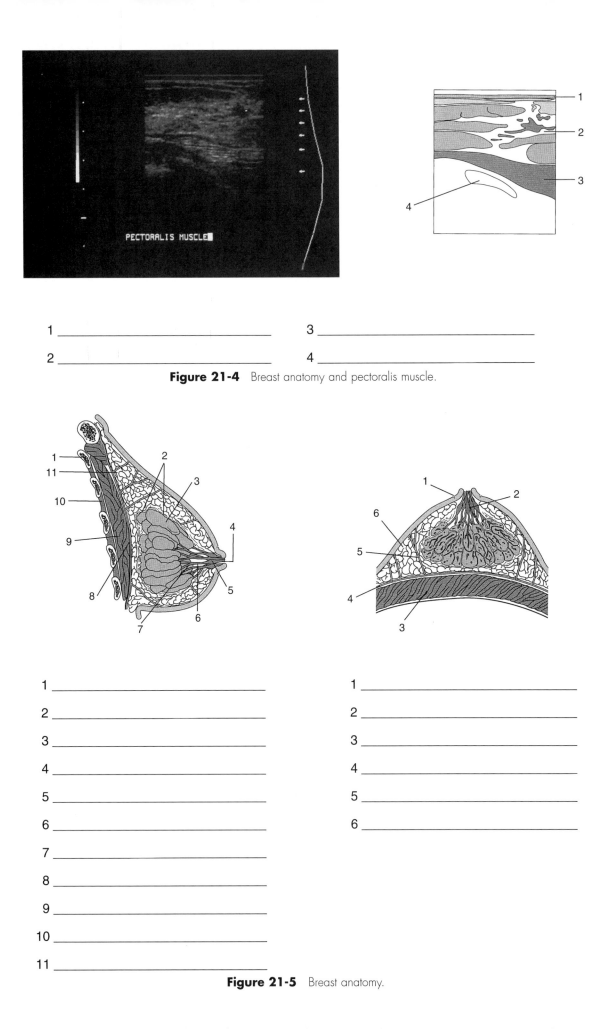

PECTORALIS MUSCLE

1 _____   3 _____

2 _____   4 _____

Figure 21-4 Breast anatomy and pectoralis muscle.

1 _____   1 _____

2 _____   2 _____

3 _____   3 _____

4 _____   4 _____

5 _____   5 _____

6 _____   6 _____

7 _____

8 _____

9 _____

10 _____

11 _____

Figure 21-5 Breast anatomy.

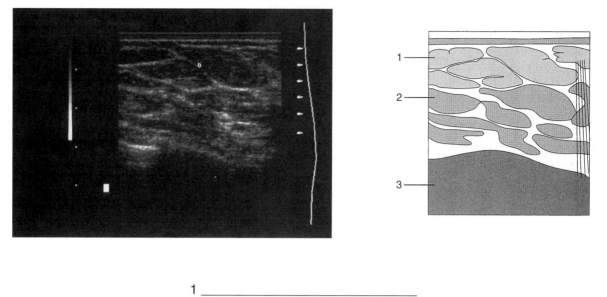

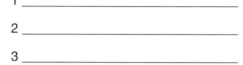

1 _____

2 _____

3 _____

Figure 21-6 Anatomic layers of the breast. (Half-tone image courtesy Acoustic Imaging, Inc., Phoenix, AZ.)

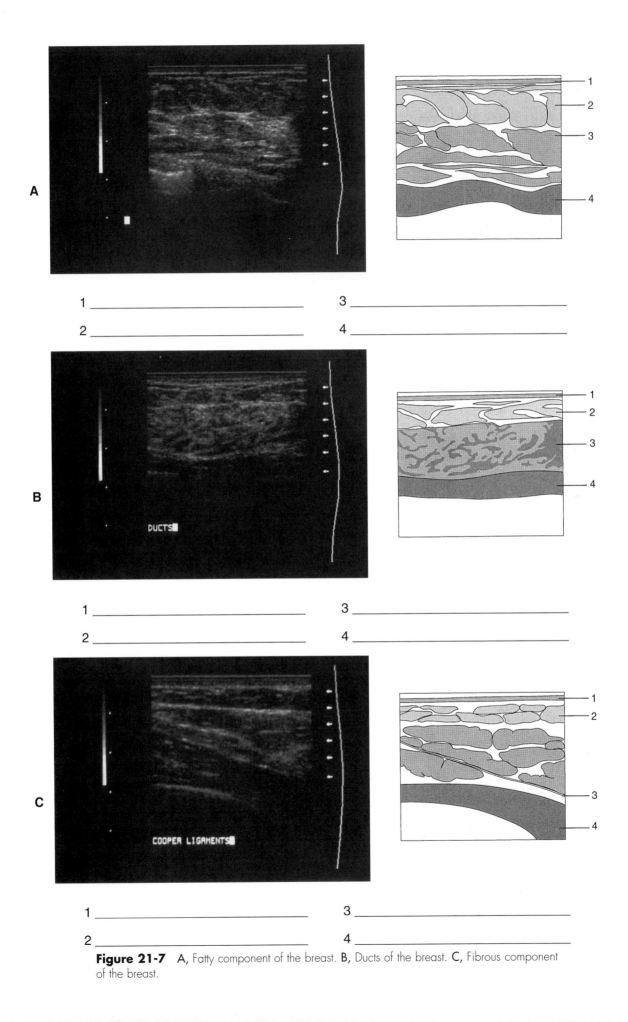

A

1 _____   3 _____

2 _____   4 _____

B

DUCTS

1 _____   3 _____

2 _____   4 _____

C

COOPER LIGAMENTS

1 _____   3 _____

2 _____   4 _____

Figure 21-7 A, Fatty component of the breast. B, Ducts of the breast. C, Fibrous component of the breast.

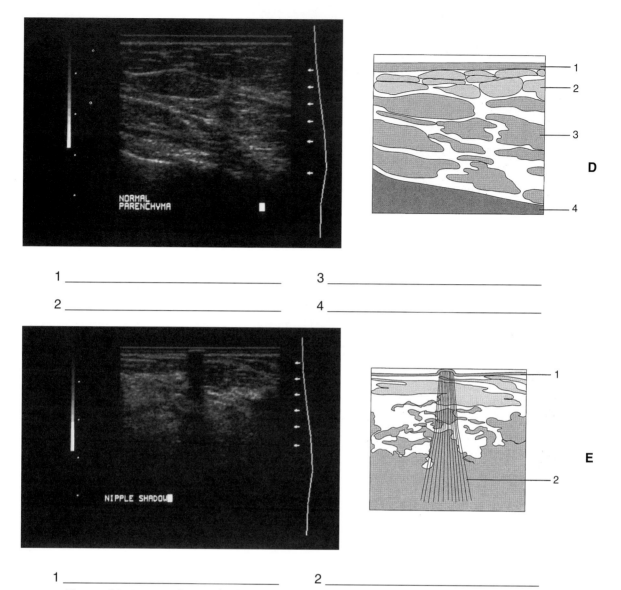

1 _____   3 _____

2 _____   4 _____

1 _____   2 _____

Figure 21-7, cont'd   D, Glandular components of the breast. E, Nipple shadow. (Half-tone images courtesy Acoustic Imaging, Inc., Phoenix, AZ.)

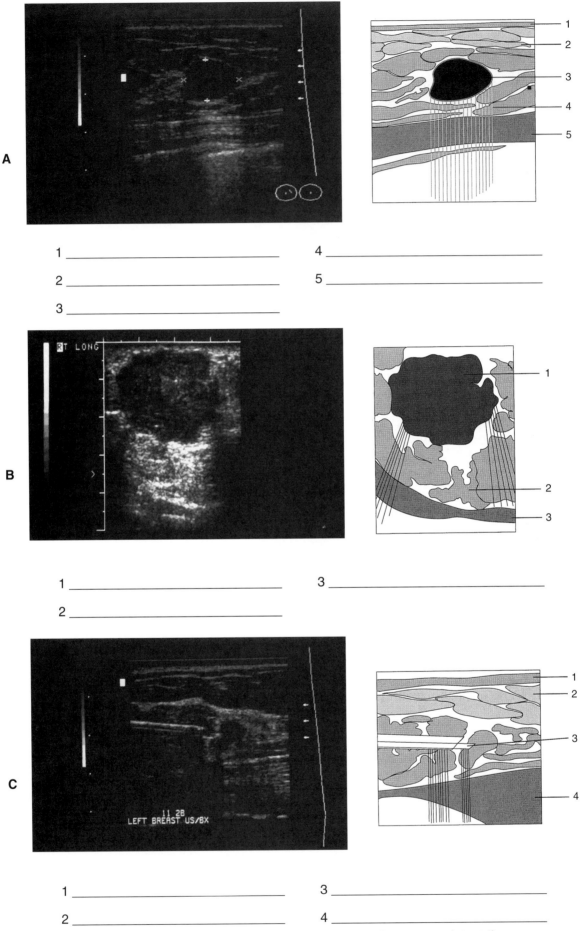

A

1 _____ 4 _____

2 _____ 5 _____

3 _____

B

1 _____ 3 _____

2 _____

C

1 _____ 3 _____

2 _____ 4 _____

Figure 21-8 A, Breast cyst. B, Solid breast mass. C, Breast biopsy. (A and C, Half-tone images courtesy Acoustic Imaging, Inc., Phoenix, AZ. B, Half-tone image courtesy Acuson Corp., Mountain View, CA.)

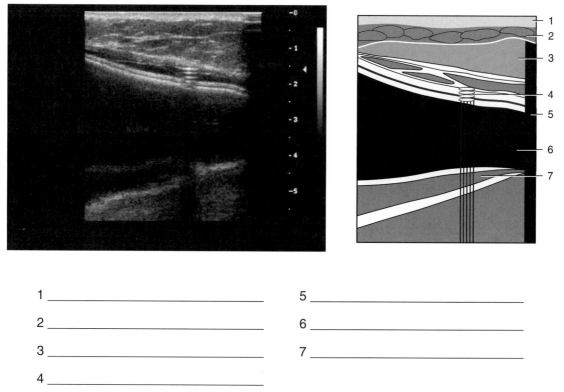

1 _____   5 _____

2 _____   6 _____

3 _____   7 _____

4 _____

Figure 21-8, cont'd D, Breast implant. (D, Half-tone image courtesy Johns Hopkins Hospital, Baltimore, MD.)

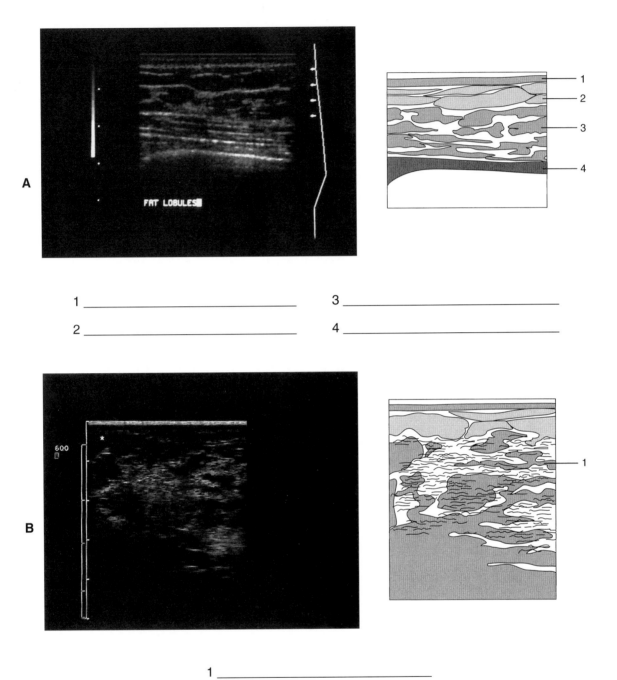

1 _____   3 _____

2 _____   4 _____

1 _____

Figure 21-9 **A,** Fatty breast. **B,** Fibrous breast. (**A,** Half-tone image courtesy Acoustic Imaging, Inc., Phoenix, AZ. **B,** Half-tone image courtesy DePaul Medical Center, Norfolk, VA.)

■ CHAPTER 22

The Neonatal Brain

REVIEW QUESTIONS

1. Sonographically, the cisterna magna appears as an
   a. anechoic space inferior to the cerebellum
   b. anechoic space superior to the cerebellum
   c. echogenic space inferior to the cerebellum
   d. echogenic space superior to the cerebellum

2. The channel that connects the third and fourth ventricles is called
   a. foramen of Luschka
   b. foramen of Magendie
   c. aqueduct of Sylvius
   d. foramen of Monro

3. The moderately echogenic structure that marks the inferior and lateral margins of the frontal horns of the lateral ventricles is the
   a. choroid plexus
   b. massa intermedia
   c. cavum septum pellucidum
   d. head of the caudate nucleus

4. Located between the frontal horns of the lateral ventricles, and lying superior and anterior to the third ventricle, this midline, fluid-filled structure (i.e., anechoic) is considered a normal variant.
   a. corpus callosum
   b. foramen of Monro
   c. cavum septum pellucidum
   d. cavum velum interpositum

5. Anatomically, which vessels lie within the lateral sylvian fissures and are frequently seen pulsating during a real-time examination?
   a. anterior cerebral arteries
   b. middle cerebral arteries
   c. posterior cerebral arteries
   d. basilar arteries

6. Which of the following best describes the position of the choroid plexus within the ventricles? It is located within
   a. the occipital horns of the lateral ventricles only
   b. the frontal, occipital, and temporal horns and bodies of the lateral ventricles only
   c. the roof of the third and fourth ventricles only
   d. the trigone region of the lateral ventricles, the medial aspects of the temporal horns, and the roof of both the third and fourth ventricles

7. Which of the following structures is *not* sonographically echogenic?
   a. fourth ventricle
   b. cerebellar vermis
   c. choroid plexus
   d. quadrigeminal plate cistern

8. Congenital malformations frequently result from an alteration of the normal events of
   a. histogenesis
   b. homeostasis
   c. cytogenesis
   d. organogenesis

9. The four major regions of the brain are
   a. cerebral hemispheres, diencephalon, brain stem, and cerebellum
   b. cerebral hemispheres, brain stem, cerebellum, and medulla oblongata
   c. cerebellum, interhemispheric fissure, brain stem, and medulla oblongata
   d. cerebral hemispheres, diencephalon, interhemispheric fissure, and medulla oblongata

10. The sonographic appearance of the thalami is
    a. anechoic
    b. homogeneous
    c. heterogeneous
    d. highly echogenic

11. What is the longitudinal echogenic line seen extending from the superior edge of the brain in the midline?
    a. caudate nucleus
    b. falx cerebri
    c. cavum septum pellucidum
    d. interpeduncular cistern

12. The sonographic appearance of the choroid plexus is
    a. highly echogenic
    b. homogenous
    c. heterogeneous
    d. anechoic

13. The falx cerebri is within the
    a. interhemispheric fissure
    b. body of the lateral ventricles
    c. foramen of Monro
    d. trigone

14. Normal ventricular size is
    a. 12 mm
    b. 2 mm or less
    c. 4 mm or less
    d. 1 mm

15. The normal midline to lateral dimension is
    a. 12 mm
    b. 2 mm or less
    c. 4 mm or less
    d. 1 mm

16. Asymmetry in the size of the lateral ventricles
    a. is abnormal
    b. is a common normal variant
    c. does not occur
    d. cannot be appreciated sonographically

17. The trigone region of the lateral ventricles is where the
    a. lateral and third ventricles communicate
    b. bodies, occipital horns, and temporal horns converge
    c. bodies, anterior horns, and temporal horns converge
    d. bodies, anterior horns, and germinal matrix converge

18. What marks the communication between the lateral and third ventricles?
    a. foramen of Luschka
    b. foramen of Magendie
    c. aqueduct of Sylvius
    d. foramen of Monro

19. On a sagittal view, the caudothalamic groove is seen as
    a. a thin, highly echogenic arc between the head of the caudate nucleus and the lateral ventricle
    b. an anechoic space between the right and left frontal lobes of the brain
    c. a thin, highly echogenic arc between the head of the caudate nucleus and the thalamus
    d. a thin, hyperechoic arc between the cavum septum pellucidum and third ventricle

20. On a coronal view, what is the echogenic, star-shaped structure inferior to the lateral ventricular bodies?
    a. fourth ventricle
    b. vermis
    c. quadrigeminal plate cistern
    d. glomus of the choroid plexus

Identify the structures indicated in the following illustrations. These figures duplicate those found in *Sonography: Introduction to Normal Structure and Function.* Refer to the textbook if you need help.

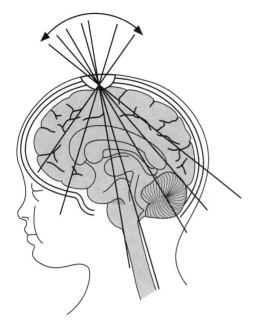

Figure 22-1 Name survey plane: _____

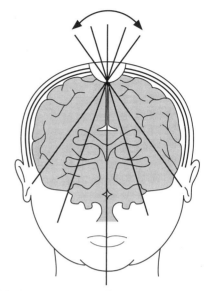

Figure 22-2 Name survey plane: _____

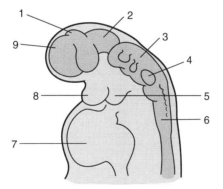

1 _____   6 _____

2 _____   7 _____

3 _____   8 _____

4 _____   9 _____

5 _____

Figure 22-3 3½ weeks' brain development.

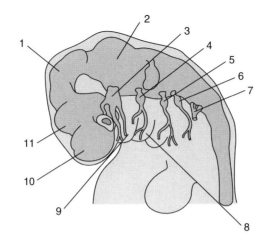

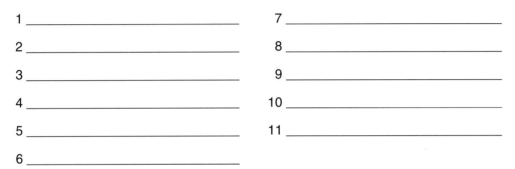

1 _____   7 _____

2 _____   8 _____

3 _____   9 _____

4 _____   10 _____

5 _____   11 _____

6 _____

Figure 22-4 5½ weeks' brain development.

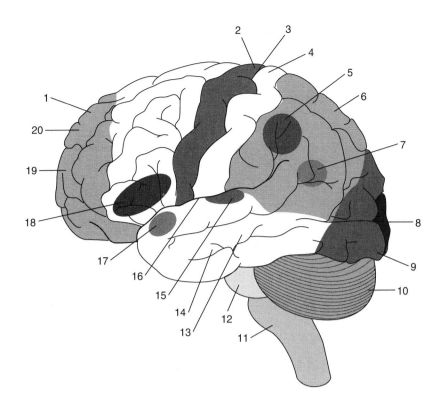

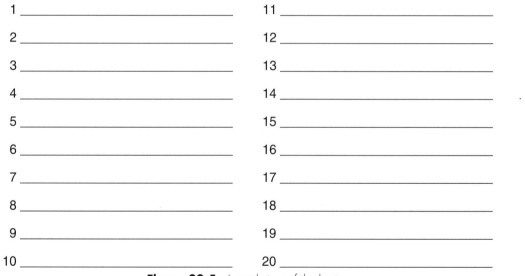

1 _____   11 _____

2 _____   12 _____

3 _____   13 _____

4 _____   14 _____

5 _____   15 _____

6 _____   16 _____

7 _____   17 _____

8 _____   18 _____

9 _____   19 _____

10 _____   20 _____

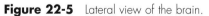

Figure 22-5 Lateral view of the brain.

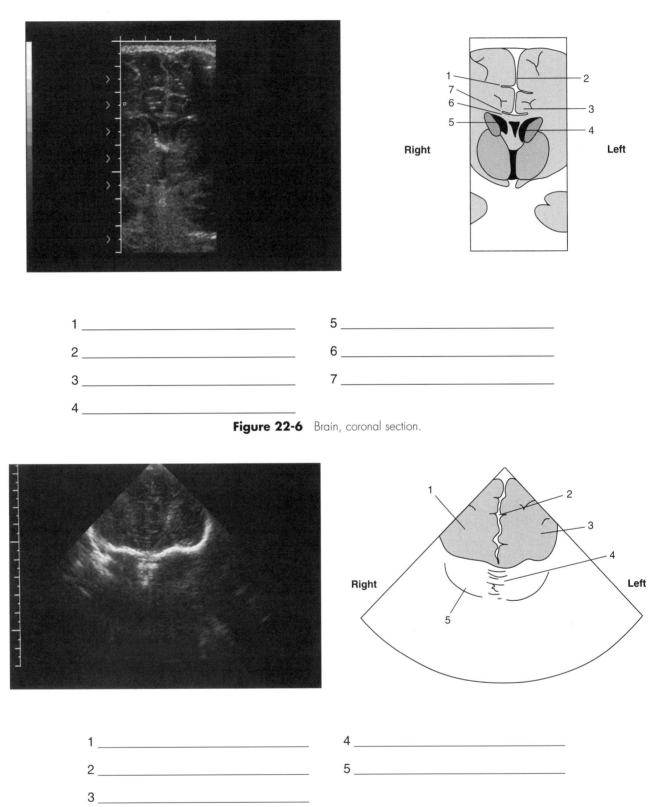

1 _____   5 _____

2 _____   6 _____

3 _____   7 _____

4 _____

Figure 22-6 Brain, coronal section.

1 _____   4 _____

2 _____   5 _____

3 _____

Figure 22-7 Brain, coronal section.

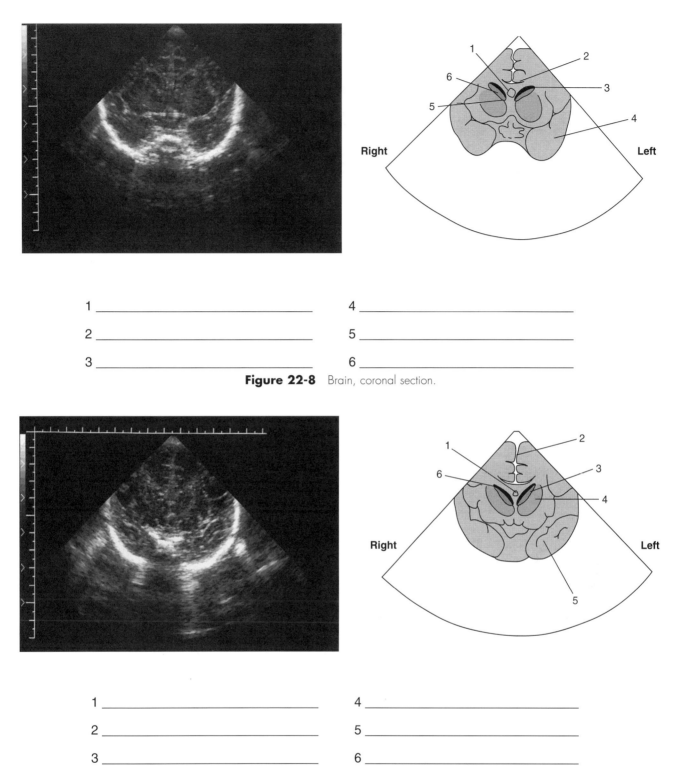

1 _____   4 _____

2 _____   5 _____

3 _____   6 _____

Figure 22-8 Brain, coronal section.

1 _____   4 _____

2 _____   5 _____

3 _____   6 _____

Figure 22-9 Brain, coronal section.

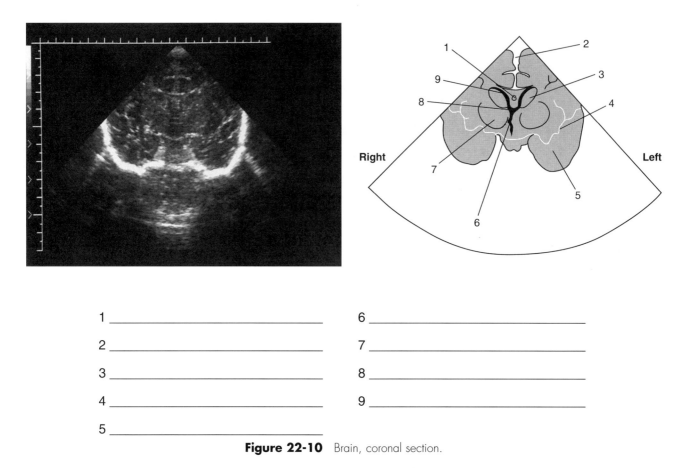

1 _____   6 _____
2 _____   7 _____
3 _____   8 _____
4 _____   9 _____
5 _____

Figure 22-10 Brain, coronal section.

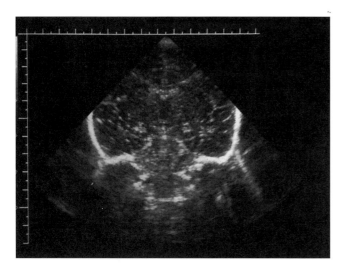

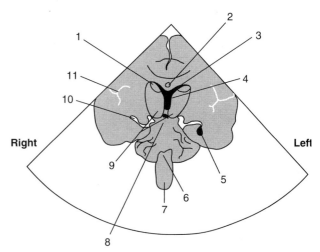

1 _____   7 _____
2 _____   8 _____
3 _____   9 _____
4 _____   10 _____
5 _____   11 _____
6 _____

Figure 22-11 Brain, coronal section.

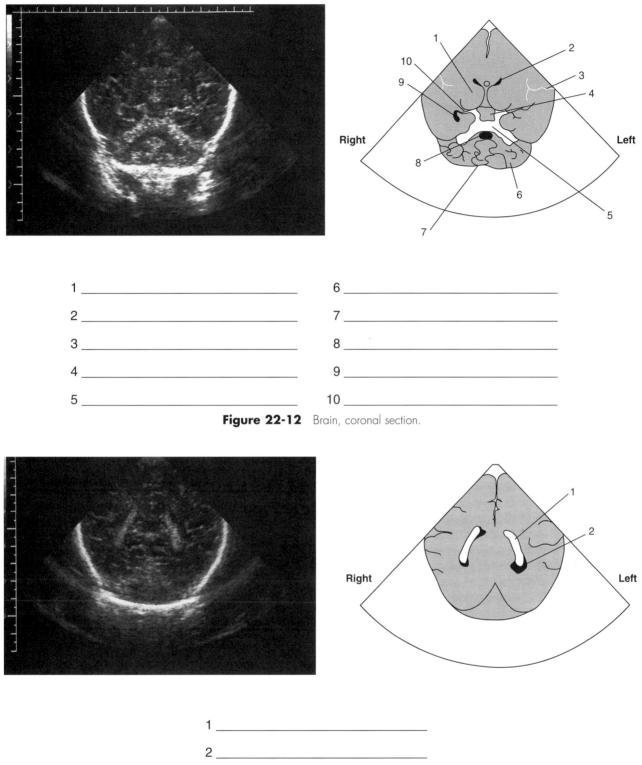

1 _____   6 _____

2 _____   7 _____

3 _____   8 _____

4 _____   9 _____

5 _____   10 _____

Figure 22-12   Brain, coronal section.

1 _____

2 _____

Figure 22-13   Brain, coronal section.

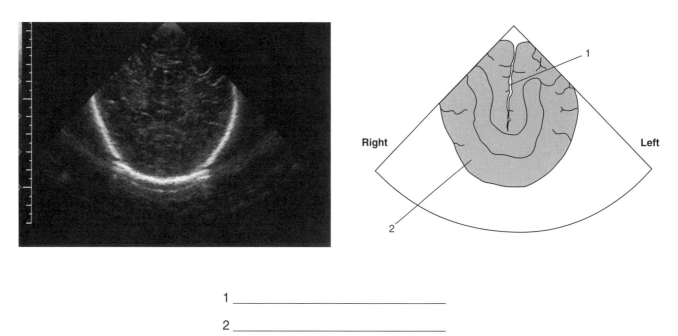

Right   Left

1 _____

2 _____

Figure 22-14 Brain, coronal section.

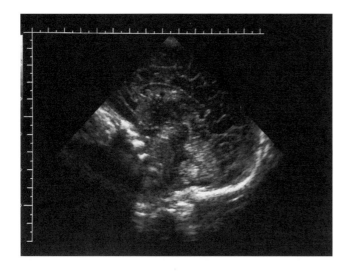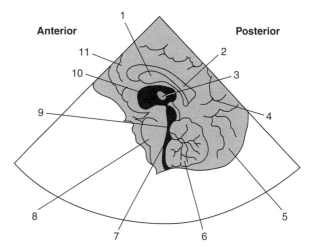

Anterior   Posterior

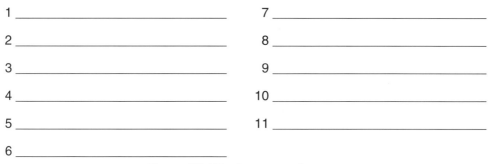

1 _____   7 _____

2 _____   8 _____

3 _____   9 _____

4 _____   10 _____

5 _____   11 _____

6 _____

Figure 22-15 Brain, sagittal section.

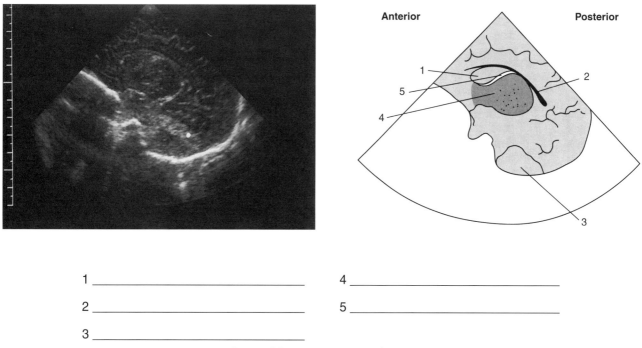

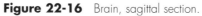

1 _____   4 _____

2 _____   5 _____

3 _____

Figure 22-16 Brain, sagittal section.

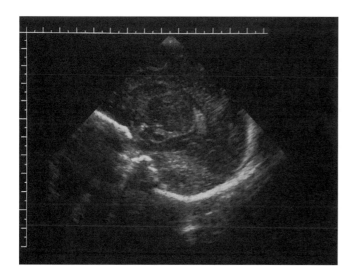

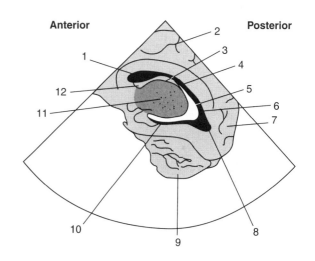

1 _____   7 _____

2 _____   8 _____

3 _____   9 _____

4 _____   10 _____

5 _____   11 _____

6 _____   12 _____

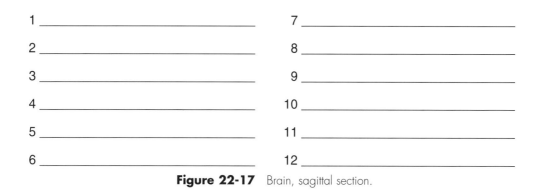

Figure 22-17 Brain, sagittal section.

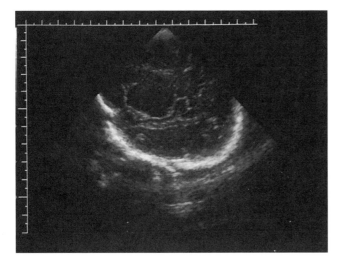
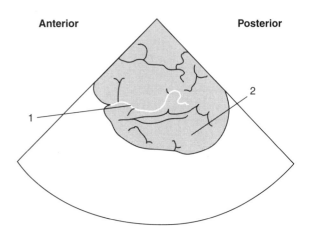

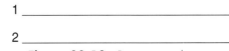

1 _____

2 _____

Figure 22-18 Brain, sagittal section.

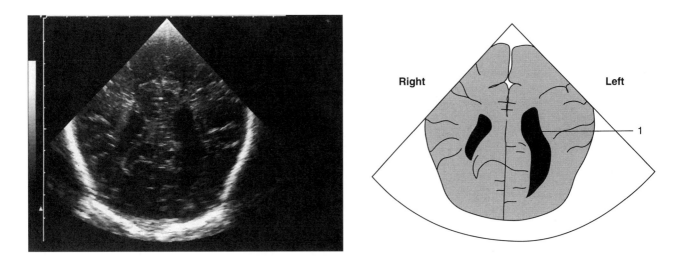

1 _____

Figure 22-19 Brain, coronal section.

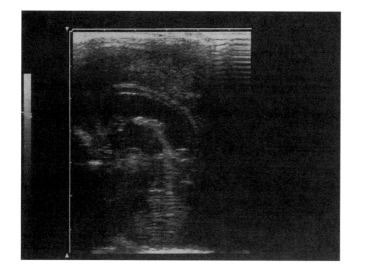
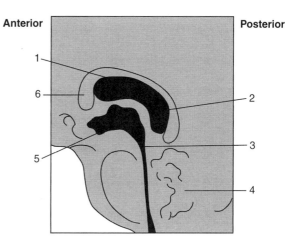

1 _____   4 _____

2 _____   5 _____

3 _____   6 _____

Figure 22-20 Brain, sagittal section.

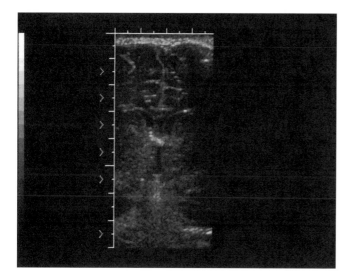
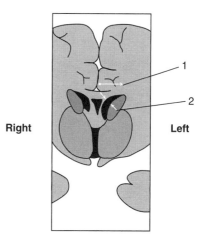

1 _____

2 _____

Figure 22-21 Brain, coronal section.

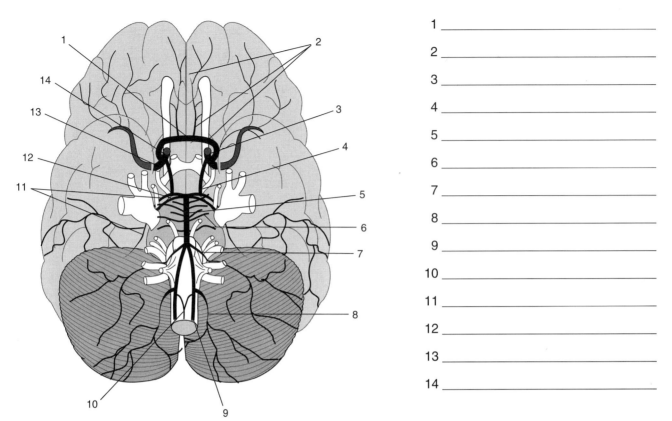

Figure 22-22 Brain arterial supply.

1 _____
2 _____
3 _____
4 _____
5 _____
6 _____
7 _____
8 _____
9 _____
10 _____
11 _____
12 _____
13 _____
14 _____

1 _____
2 _____
3 _____
4 _____
5 _____
6 _____
7 _____
8 _____
9 _____
10 _____
11 _____
12 _____

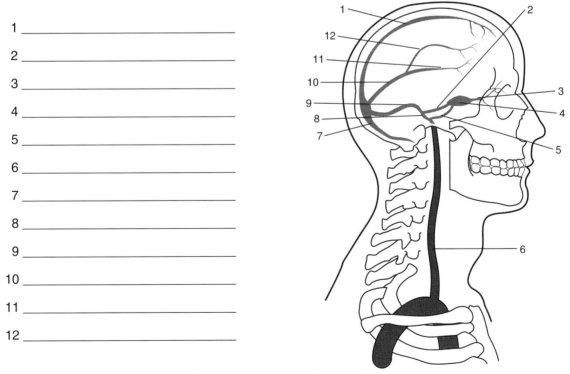

Figure 22-23 Major venous drainage of the brain.

CHAPTER 23

Pediatric Echocardiography

REVIEW QUESTIONS

1. Describe the function of the heart.

2. Describe the location of the heart and the surrounding structures.

3. Describe the blood flow through the heart.

4. What is defined as the pulmonary circulation?

5. What is defined as the systemic circulation?

6. Describe the parts of the heart and their sonographic appearance.

7. Describe the cardiac conduction system.

8. Briefly describe cardiac perfusion and drainage.

9. Which physician specializes in managing diseases of the heart?

10. Name two diagnostic tests of the heart and the personnel who perform and interpret these tests.

11. Describe the relative differences in oxygen content and pressures between the right heart and the left heart.

12. Name the six echocardiographic "windows" used to visualize the heart from the transthoracic approach.

13. What are the three levels examined in the parasternal short axis view?

14. In the true parasternal long axis view, the apex is not visualized.
    a. true
    b. false

15. What are the characteristics used to distinguish the right ventricle from the left ventricle?

16. Name the two papillary muscles of the left ventricle and their most common position.

17. The pacemaker of the heart is the _____ node.

18. What, on the ECG, do the following waves or deflections represent?

    P-wave:

    QRS-wave:

    T-wave:

19. The aortic valve is seen in the apical four-chamber view.

   a. true
   b. false

20. The inner lining of the myocardium facing the cavity is called the _____.

21. The outer lining of the myocardium is called the _____ and is composed of two linings, the _____ and the _____.

22. What is the pericardial cavity and what does it contain?

23. There is a normal splitting of the second heart sound.

   a. true
   b. false

24. What is a stress echocardiogram?

25. What is a TEE?

26. The left main coronary artery branches into what two coronary arteries?

27. What effect does epinephrine have on the heart?

28. The pressures in the right heart are normally higher than in the left heart.

   a. true
   b. false

29. The oxygen content in the left heart is normally lower than in the right heart.

   a. true
   b. false

Identify the structures indicated in the following illustrations. These figures duplicate those found in *Sonography: Introduction to Normal Structure and Function.* Refer to the textbook if you need help.

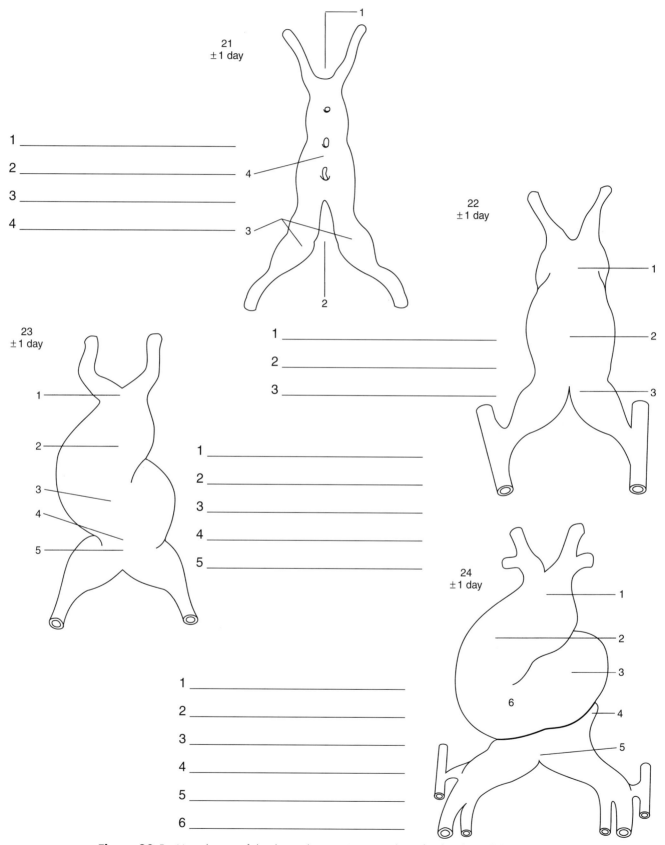

1 _____

2 _____

3 _____

4 _____

1 _____

2 _____

3 _____

1 _____

2 _____

3 _____

4 _____

5 _____

1 _____

2 _____

3 _____

4 _____

5 _____

6 _____

Figure 23-1 Ventral views of developing heart at 20 to 25 days of embryological development.

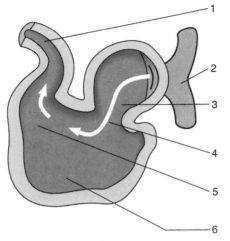

Developing heart, sagittal section.

1 _____

2 _____

3 _____

4 _____

5 _____

6 _____

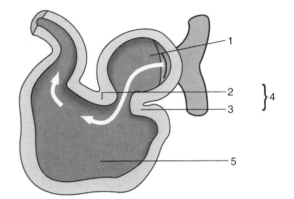

Developing heart, sagittal section.

1 _____

2 _____

3 _____

4 _____

5 _____

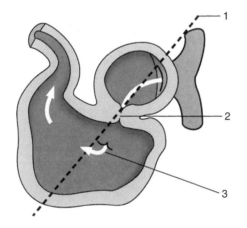

Developing heart, sagittal section.

1 _____

2 _____

3 _____

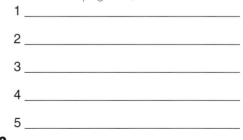

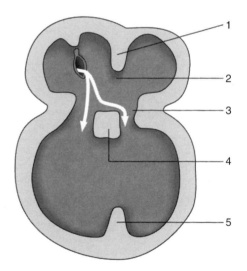

Developing heart, coronal section.

1 _____

2 _____

3 _____

4 _____

5 _____

Figure 23-2

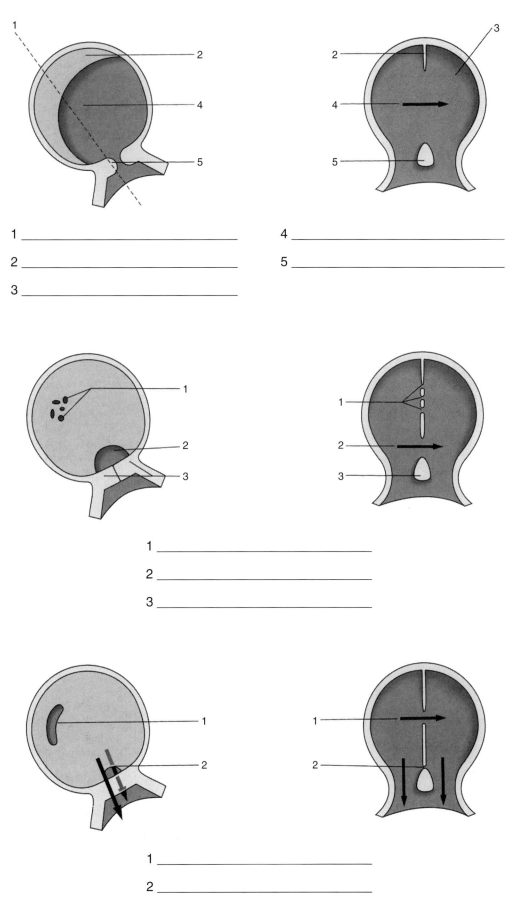

1 _____   4 _____

2 _____   5 _____

3 _____

1 _____

2 _____

3 _____

1 _____

2 _____

Figure 23-3 Developing heart, coronal sections.   *continued*

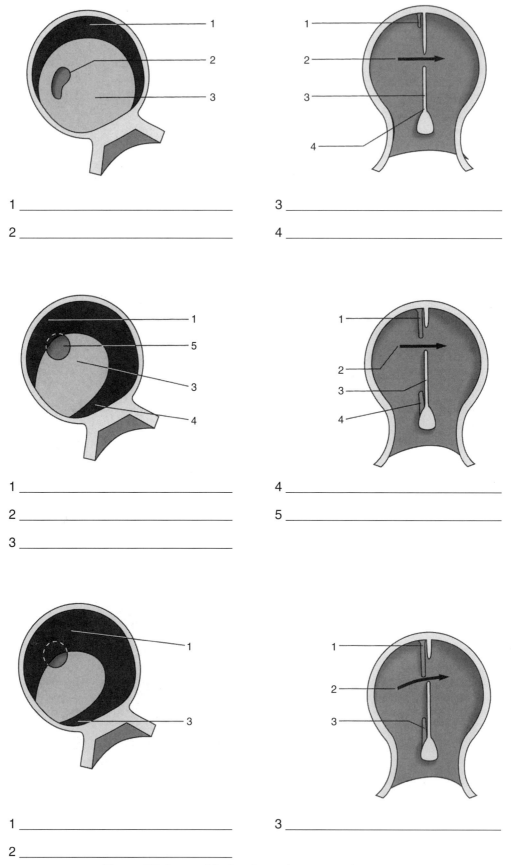

1 _____   3 _____
2 _____   4 _____

1 _____   4 _____
2 _____   5 _____
3 _____

1 _____   3 _____
2 _____

Figure 23-3, cont'd Developing heart, coronal sections.

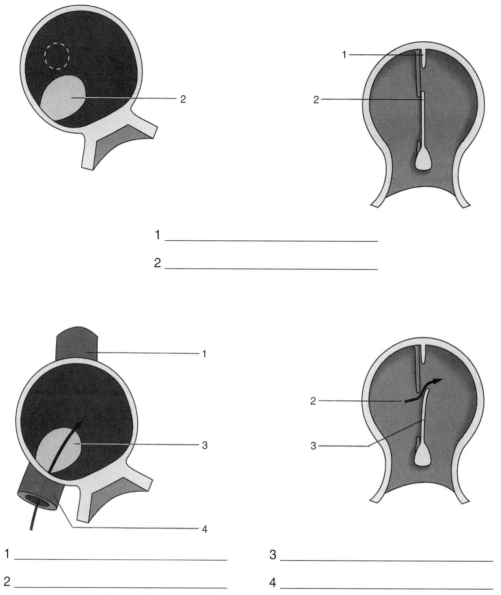

1 _____

2 _____

1 _____ 3 _____

2 _____ 4 _____

Figure 23-3, cont'd Developing heart, coronal sections.

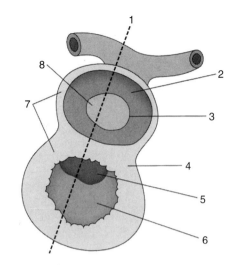

Developing heart, fifth week, sagittal section.

1 _____   5 _____

2 _____   6 _____

3 _____   7 _____

4 _____   8 _____

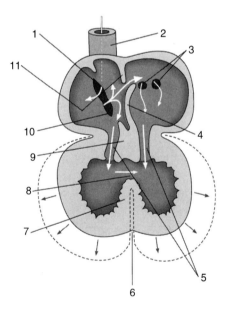

Developing heart, coronal section.

1 _____   7 _____

2 _____   8 _____

3 _____   9 _____

4 _____   10 _____

5 _____   11 _____

6 _____

Figure 23-4

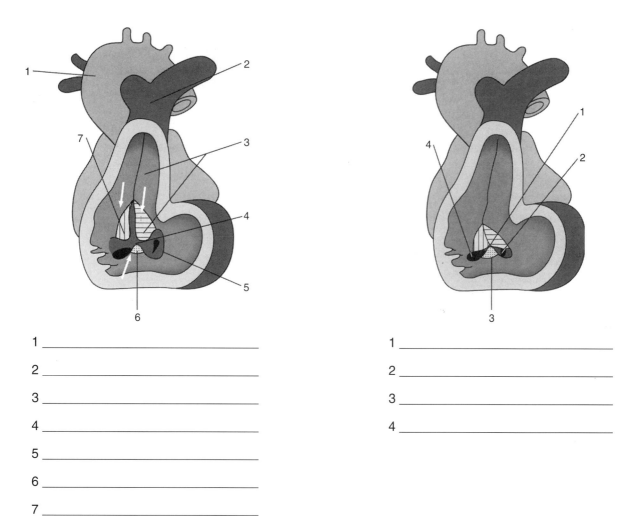

1 _____

2 _____

3 _____

4 _____

5 _____

6 _____

7 _____

1 _____

2 _____

3 _____

4 _____

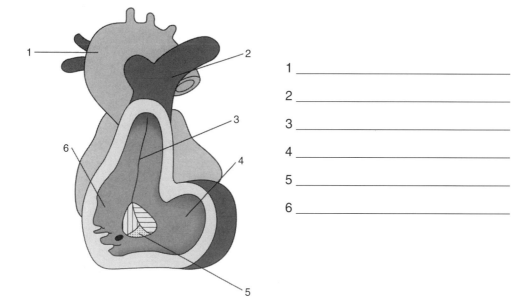

1 _____

2 _____

3 _____

4 _____

5 _____

6 _____

Figure 23-5 Developing heart.

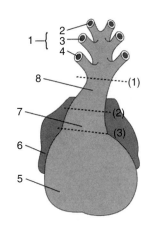

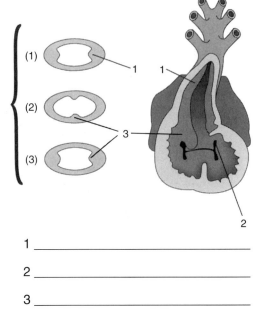

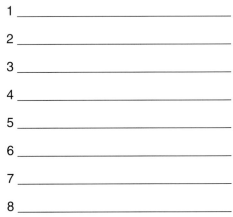

1 _____

2 _____

3 _____

4 _____

5 _____

6 _____

7 _____

8 _____

1 _____

2 _____

3 _____

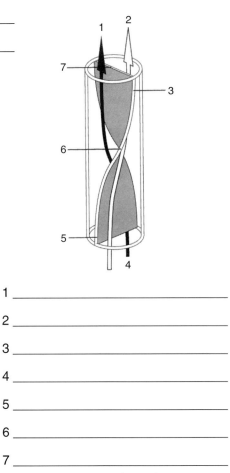

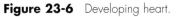

1 _____

2 _____

3 _____

4 _____

5 _____

6 _____

7 _____

Figure 23-6 Developing heart.

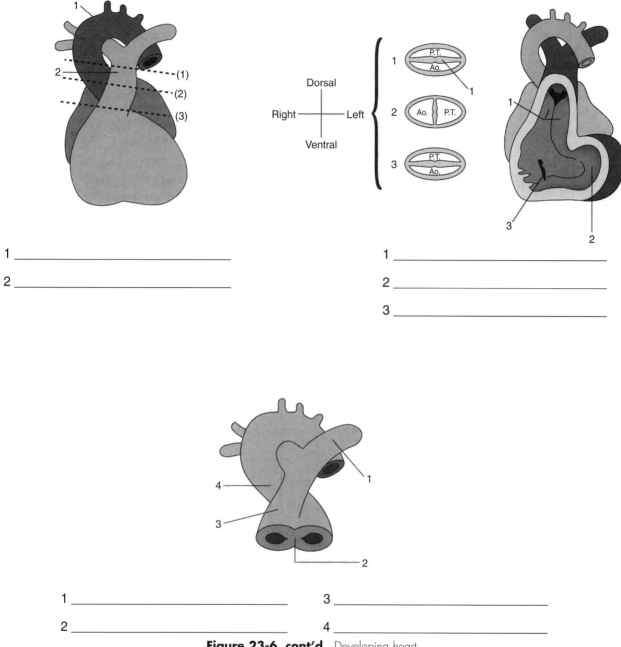

1 _____

2 _____

1 _____

2 _____

3 _____

1 _____   3 _____

2 _____   4 _____

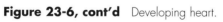

Figure 23-6, cont'd Developing heart.

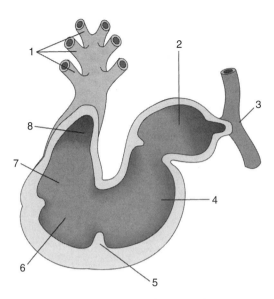

Developing heart, 5 weeks, sagittal section.

1 _____   5 _____

2 _____   6 _____

3 _____   7 _____

4 _____   8 _____

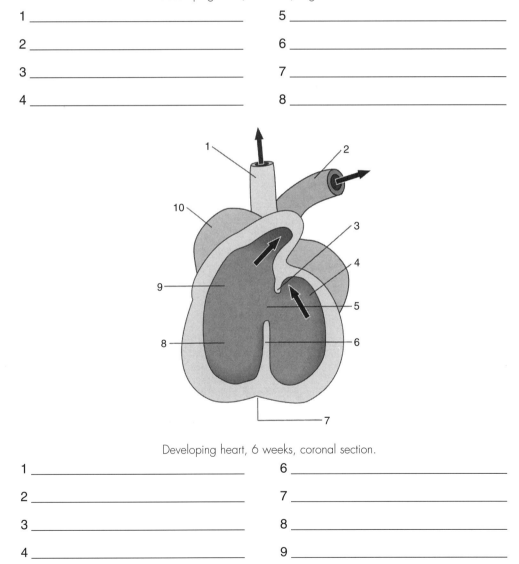

Developing heart, 6 weeks, coronal section.

1 _____   6 _____

2 _____   7 _____

3 _____   8 _____

4 _____   9 _____

5 _____   10 _____

Figure 23-7

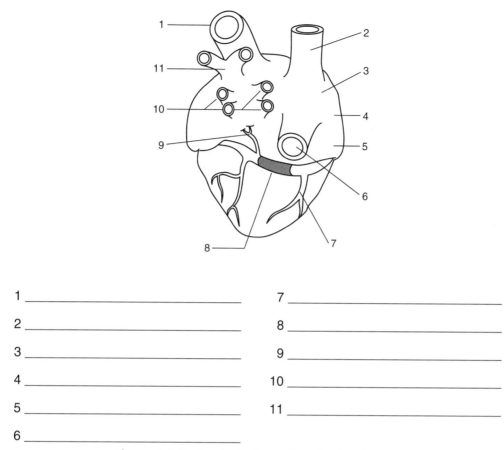

1 _____	7 _____
2 _____	8 _____
3 _____	9 _____
4 _____	10 _____
5 _____	11 _____
6 _____	

Figure 23-8 Developing heart, 8 weeks, dorsal view.

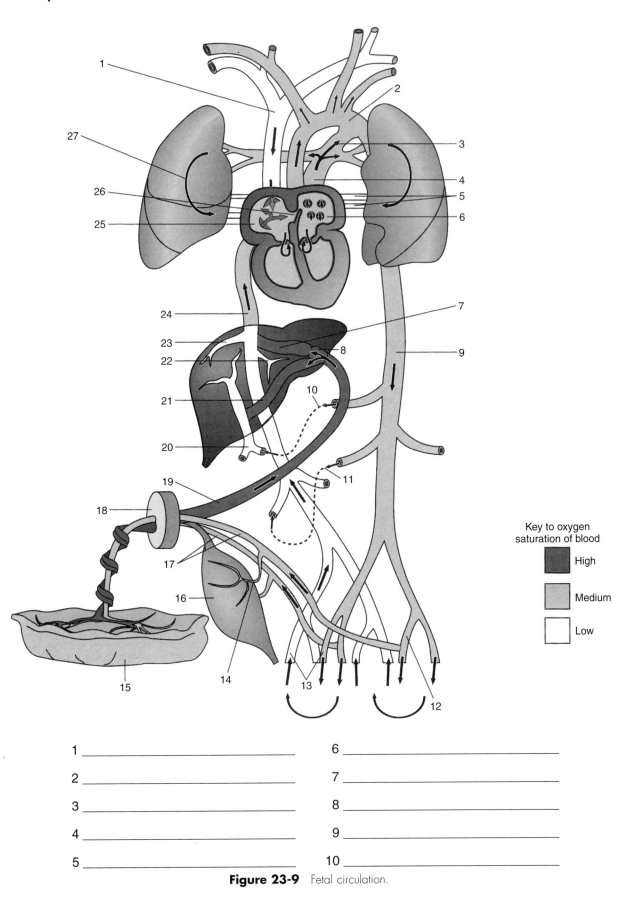

Figure 23-9 Fetal circulation.

1 _____   6 _____

2 _____   7 _____

3 _____   8 _____

4 _____   9 _____

5 _____   10 _____

Key to oxygen
saturation of blood

High

Medium

Low

1 _____

2 _____

3 _____

4 _____

5 _____

6 _____

Note: blocks denote
transducer position.

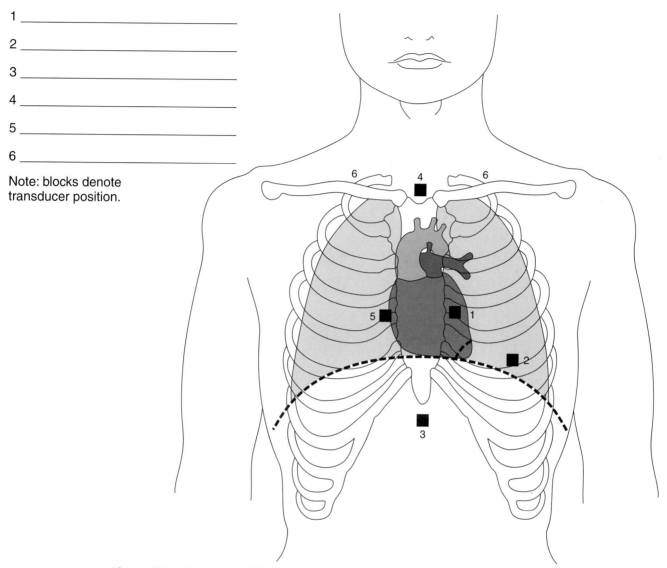

Figure 23-10 Position of the heart with respect to other organs within the chest cavity.

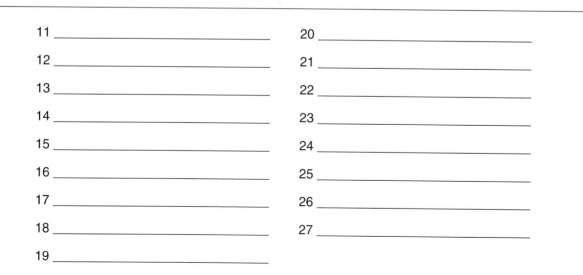

11 _____

12 _____

13 _____

14 _____

15 _____

16 _____

17 _____

18 _____

19 _____

20 _____

21 _____

22 _____

23 _____

24 _____

25 _____

26 _____

27 _____

1 _____   16 _____

2 _____   17 _____

3 _____   18 _____

4 _____   19 _____

5 _____   20 _____

6 _____   21 _____

7 _____   22 _____

8 _____   23 _____

9 _____   24 _____

10 _____   25 _____

11 _____   26 _____

12 _____   27 _____

13 _____   28 _____

14 _____   29 _____

15 _____

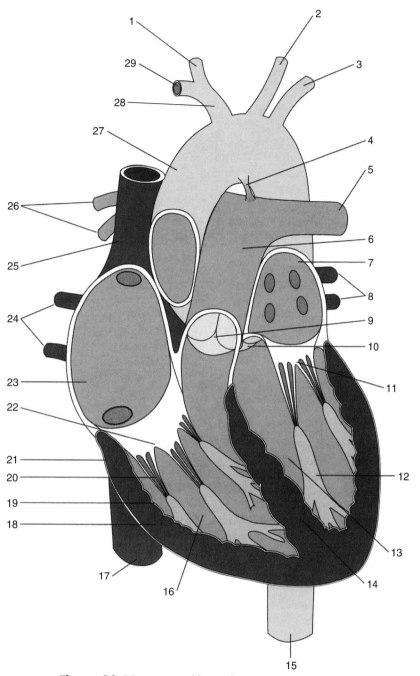

Figure 23-11 Neonatal heart showing cardiac structures.

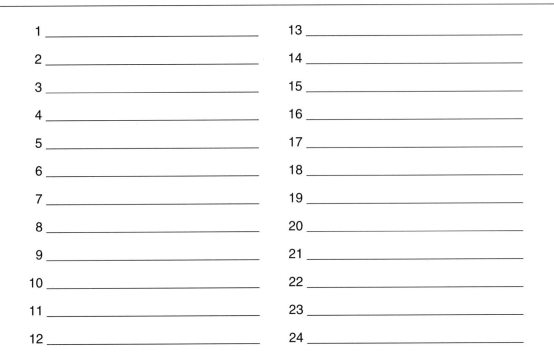

1 _____

2 _____

3 _____

4 _____

5 _____

6 _____

7 _____

8 _____

9 _____

10 _____

11 _____

12 _____

13 _____

14 _____

15 _____

16 _____

17 _____

18 _____

19 _____

20 _____

21 _____

22 _____

23 _____

24 _____

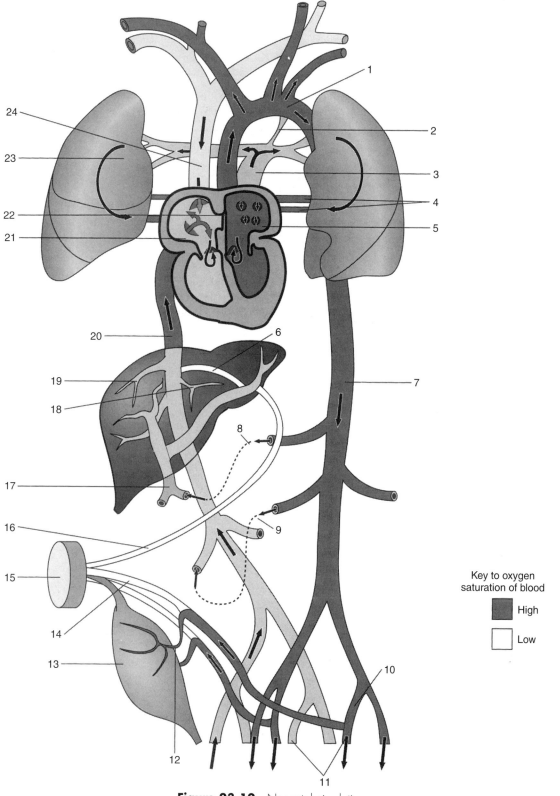

Figure 23-12 Neonatal circulation.

1 _____

2 _____

3 _____

4 _____

5 _____

6 _____

7 _____

8 _____

9 _____

10 _____

11 _____

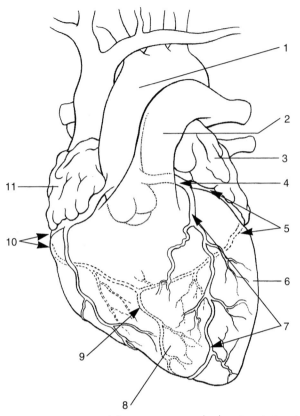
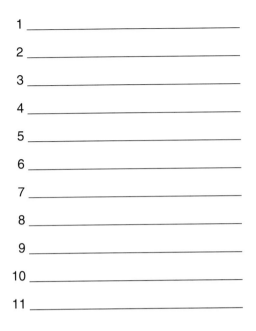

Coronary arteries and their positions on the heart, anterior view.

1 _____

2 _____

3 _____

4 _____

5 _____

6 _____

7 _____

8 _____

9 _____

10 _____

11 _____

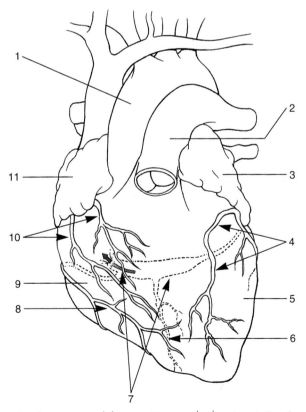
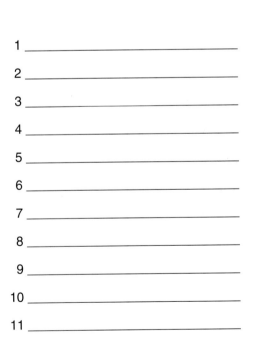

Cardiac veins and their positions on the heart, anterior view.

Figure 23-13

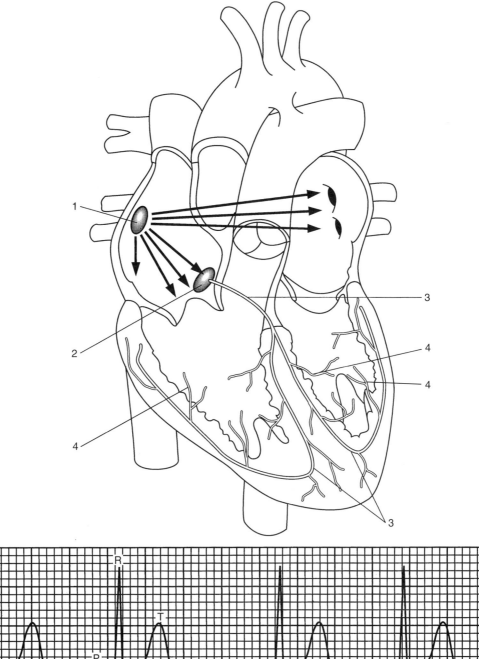

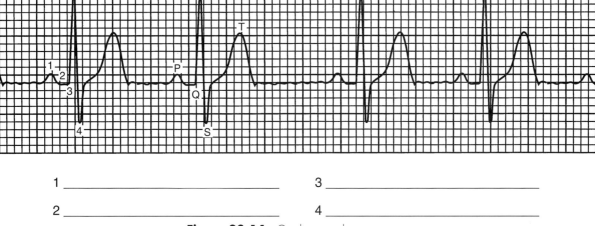

1 _____   3 _____

2 _____   4 _____

Figure 23-14 Cardiac conduction system.

1 _____

2 _____

3 _____

4 _____

1 _____

2 _____

3 _____

4 _____

5 _____

6 _____

7 _____

1 _____

2 _____

3 _____

4 _____

5 _____

6 _____

7 _____

1 _____

2 _____

3 _____

1 _____

2 _____

3 _____

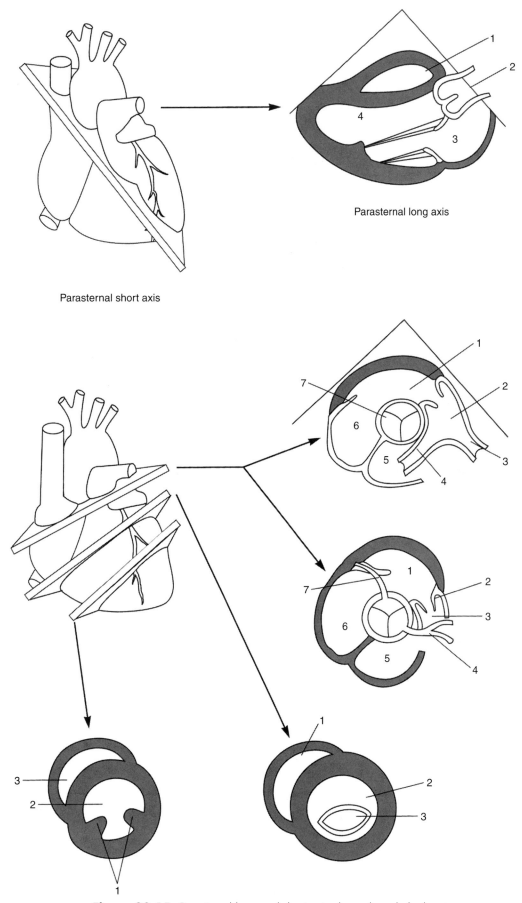

Parasternal long axis

Parasternal short axis

Figure 23-15 Parasternal long and short axis planes through the heart.

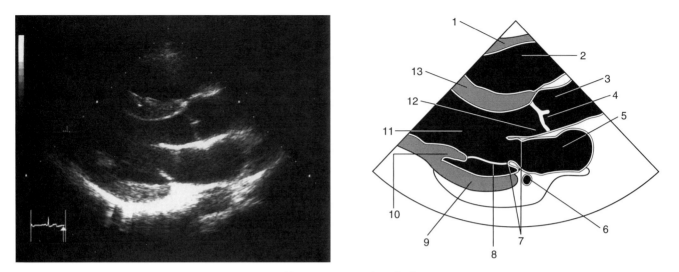

Parasternal long axis view, diastolic frame.

1 _____   8 _____

2 _____   9 _____

3 _____   10 _____

4 _____   11 _____

5 _____   12 _____

6 _____   13 _____

7 _____

Figure 23-16

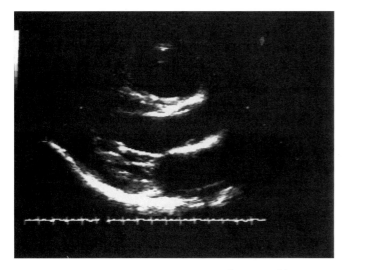
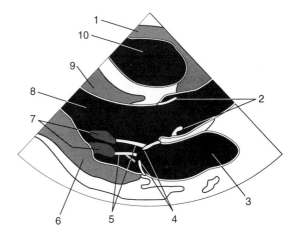

Parasternal long axis view, systolic frame.

1 _____   6 _____

2 _____   7 _____

3 _____   8 _____

4 _____   9 _____

5 _____   10 _____

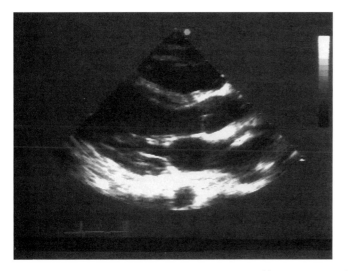
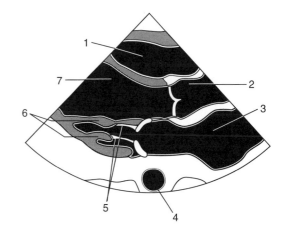

Parasternal long axis view, late diastolic frame.

1 _____   5 _____

2 _____   6 _____

3 _____   7 _____

4 _____

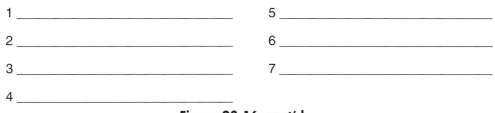

Figure 23-16, cont'd

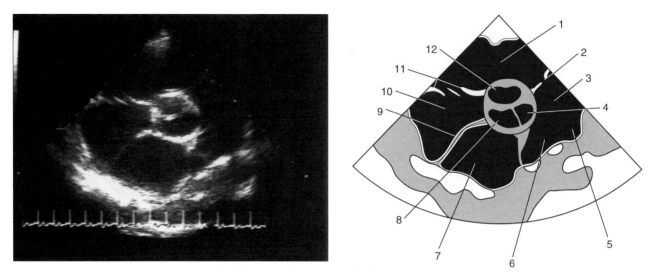

Closed aortic valve, parasternal short axis section.

1 _____   7 _____

2 _____   8 _____

3 _____   9 _____

4 _____   10 _____

5 _____   11 _____

6 _____   12 _____

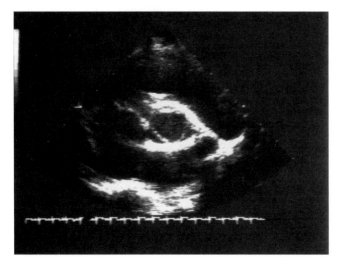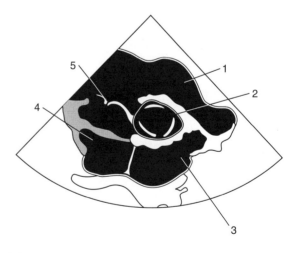

Open aortic valve, parasternal short axis section.

1 _____   4 _____

2 _____   5 _____

3 _____

Figure 23-21

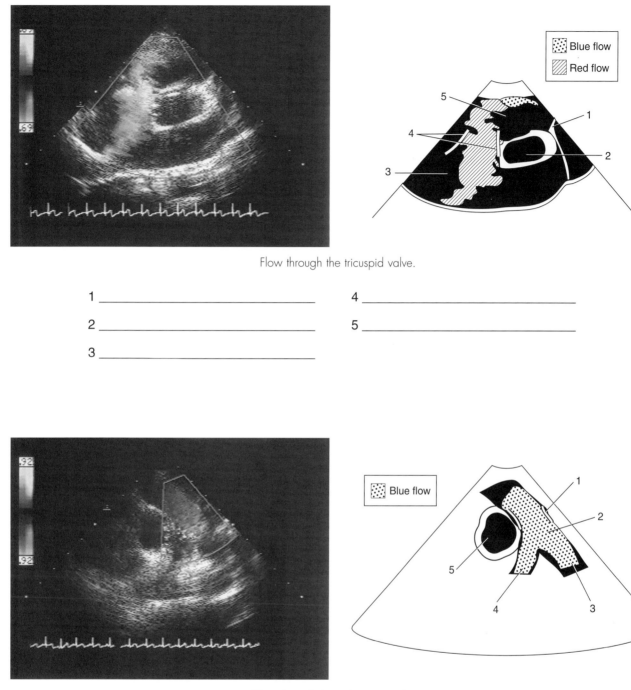

Flow through the tricuspid valve.

1 _____   4 _____

2 _____   5 _____

3 _____

Flow through the pulmonary valve.

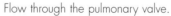

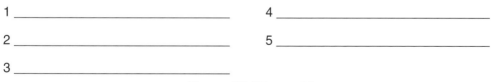

1 _____   4 _____

2 _____   5 _____

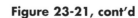

3 _____

Figure 23-21, cont'd

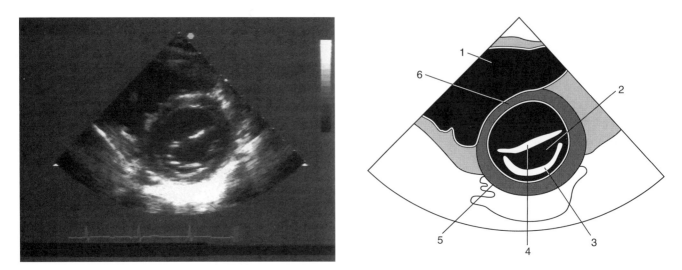

Mitral valve, short axis plane.

1 _____ 4 _____

2 _____ 5 _____

3 _____ 6 _____

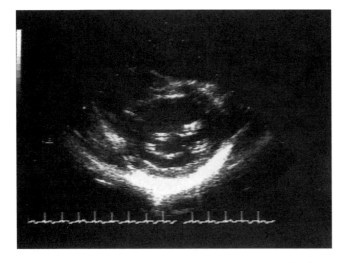 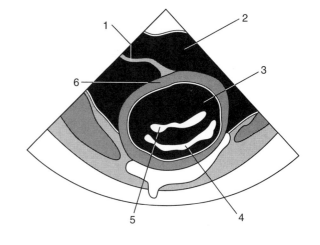

Mitral valve, short axis plane.

1 _____ 4 _____

2 _____ 5 _____

3 _____ 6 _____

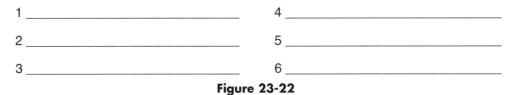

Figure 23-22

1 _____

2 _____

3 _____

4 _____

5 _____

6 _____

7 _____

8 _____

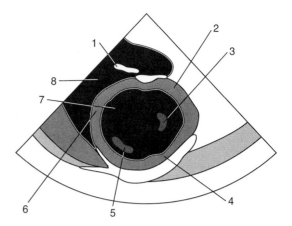

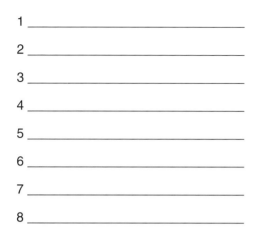

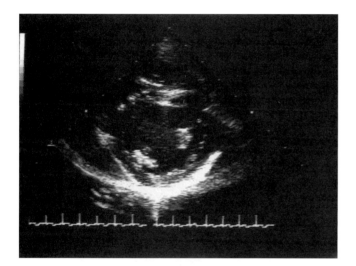

1 _____

2 _____

3 _____

4 _____

5 _____

6 _____

7 _____

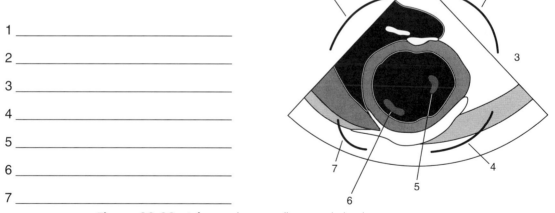

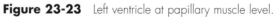

Figure 23-23 Left ventricle at papillary muscle level.

1 _____

2 _____

3 _____

4 _____

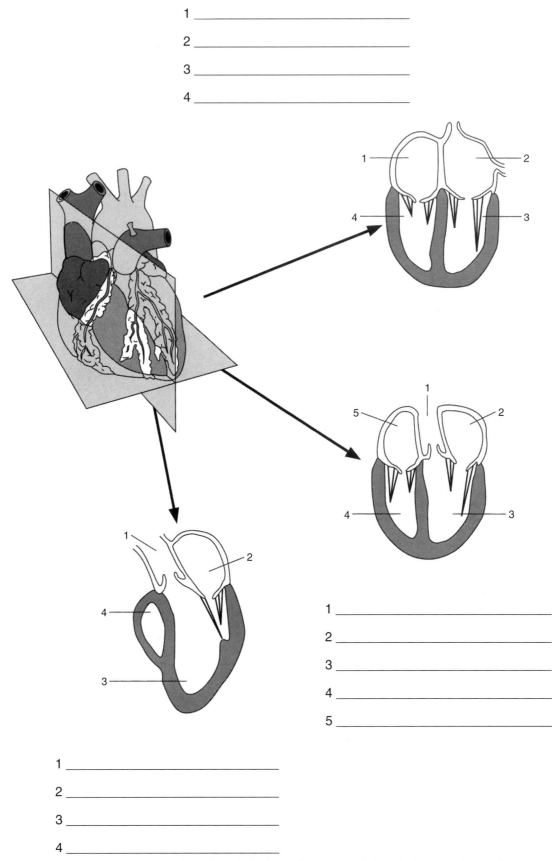

1 _____

2 _____

3 _____

4 _____

5 _____

1 _____

2 _____

3 _____

4 _____

Figure 23-24 Apical planes through the heart. (Courtesy Park MK: *Pediatric cardiology for practitioners,* Chicago, 1988, Year Book.)

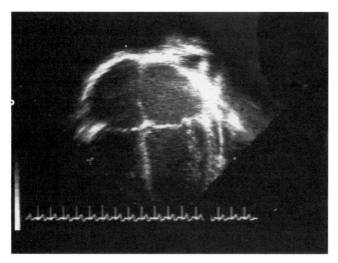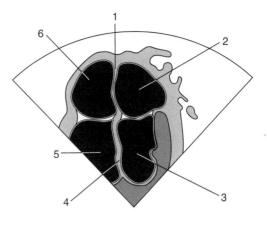

Apical four-chamber sections.

1 _____   4 _____

2 _____   5 _____

3 _____   6 _____

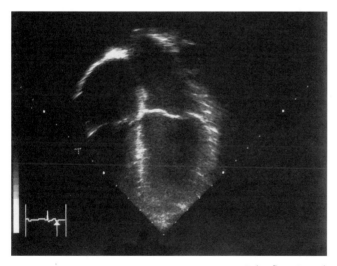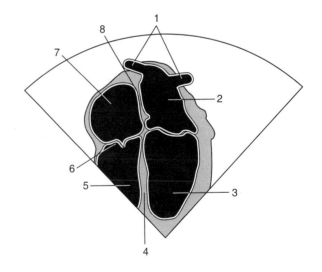

Color flow Doppler of the mitral valve.

1 _____   5 _____

2 _____   6 _____

3 _____   7 _____

4 _____   8 _____

Figure 23-25

continued

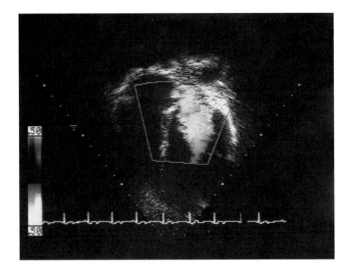
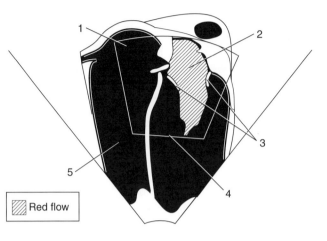

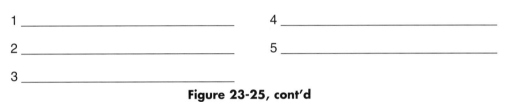

1 _____   4 _____

2 _____   5 _____

3 _____

Figure 23-25, cont'd

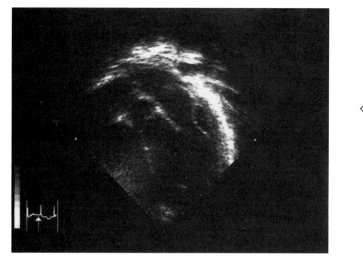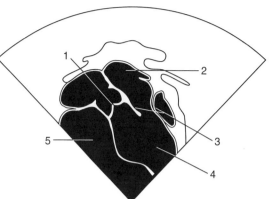

Apical long axis sections.

1 _____   4 _____

2 _____   5 _____

3 _____

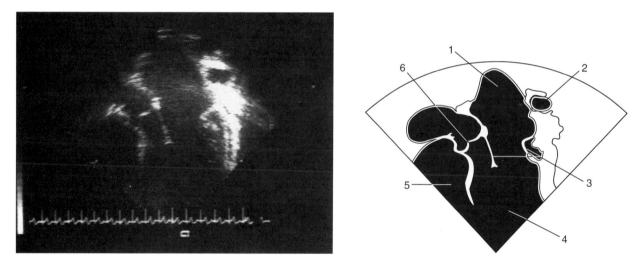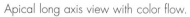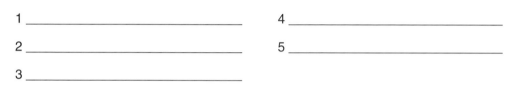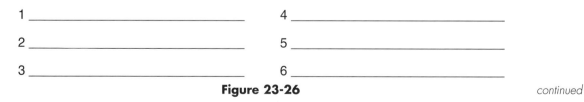

Apical long axis view with color flow.

1 _____   4 _____

2 _____   5 _____

3 _____   6 _____

Figure 23-26

continued

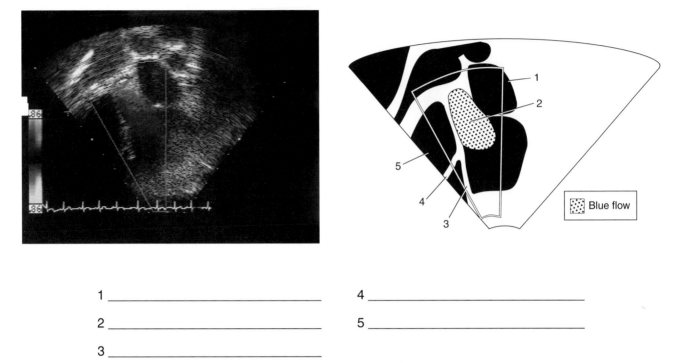

1 _____   4 _____

2 _____   5 _____

3 _____

Figure 23-26, cont'd

1 _____
2 _____
3 _____
4 _____
5 _____
6 _____

1 _____
2 _____
3 _____
4 _____
5 _____

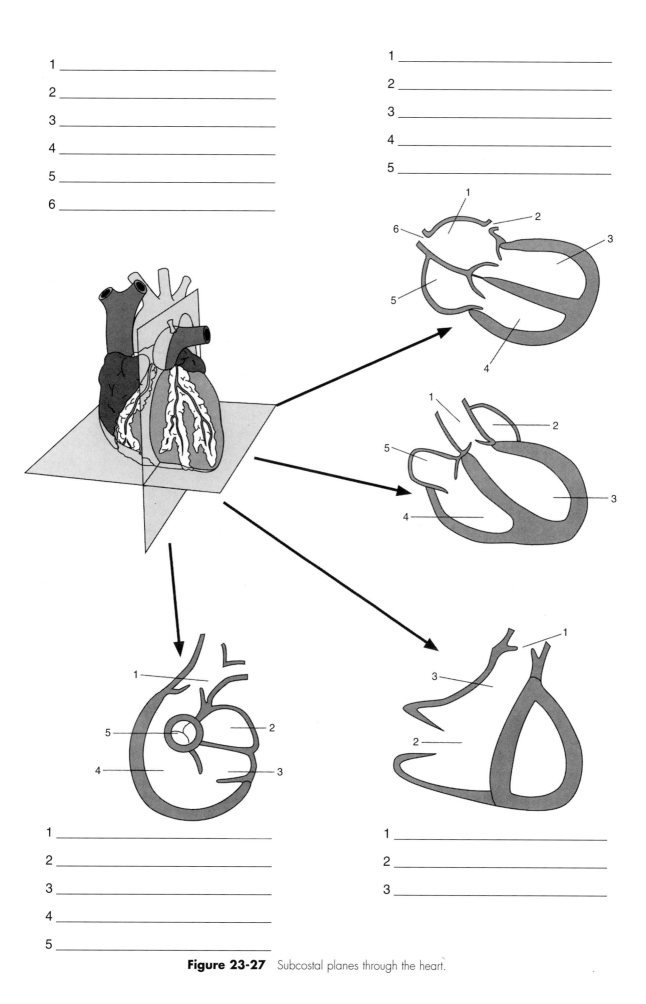

1 _____
2 _____
3 _____
4 _____
5 _____

1 _____
2 _____
3 _____

Figure 23-27 Subcostal planes through the heart.

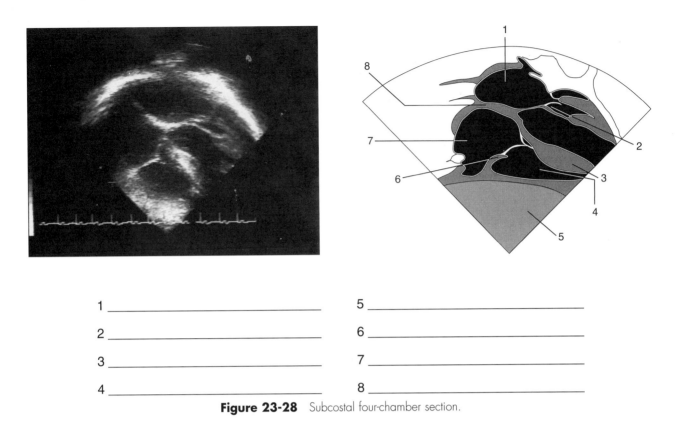

1 _____   5 _____

2 _____   6 _____

3 _____   7 _____

4 _____   8 _____

Figure 23-28 Subcostal four-chamber section.

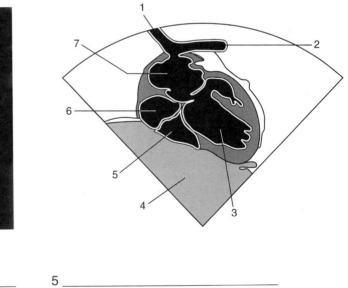

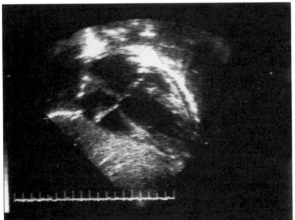

1 _____   5 _____

2 _____   6 _____

3 _____   7 _____

4 _____

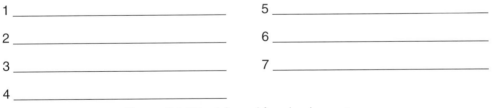
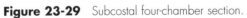

Figure 23-29 Subcostal four-chamber section.

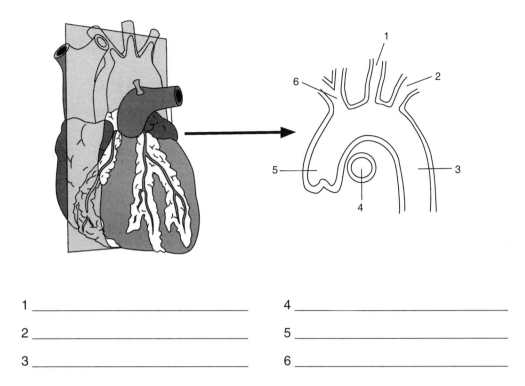

1 _____   4 _____

2 _____   5 _____

3 _____   6 _____

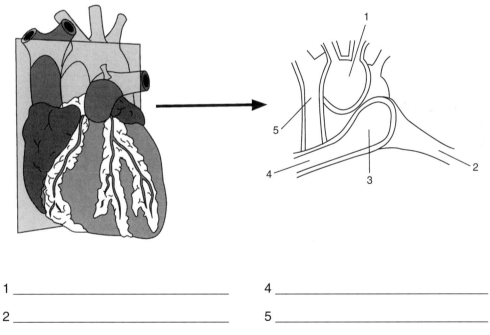

1 _____   4 _____

2 _____   5 _____

3 _____

Figure 23-30   Suprasternal planes through the heart. (Courtesy Park MK: *Pediatric cardiology for practitioners,* Chicago, 1988, Year Book.)

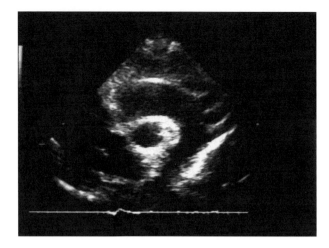
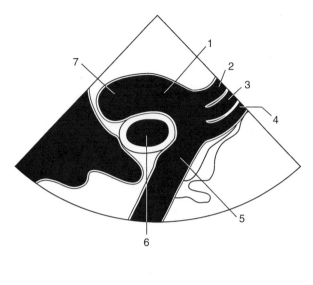

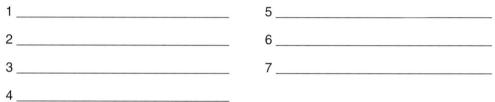

1 _____   5 _____

2 _____   6 _____

3 _____   7 _____

4 _____

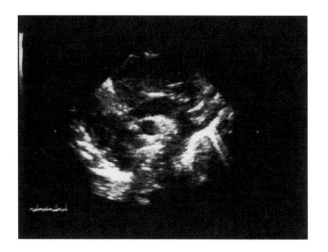
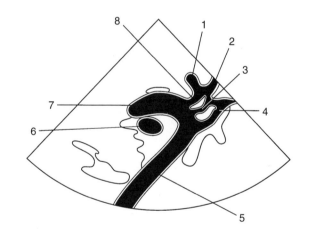

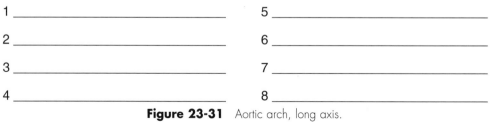

1 _____   5 _____

2 _____   6 _____

3 _____   7 _____

4 _____   8 _____

Figure 23-31 Aortic arch, long axis.

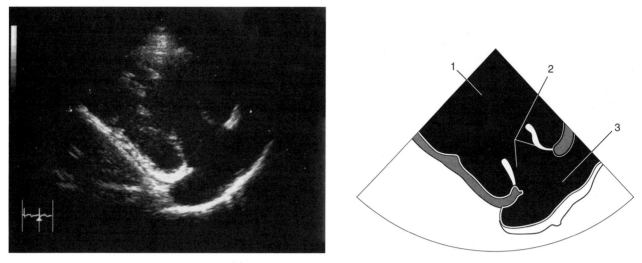

Right ventricular inflow tract, long axis, diastolic image.

1 _____   3 _____

2 _____

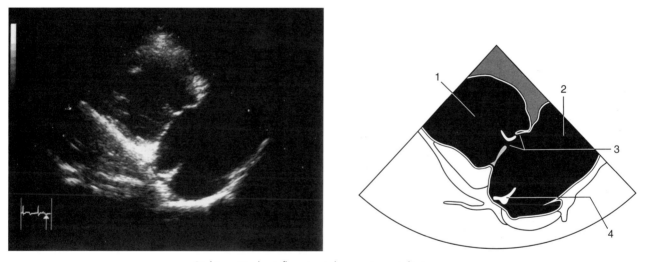

Right ventricular inflow tract, long axis, systolic image.

1 _____   3 _____

2 _____   4 _____

Figure 23-32

continued

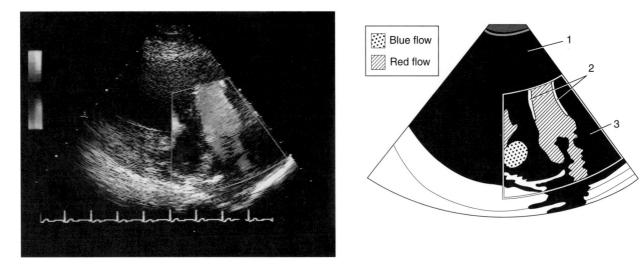

Color flow Doppler of the right ventricular inflow tract.

1 _____   3 _____

2 _____

Figure 23-32, cont'd

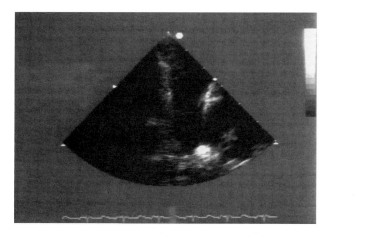
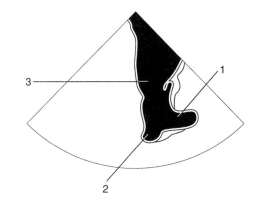

Right ventricular outflow tract, parasternal long axis, systolic image.

1 _____   3 _____

2 _____

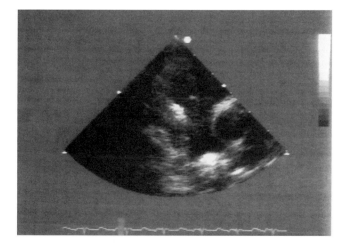
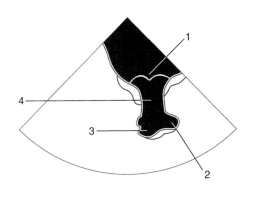

Right ventricular outflow tract, parasternal long axis, diastolic image.

1 _____   3 _____

2 _____   4 _____

Figure 23-33

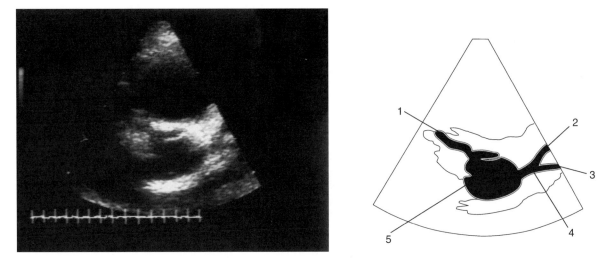

Proximal coronary arteries as they exit the aorta.

1 _____   4 _____

2 _____   5 _____

3 _____

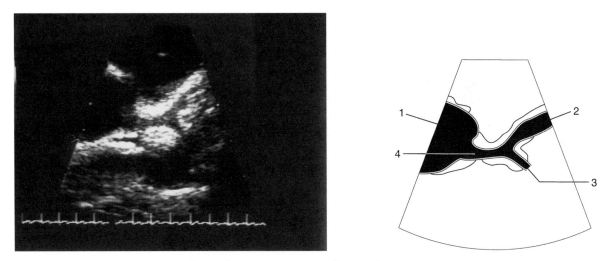

Proximal coronary arteries as they exit the aorta.

1 _____   3 _____

2 _____   4 _____

Figure 23-34

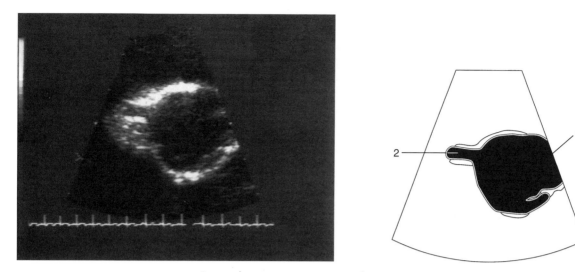

Proximal coronary artery exiting the aorta.

1 _____   2 _____

Figure 23-34, cont'd

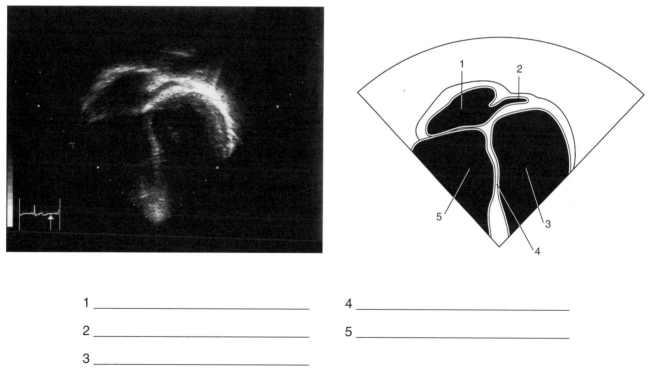

1 _____   4 _____

2 _____   5 _____

3 _____

Figure 23-35 Coronary sinus, apical four-chamber section.

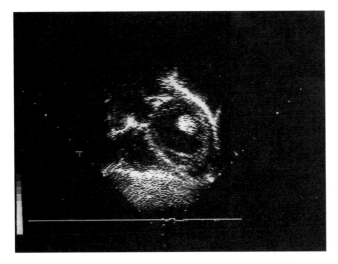

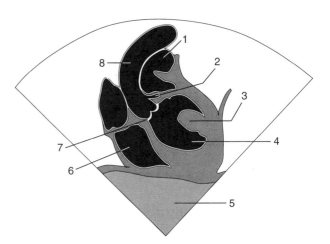

Heart, sagittal section.

1 _____   5 _____

2 _____   6 _____

3 _____   7 _____

4 _____   8 _____

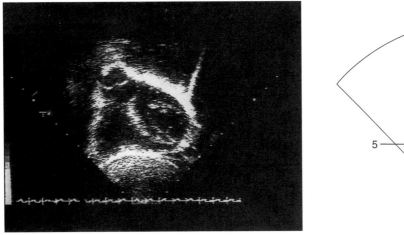

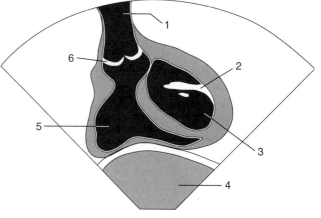

Heart, short axis section.

1 _____   4 _____

2 _____   5 _____

3 _____   6 _____

Figure 23-36

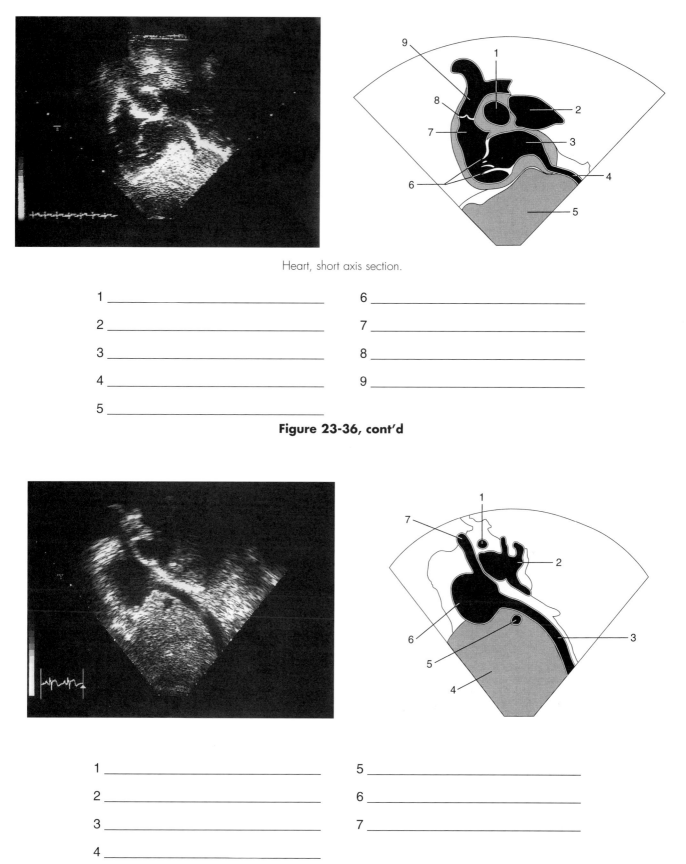

Heart, short axis section.

1 _____   6 _____

2 _____   7 _____

3 _____   8 _____

4 _____   9 _____

5 _____

Figure 23-36, cont'd

1 _____   5 _____

2 _____   6 _____

3 _____   7 _____

4 _____

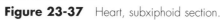

Figure 23-37 Heart, subxiphoid section.

CHAPTER 24

Adult Echocardiography

REVIEW QUESTIONS

1. The anterior surface of the heart is made up almost entirely of the
   a. left ventricle
   b. right ventricle
   c. left atrium
   d. right atrium
   e. aorta

2. All of the following are found in the right atrium except the
   a. Chiari network
   b. superior vena cava
   c. coronary sinus
   d. eustachian valve
   e. moderator band

3. The interventricular septum runs continuous with the
   a. posterior aortic root
   b. anterior aortic root
   c. posteromedial papillary muscle
   d. posterior mitral valve leaflet
   e. anterior mitral valve leaflet

4. All of the following are true about the mitral valve except
   a. it is a bicuspid valve
   b. the valve is open in diastole and closed in systole
   c. the mitral valve helps to control the flow of oxygenated blood in the left heart
   d. the mitral valve is a semilunar valve that controls blood flow from the left atrium to the left ventricle
   e. the valve leaflets are the anterior and posterior leaflets

5. Normally the dominant pacemaker of the heart is the
   a. Purkinje fibers
   b. bundle of His
   c. AV node
   d. SA node
   e. electrical impulse

6. Atrial contraction corresponds to which portion of the ECG?
   a. P wave
   b. Q wave
   c. R wave
   d. S wave
   e. T wave

7. Left heart circulation is as follows
   a. pulmonary veins, left atrium, tricuspid valve, left ventricle, aortic valve
   b. pulmonary veins, left atrium, mitral valve, left ventricle, aortic valve
   c. pulmonary artery, left atrium, mitral valve, left ventricle, aortic valve
   d. pulmonary artery, left atrium, tricuspid valve, left ventricle, aortic valve
   e. none of the above

8. The right atrium can be seen in all of the following views except the

a. parasternal long axis

b. parasternal short axis (atrioventricular level)

c. apical four chamber

d. subxiphoid four chamber

9. The aortic arch is visualized from which orientation?

a. parasternal

b. apical

c. subxiphoid

d. suprasternal

e. right parasternal

10. Where should the left atrium be measured on the M-mode?

a. Q wave

b. midsystole

c. T wave

d. largest dimension

e. QRS complex

11. Normal flow across the aortic valve appears as

a. flow toward the transducer, in the shape of a bullet during systole

b. flow away from the transducer, in the shape of a bullet during systole

c. flow toward the transducer, in the shape of letter M during systole

d. flow away from the transducer, in the shape of letter M during diastole

e. flow away from the transducer, in the shape of a bullet during diastole

12. Which point on the image shown below corresponds to atrial contraction?

a. D point

b. E point

c. F point

d. A point

e. C point

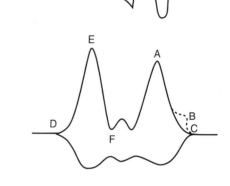

13. Name the view shown below.

a. parasternal long axis

b. parasternal short axis (mitral level)

c. right ventricular inflow view

d. apical two chamber

e. apical long axis

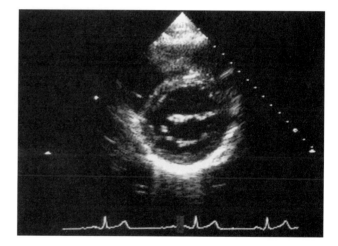

14. Which structure is seen posterior to the aortic root
    in the image shown at right?
    a. left atrium
    b. right atrium
    c. left ventricle
    d. right ventricle
    e. pulmonary artery

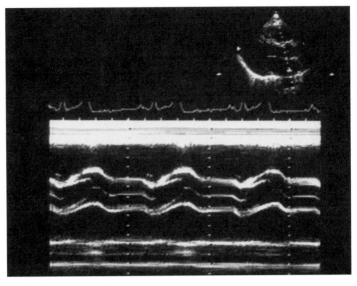

15. Label the structures in the image shown below.

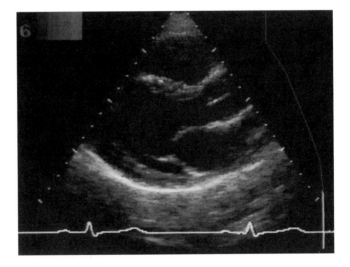

16. Transesophageal echocardiogram (TEE) is indicated the most for a
    a. 45-year-old patient with cerebrovascular accident
    b. 80-year-old patient with cerebrovascular accident
    c. 20-year-old patient with mitral valve prolapse and occasional palpitations
    d. 40-year-old patient with large atrial secundum defect seen on TEE

17. In evaluation of prosthetic valves, the following statements are true with the exception of
    a. TEE is ideal for evaluation of prosthetic mitral regurgitation
    b. TEE is better than TTE for evaluation of Doppler flow through the prosthetic valves
    c. TEE is more sensitive than TTE for detecting paravalvular leaks
    d. TEE is more sensitive than TTE for detecting prosthetic valve endocarditis

18. In most laboratories, the most common reason for obtaining a TEE is
    a. native valve function
    b. detection of endocarditis
    c. cardiac source of embolus
    d. congenital heart disease

19. Suspected aortic dissection may be diagnosed with confidence with
    a. an ECG
    b. chest x-ray
    c. nuclear interrogation
    d. TEE

20. Patient preparation for TEE examination includes all the following except
    a. fasting 4-hour period
    b. patient medication
    c. patient history
    d. complete blood count (CBC)

21. Intraoperative TEE can be used to
    a. evaluate valve repair
    b. detect air or fat embolisms
    c. monitor high-risk coronary artery disease
    d. all of the above
    e. none of the above

Identify the structures indicated in the following illustrations. These figures duplicate those found in *Sonography: Introduction to Normal Structure and Function.* Refer to the textbook if you need help.

1 _____   13 _____

2 _____   14 _____

3 _____   15 _____

4 _____   16 _____

5 _____   17 _____

6 _____   18 _____

7 _____   19 _____

8 _____   20 _____

9 _____   21 _____

10 _____   22 _____

11 _____   23 _____

12 _____   24 _____

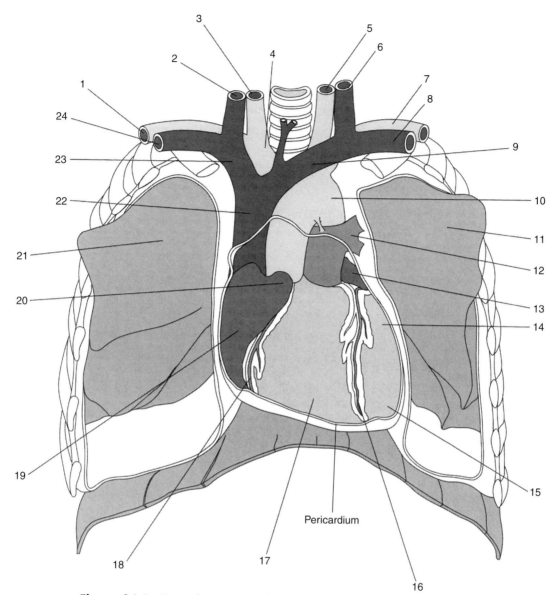

Figure 24-1 External structures and location of the heart in the thoracic cavity.

1 _____

2 _____

3 _____

4 _____

5 _____

6 _____

7 _____

8 _____

9 _____

10 _____

11 _____

12 _____

13 _____

14 _____

15 _____

16 _____

17 _____

18 _____

19 _____

20 _____

21 _____

22 _____

23 _____

24 _____

25 _____

26 _____

27 _____

28 _____

29 _____

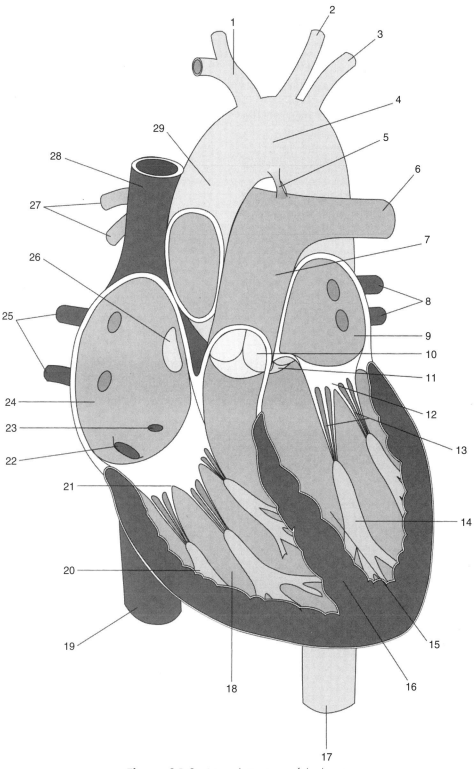

Figure 24-2 Internal structures of the heart.

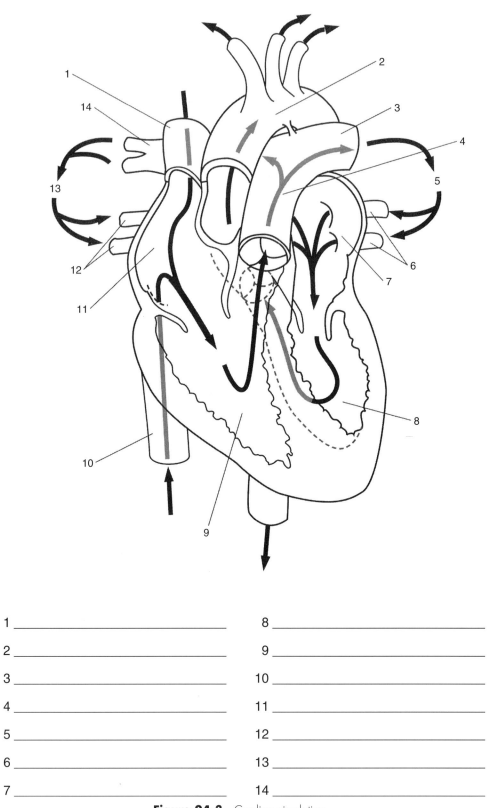

1 _____   8 _____

2 _____   9 _____

3 _____   10 _____

4 _____   11 _____

5 _____   12 _____

6 _____   13 _____

7 _____   14 _____

Figure 24-3 Cardiac circulation.

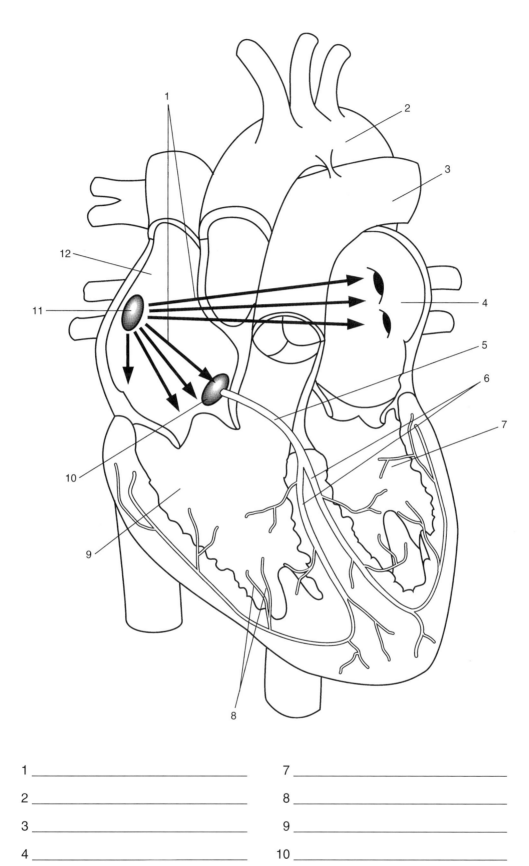

Figure 24-4 Conduction system of the heart.

1 _____   7 _____

2 _____   8 _____

3 _____   9 _____

4 _____   10 _____

5 _____   11 _____

6 _____   12 _____

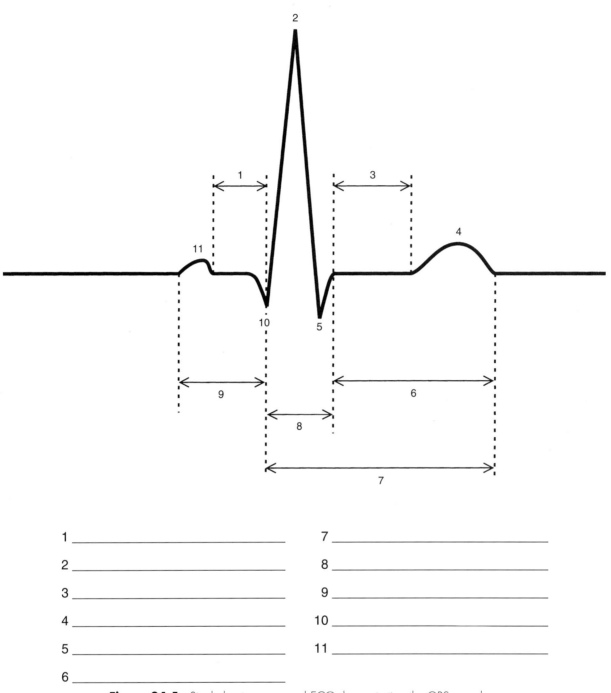

1 _____   7 _____

2 _____   8 _____

3 _____   9 _____

4 _____   10 _____

5 _____   11 _____

6 _____

Figure 24-5 Single beat on a normal ECG demonstrating the QRS complex.

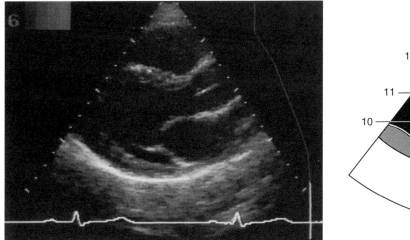
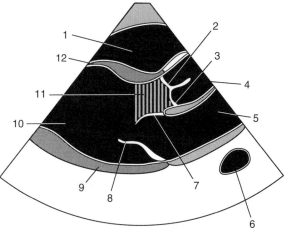

1 _____   7 _____

2 _____   8 _____

3 _____   9 _____

4 _____   10 _____

5 _____   11 _____

6 _____   12 _____

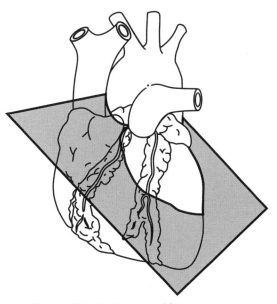

Figure 24-6 Parasternal long axis view.

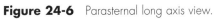

A

B

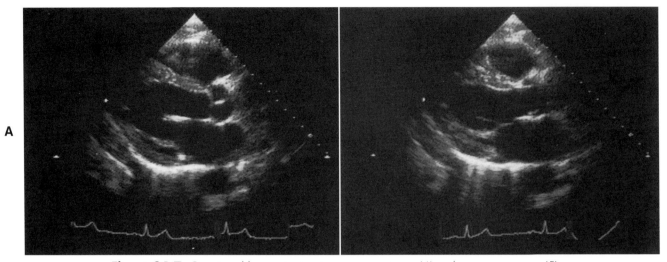

Figure 24-7 Parasternal long axis view in _____ (A) and _____ (B).

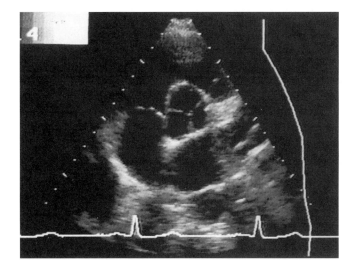
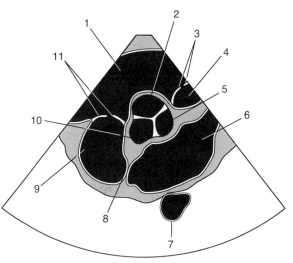

1 _____	7 _____
2 _____	8 _____
3 _____	9 _____
4 _____	10 _____
5 _____	11 _____
6 _____	

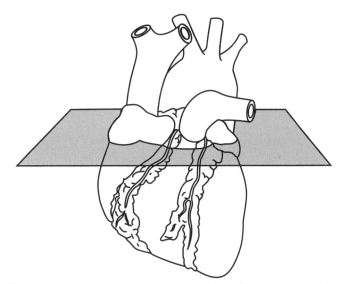

Figure 24-8 Parasternal short axis view at the level of the aortic valve during diastole.

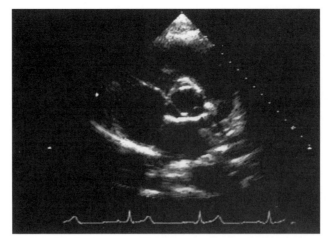

Figure 24-9 Parasternal long axis view at the level of the aortic valve during _____ .

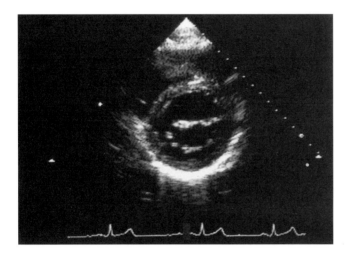

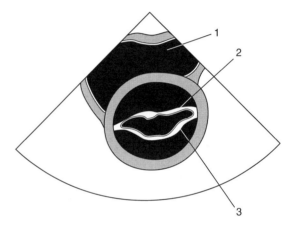

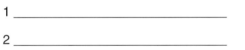

1 _____   3 _____

2 _____

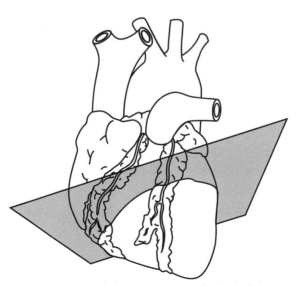

Figure 24-10 Parasternal short axis view at the level of the mitral valve.

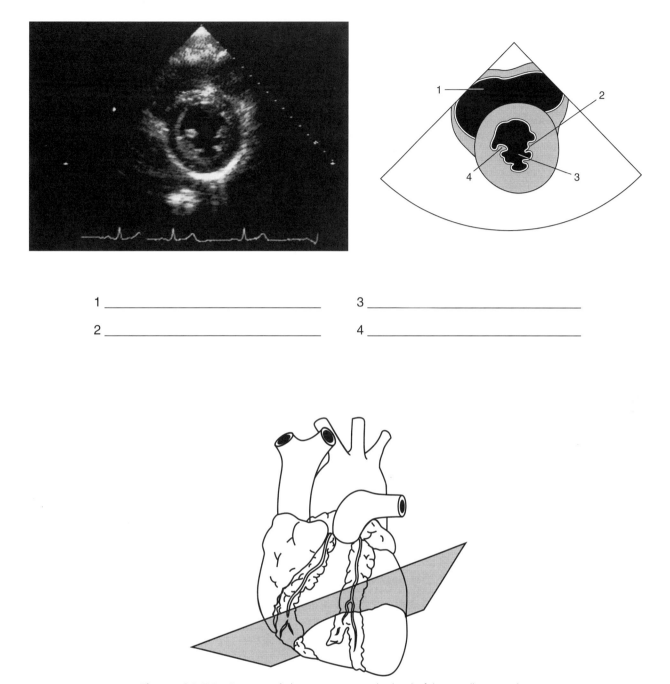

1 _____   3 _____

2 _____   4 _____

Figure 24-11 Parasternal short axis view at the level of the papillary muscles.

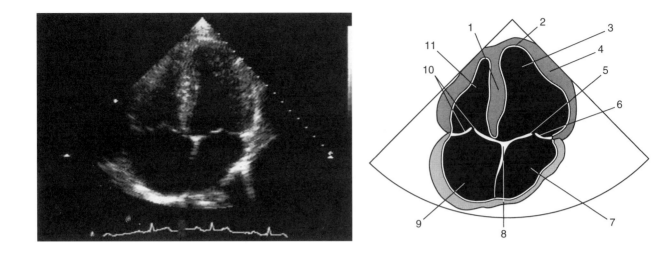

1 _____   7 _____

2 _____   8 _____

3 _____   9 _____

4 _____   10 _____

5 _____   11 _____

6 _____

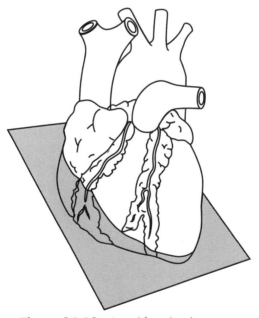

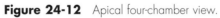

Figure 24-12 Apical four-chamber view.

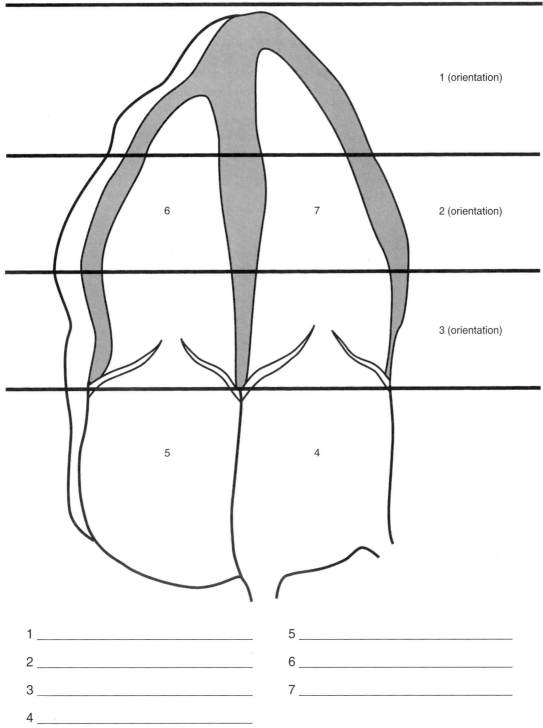

1 (orientation)

2 (orientation)

3 (orientation)

1 _____   5 _____

2 _____   6 _____

3 _____   7 _____

4 _____

Figure 24-13 Subdivisions of the left ventricular walls from an apical four-chamber view.

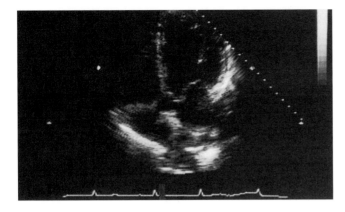
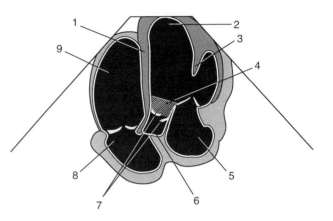

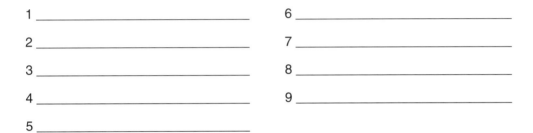

1 _____   6 _____

2 _____   7 _____

3 _____   8 _____

4 _____   9 _____

5 _____

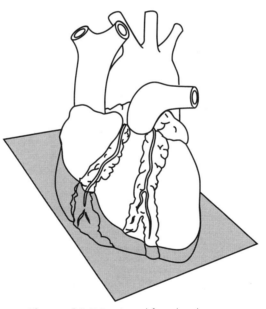

Figure 24-14 Apical five-chamber view.

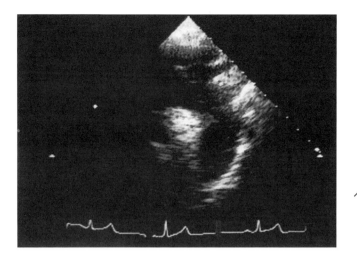 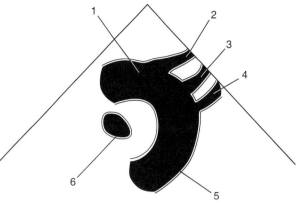

1 _____   4 _____

2 _____   5 _____

3 _____   6 _____

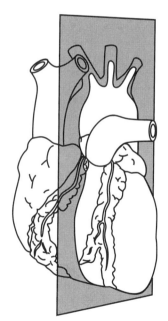

Figure 24-15 Aortic arch from the suprasternal notch.

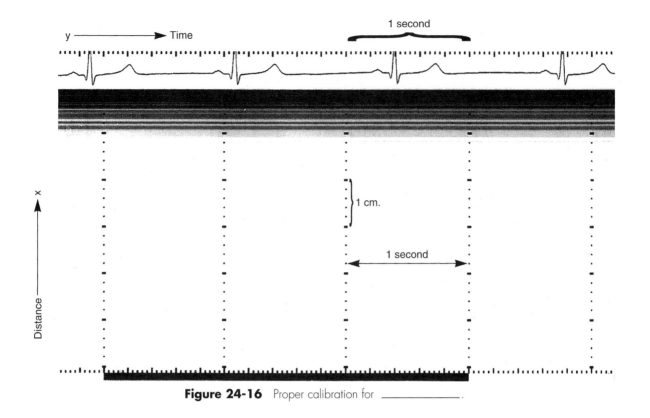

Figure 24-16 Proper calibration for _____.

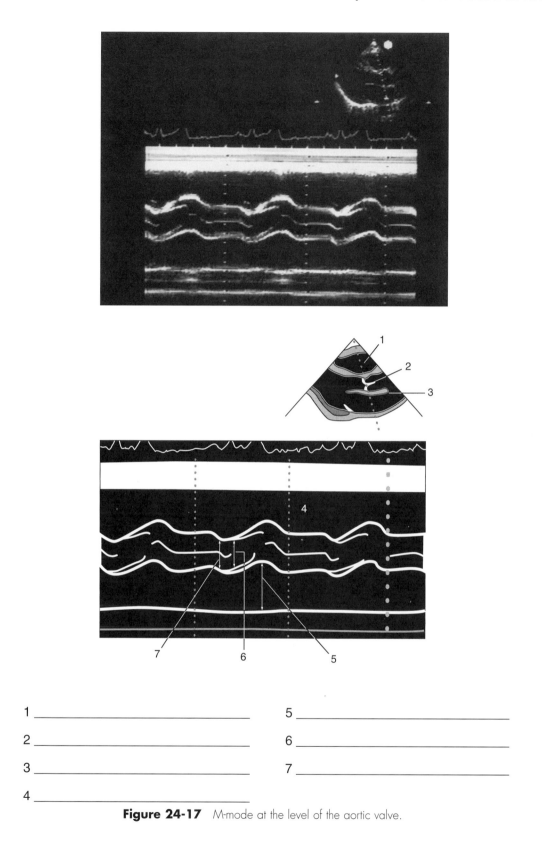

1 _____	5 _____
2 _____	6 _____
3 _____	7 _____
4 _____	

Figure 24-17 M-mode at the level of the aortic valve.

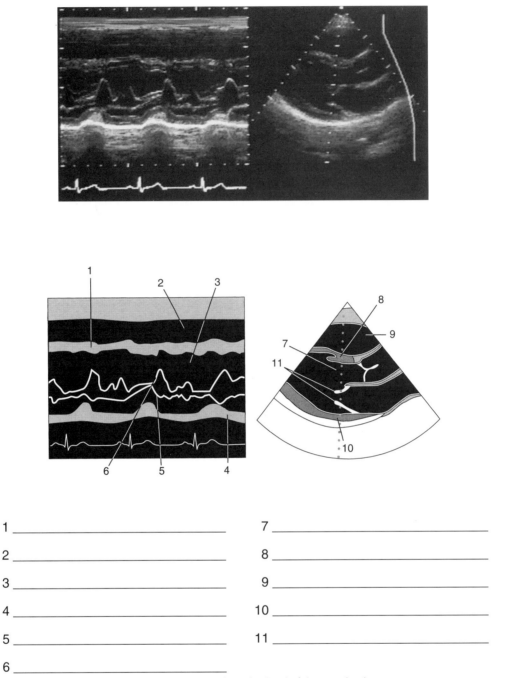

1		7	
2		8	
3		9	
4		10	
5		11	
6			

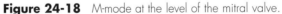

Figure 24-18 M-mode at the level of the mitral valve.

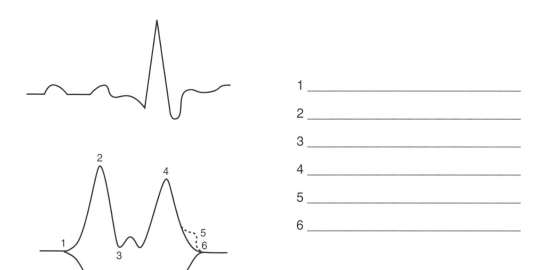

1 _____

2 _____

3 _____

4 _____

5 _____

6 _____

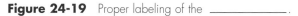

Figure 24-19 Proper labeling of the _____.

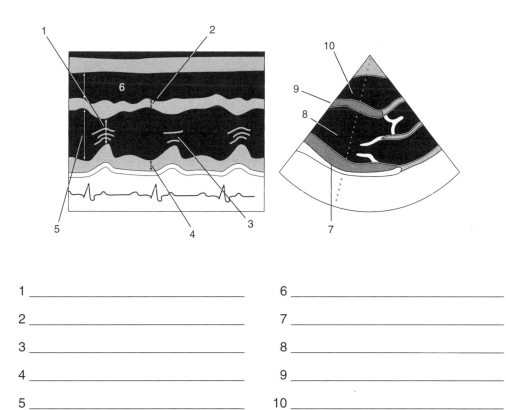

1 _____   6 _____

2 _____   7 _____

3 _____   8 _____

4 _____   9 _____

5 _____   10 _____

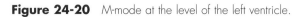

Figure 24-20 M-mode at the level of the left ventricle.

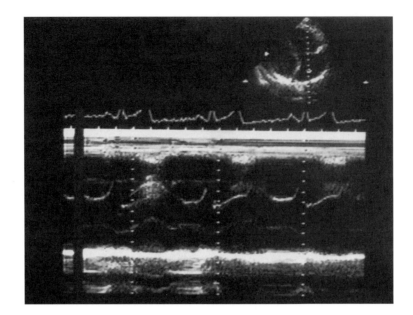

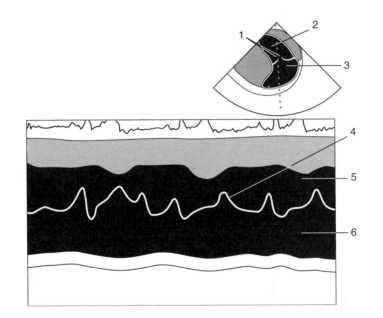

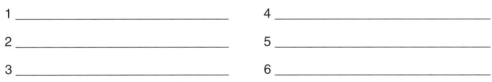

1 _____   4 _____

2 _____   5 _____

3 _____   6 _____

Figure 24-21 M-mode through the tricuspid valve.

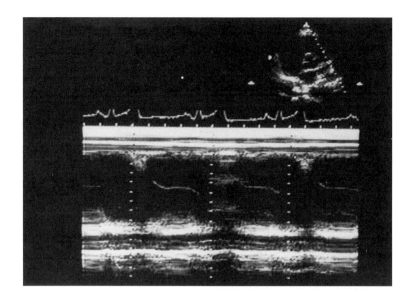

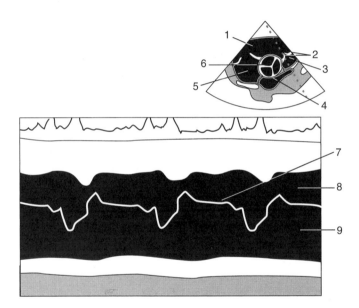

1 _____   6 _____

2 _____   7 _____

3 _____   8 _____

4 _____   9 _____

5 _____

Figure 24-22 M-mode through the pulmonic valve with its proper alphabetical labels.

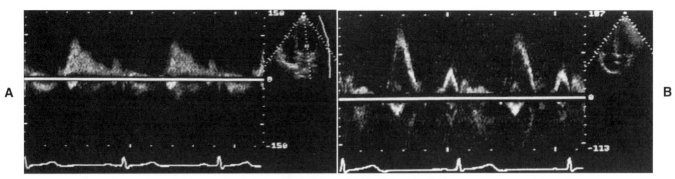

Figure 24-23 Doppler flow profiles of the mitral valve in both _____ (*A*) and _____ (*B*).

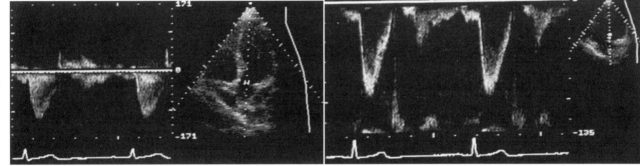

Figure 24-24 Doppler flow profiles of the aortic valve in both _____ (*A*) and _____ (*B*).

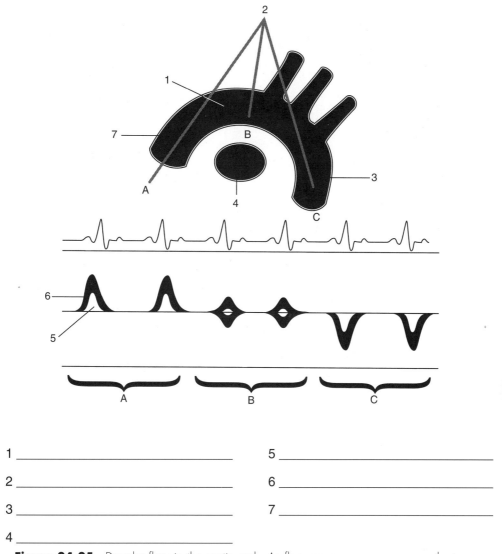

1 _____   5 _____

2 _____   6 _____

3 _____   7 _____

4 _____

Figure 24-25 Doppler flow in the aortic arch. As flow moves _____ the transducer in the ascending aorta, it appears _____ the baseline; as the flow moves _____ in the descending aorta, it falls _____ the baseline.

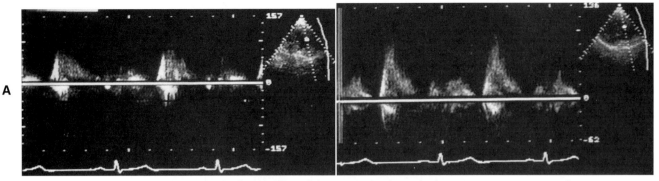

Figure 24-26 Doppler flow profiles of the tricuspid valve in both _____ (A) and _____ (B).

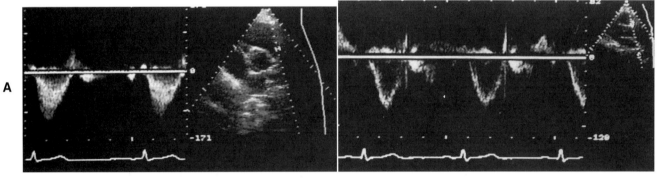

Figure 24-27 Doppler flow profiles of the pulmonic valve in both _____ (A) and _____ (B).

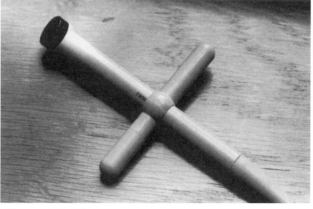

Figure 24-28 _____ probe.

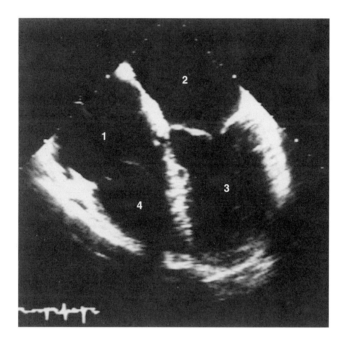

1 _____   3 _____

2 _____   4 _____

Figure 24-29 TEE midesophageal view.

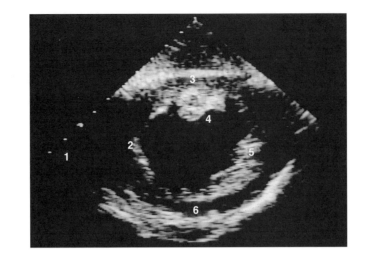

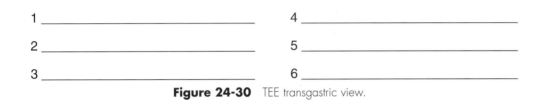

1 _____   4 _____

2 _____   5 _____

3 _____   6 _____

Figure 24-30 TEE transgastric view.

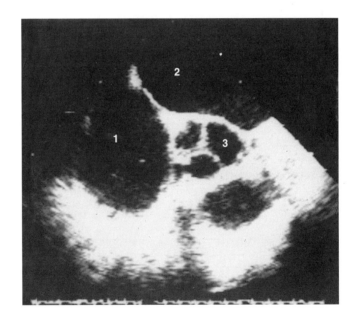

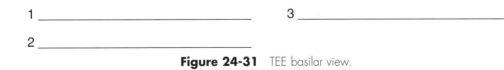

1 _____   3 _____

2 _____

Figure 24-31 TEE basilar view.

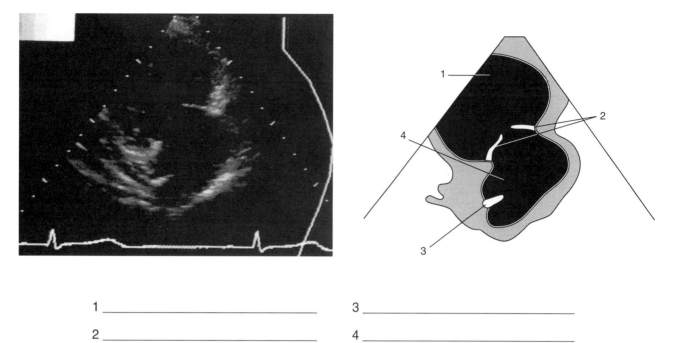

1 _____   3 _____
2 _____   4 _____

Figure 24-32 Right ventricular inflow view.

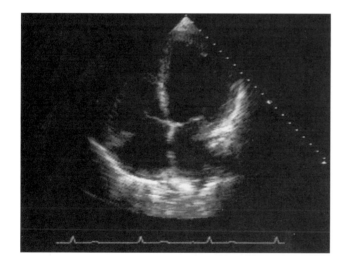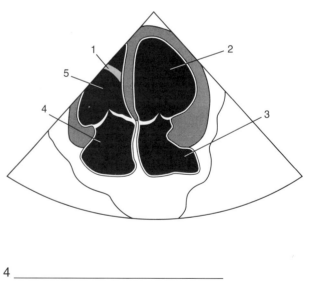

1 _____   4 _____
2 _____   5 _____
3 _____

Figure 24-33 Apical four-chamber view.

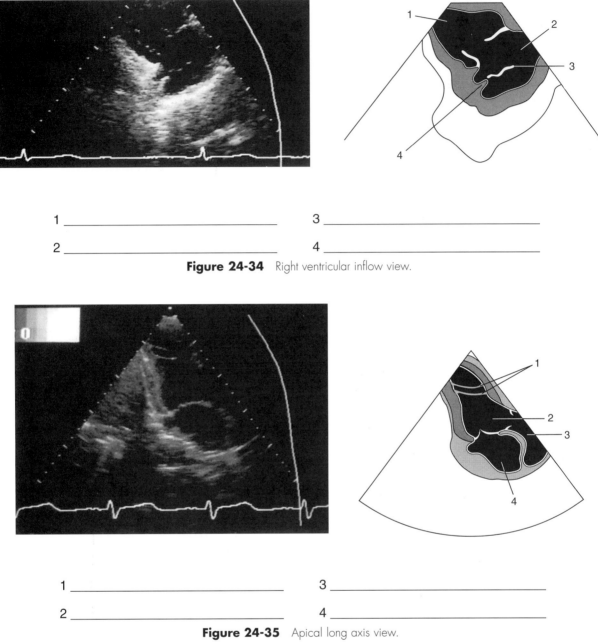

1 _____   3 _____

2 _____   4 _____

Figure 24-34 Right ventricular inflow view.

1 _____   3 _____

2 _____   4 _____

Figure 24-35 Apical long axis view.

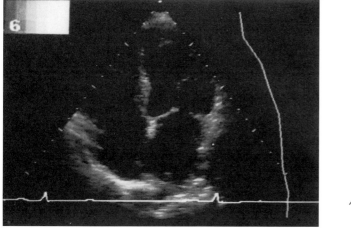

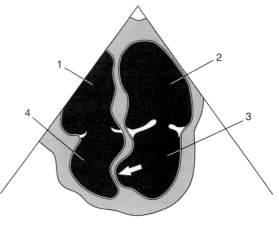

1 _____   3 _____

2 _____   4 _____

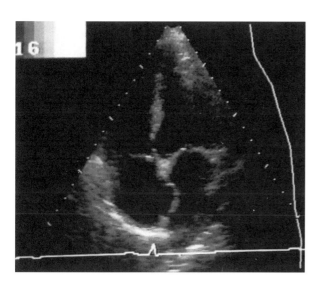

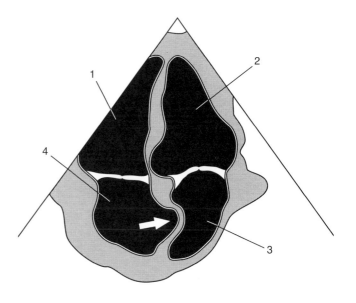

1 _____   3 _____

2 _____   4 _____

Figure 24-36 Apical four-chamber view.

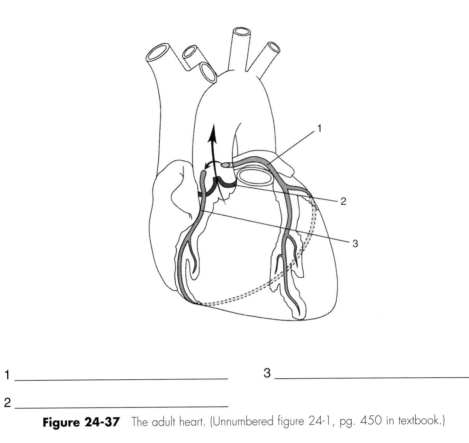

1 _____   3 _____

2 _____

Figure 24-37 The adult heart. (Unnumbered figure 24-1, pg. 450 in textbook.)

CHAPTER 25

Vascular Technology

REVIEW QUESTIONS

1. Indirect vascular laboratory evaluations are best defined as
   a. B-mode imaging combined with Doppler velocity spectral analysis
   b. tests that examine blood vessels at the site of disease
   c. physiologic test procedures that demonstrate pressure and/or volume changes in vessels distal to the location of disease
   d. duplex evaluations that examine the velocity spectral patterns distal to the location of disease

2. Which of the following vessels is not a part of the cerebrovascular system?
   a. common carotid artery
   b. vertebral artery
   c. internal iliac artery
   d. internal carotid artery

3. The internal carotid artery supplies the high resistance vascular beds of the brain and eye.
   a. true
   b. false

4. Which of the following is not a component of the Doppler equation?
   a. angle of the Doppler beam with respect to the path of blood flow
   b. the speed of sound in soft tissue
   c. the Doppler peak diastolic frequency
   d. the velocity of blood flow

5. The Doppler time velocity waveform from the normal common carotid artery is characterized by all of the following except
   a. rapid systolic deceleration
   b. systolic window
   c. spectral broadening
   d. constant forward diastolic flow

6. Which of the following does not accurately define the left common iliac artery?
   a. the vessel lies posterior to the ureter and anterior to the peritoneum
   b. the left common iliac vein is posterior to the artery
   c. the psoas magnus muscle borders the artery laterally
   d. the vessel is the first segment of the peripheral arterial tree distal to the aorta

7. In the absence of peripheral arterial occlusive disease, systolic pressure is greater in the tibial arteries than in the abdominal aorta.
   a. true
   b. false

8. Which of the following is not a characteristic of a normal peripheral artery?
   a. narrow systolic Doppler spectral bandwidth
   b. reversed diastolic flow
   c. blunted systolic peak
   d. systolic window

9. Which of the following vessels is not a part of the deep venous system of the lower extremities?
   a. profunda femoris vein
   b. perforator vein
   c. superficial femoral vein
   d. anterior tibial vein

10. The gastrocnemius veins are part of the deep venous system and normally empty into the greater saphenous vein of the thigh.
    a. true
    b. false

11. Which of the following statements is incorrect?
    a. venous flow from the legs is under control of the calf muscle pump
    b. during exercise, venous pressure at foot level will exceed 40 mm Hg
    c. the direction of venous flow is normally from the superficial venous system to the deep venous system
    d. veins can withstand tremendous volume change with little change in transmural pressure due to the small amount of elastin found in the venous wall

12. The goal of the vascular diagnostic laboratory is to answer the following questions using an array of indirect and direct noninvasive evaluations: Is vascular disease present? Where is it located? How severe is the disease process? What is the prognosis? Are medical/surgical results being obtained?
    a. true
    b. false

13. Which of the following statements best differentiates indirect noninvasive vascular test procedures from direct noninvasive vascular procedures?
    a. indirect test procedures give morphologic information that allows evaluation of degree of lesion severity
    b. indirect test procedures detect the presence of lesions that are not yet hemodynamically significant, while the direct test procedures only give information on disease that is flow reducing

    c. indirect test procedures are physiologic and indicate the presence of significant occlusive disease by demonstrating pressure or limb volume changes downstream from the site of the lesion, while direct procedures evaluate the disease at the site where it is located
    d. indirect test procedures use continuous wave Doppler as well as plethysmographic testing

14. All of the following are branches of the internal carotid artery except
    a. middle cerebral artery
    b. posterior cerebral artery
    c. anterior cerebral artery
    d. ophthalmic artery

15. Which of the following is not true of the vertebral arteries?
    a. they arise as the first branch of the subclavian arteries
    b. they course toward the brain by passing through the upper four cervical vertebrae
    c. they pass superior to the atlas, wind around the lateral mass of the atlas, and enter the vertebral cabal superior to the spinal cord
    d. they enter the skull through the foramen magnum to form the basilar artery, which supplies the structures in the posterior fossa

16. The common carotid artery supplies approximately _____ of blood flow to the internal carotid artery.
    a. 50%
    b. 60%
    c. 80%
    d. 40%

17. The Doppler spectral waveform from the low resistance internal carotid artery can be characterized by
    a. high peak systolic velocity and low diastolic flow
    b. rapid systolic upstroke, rapid deceleration to low diastolic flow
    c. cephalad flow throughout the cardiac cycle
    d. slow systolic rise time, rapid deceleration, flow reversal in late systole, and low diastolic flow

18. Which of the following statements best describes boundary layer separation in the carotid bulb?
    a. both forward and reverse flow patterns are present as a result of the dilatation of the carotid bulb and the presence of a pressure-flow gradient on the posterolateral wall of the bulb
    b. flow moves forward on the wall opposite the flow divide between the internal and external carotid arteries
    c. forward flow is seen on the wall opposite the flow divide, while reverse flow is seen on the anterolateral wall of the bulb
    d. disordered flow patterns are seen in the carotid bulb as a result of thickening of the arterial intima

19. All of the following are components of the Doppler equation except
    a. carrier Doppler frequency
    b. angle of insonation with respect to the path of blood flow
    c. constant for the speed of sound in blood
    d. velocity of red cell movement

20. Which of the following is not part of the femoral-popliteal arterial system?
    a. common femoral
    b. profunda femoris
    c. popliteal
    d. internal iliac

21. All of the following are true of the anterior tibial artery except
    a. proximally, it lies close to the inner side neck of the fibula
    b. it lies on the fibula and anterior ligament of the ankle joint in the lower third of the leg
    c. it becomes the dorsalis pedis artery in the distal portion of the leg
    d. it is almost always accompanied by two anterior tibial veins

22. Which of the following is not a true statement?
    a. the resistance to blood flow in the small tibial arteries should be greater than that in the aorta
    b. normally, at rest there is no significant pressure gradient between the aorta and the distal tibial arteries

    c. with normal arterial wall compliance, the Doppler spectral waveform from the peripheral arteries of the extremities should be triphasic
    d. during systole and left ventricular contraction, the arterial pulse pressure wave is transmitted through the aorta and into the high resistance peripheral arterial bed

23. All of the following changes may normally be found in the Doppler spectral waveform from elderly patients except
    a. loss of the reverse diastolic flow component
    b. reduction in the peak diastolic forward velocity
    c. decrease in the peak systolic velocity
    d. decrease in vessel wall elasticity

24. In the normal abdominal aorta, the peak systolic velocity averages _____ cm/sec while an average of _____ cm/sec is normally found in the popliteal artery.
    a. 60/80
    b. 80/50
    c. 100/50
    d. 90/60

25. Which of the following is not considered to be a normal Doppler spectral flow pattern found in the peripheral venous system?
    a. spontaneous flow
    b. respirophasicity
    c. pulsatility
    d. retrograde flow

26. Duplication is commonly found associated with all of the veins listed below except
    a. popliteal
    b. superficial femoral
    c. greater saphenous
    d. common iliac

27. Which of the following is not a true statement regarding the peripheral veins?
    a. they can undergo remarkable volume changes with little change in transmural pressure
    b. the percentage of smooth muscle found in the walls of veins varies with their location
    c. the venous wall is only half as thick as the arterial wall and is composed primarily of elastin fibers
    d. the venous pressure in the feet of an exercising adult is usually less than 25 mm Hg

Identify the structures indicated in the following illustrations. These figures duplicate those found in *Sonography: Introduction to Normal Structure and Function.* Refer to the textbook if you need help.

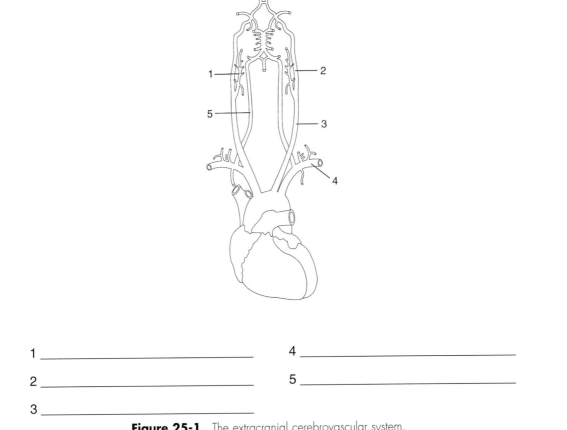

1 _____   4 _____

2 _____   5 _____

3 _____

Figure 25-1 The extracranial cerebrovascular system.

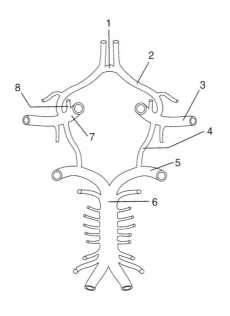

1 _____   5 _____

2 _____   6 _____

3 _____   7 _____

4 _____   8 _____

Figure 25-2 Circle of Willis.

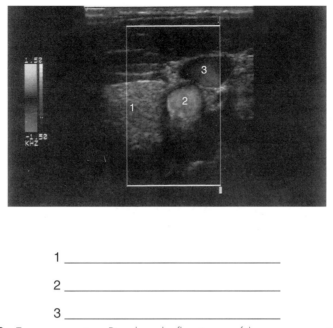

1 _____

2 _____

3 _____

Figure 25-3 Transverse section, Doppler color flow image of the common carotid artery, jugular vein, and thyroid gland.

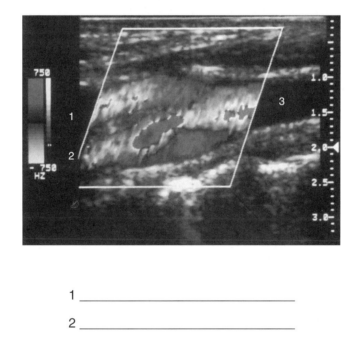

1 _____

2 _____

3 _____

Figure 25-4 Long axis section, Doppler color flow image of the carotid bifurcation demonstrates the common, external, and internal carotid arteries. Note the zone of retrograde flow in the carotid bulb caused by boundary layer.

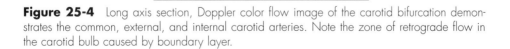

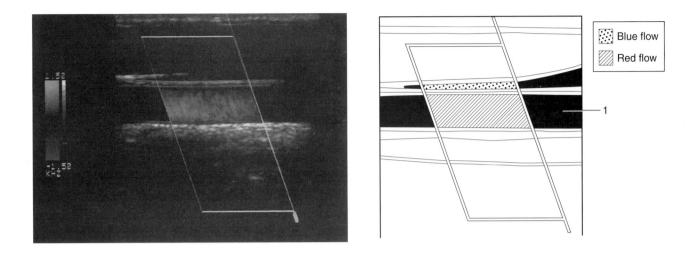

▦	Blue flow
▨	Red flow

——— 1

1 _____

Figure 25-5 Long axis section of the common carotid artery. Arterial wall definition reveals linear reflectivity resulting from the echogenicity of collagen found in the intima and media.

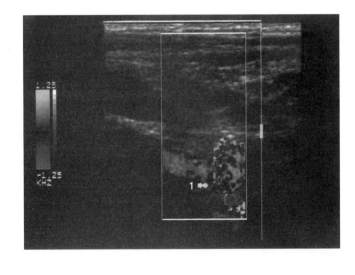

1 _____

Figure 25-6 Doppler color flow image of the vertebral artery origin. The subclavian artery is seen in the transverse plane just distal to the origin of the right common carotid artery.

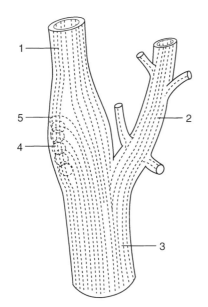

1 _____

2 _____

3 _____

4 _____

5 _____

Figure 25-7 Carotid bifurcation.

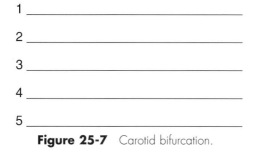

Figure 25-8 Doppler time-velocity waveform from a normal _____ .

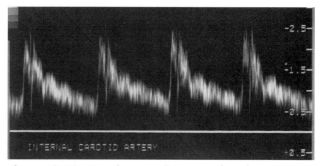

Figure 25-9 Doppler time-velocity waveform from a normal internal carotid artery demonstrating constant forward _____ flow.

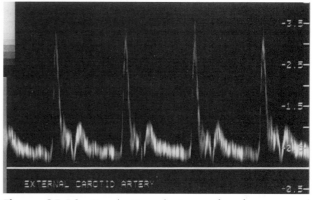

Figure 25-10 Doppler time-velocity waveform from a normal external carotid artery. Note the _____ flow component.

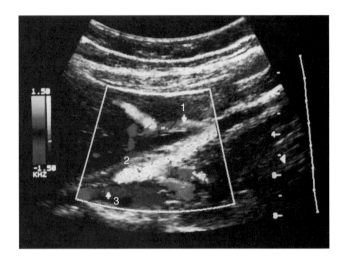

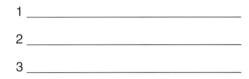

1 _____

2 _____

3 _____

Figure 25-13 Doppler color flow image of the aortic bifurcation. (Courtesy of Advanced Technology Laboratories.)

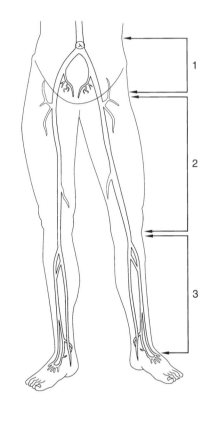

1 _____

2 _____

3 _____

Figure 25-12 Lower extremity peripheral arterial tree.

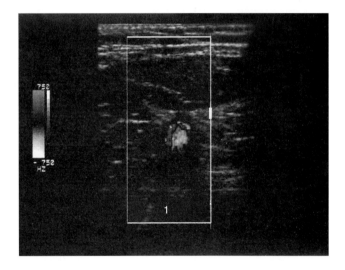

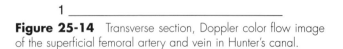

1 _____

Figure 25-14 Transverse section, Doppler color flow image of the superficial femoral artery and vein in Hunter's canal.

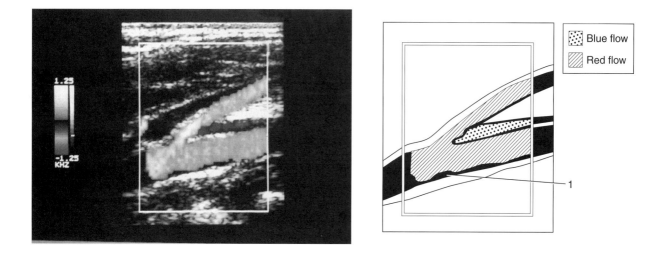

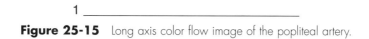

1 _____

Figure 25-15 Long axis color flow image of the popliteal artery.

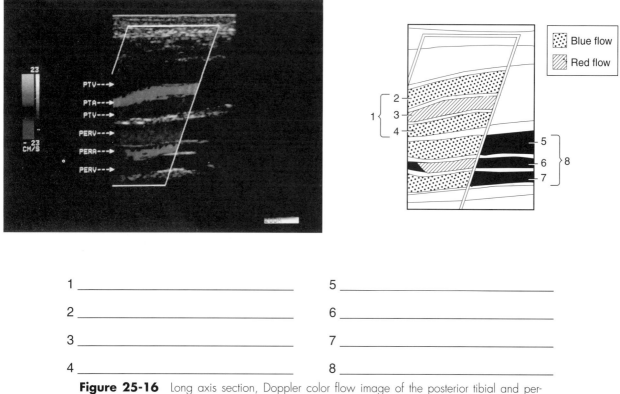

1 _____   5 _____

2 _____   6 _____

3 _____   7 _____

4 _____   8 _____

Figure 25-16 Long axis section, Doppler color flow image of the posterior tibial and peroneal arteries surrounded by their companion tibial veins of the same name. (Half-tone image courtesy Advanced Technology Laboratories.)

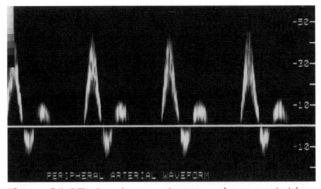

Figure 25-17 Doppler time-velocity waveform recorded from a lower extremity peripheral artery. Note the _____ pattern of flow.

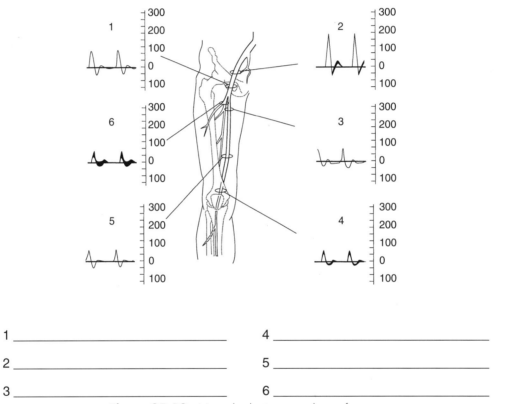

1 _____

2 _____

3 _____

4 _____

5 _____

6 _____

Figure 25-18 Normal velocity spectral waveforms.

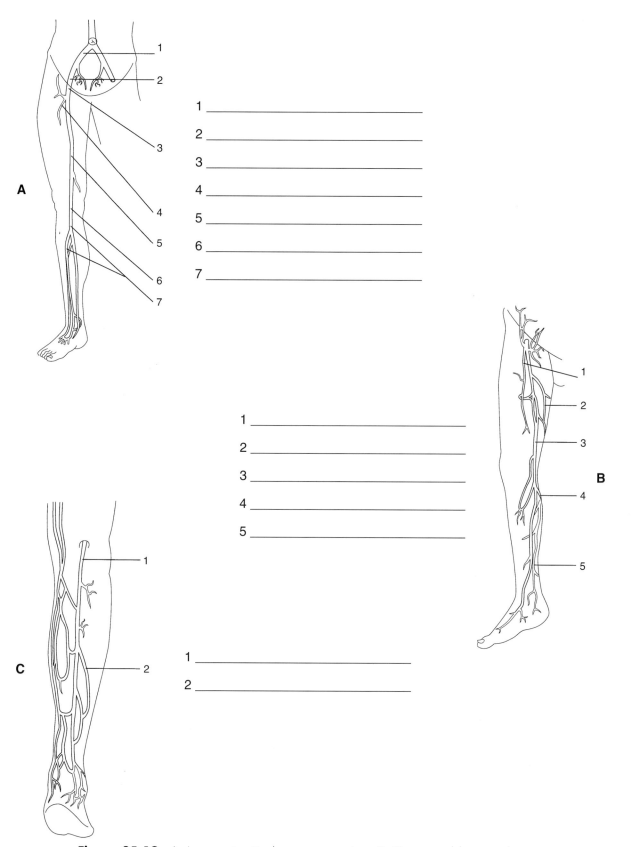

1 _____

2 _____

3 _____

4 _____

5 _____

6 _____

7 _____

1 _____

2 _____

3 _____

4 _____

5 _____

1 _____

2 _____

Figure 25-19 A, Lower extremity deep venous system. B, Greater and lesser saphenous veins. C, Greater and lesser saphenous veins.

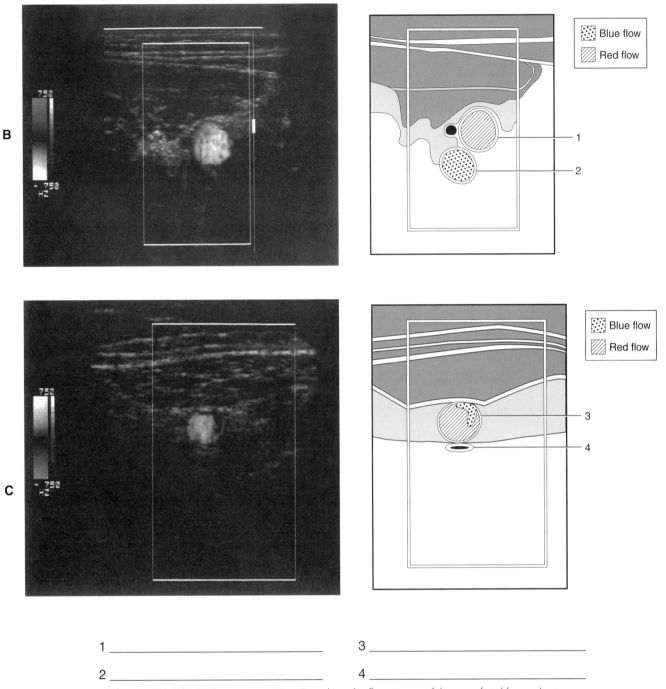

1 _____ 3 _____

2 _____ 4 _____

Figure 25-20 B, Transverse section, Doppler color flow image of the superficial femoral artery and vein. C, Transverse section, Doppler color flow image of the superficial femoral artery and vein demonstrating coaptation of the venous walls that occurs with gentle transducer pressure.

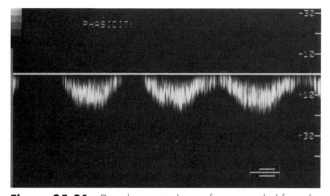

Figure 25-21 Doppler spectral waveform recorded from the normal _____. Note phasicity of flow, which varies with the respiratory cycle.

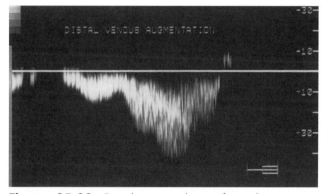

Figure 25-22 Doppler spectral waveform demonstrating augmentation of venous flow with manual _____ of the limb _____ to the transducer.

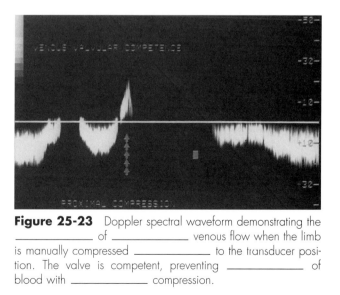

Figure 25-23 Doppler spectral waveform demonstrating the _____ of _____ venous flow when the limb is manually compressed _____ to the transducer position. The valve is competent, preventing _____ of blood with _____ compression.

CHAPTER 26

Introduction to Ultrasound of Human Disease

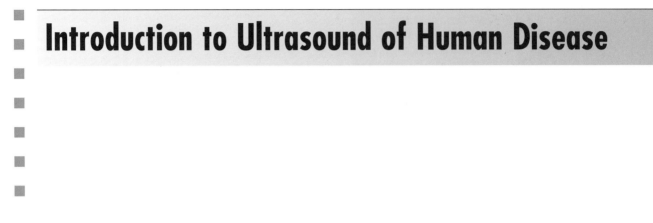

REVIEW QUESTIONS

1. The organ shown below would best be described by which term?

  a. cystic

  b. homogenous

  c. heterogeneous

  d. calcified

2. The image shown below demonstrates which type of pathology?

  a. cystic mass

  b. solid mass

  c. complex mass

  d. calcified structure

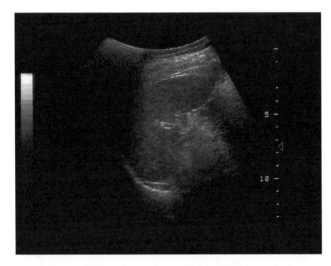

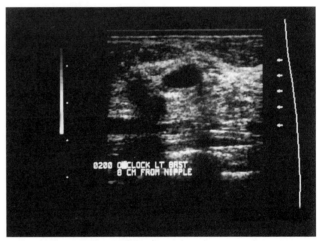

Image courtesy Acoustic Imaging, Inc., Phoenix, AZ.

3. The image shown below demonstrates which type of pathology?

a. cystic mass

b. solid mass

c. complex mass

d. calcified structure

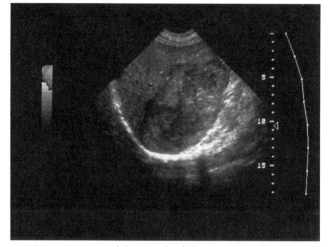

Image courtesy Philips Medical Systems, Bothell, WA.

4. The image shown below demonstrates which type of shadowing?

a. pathologic

b. regular

c. refractive

d. none of the above

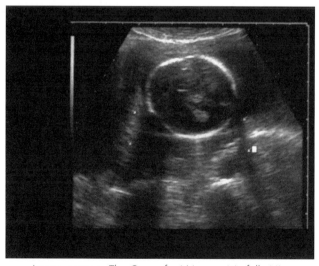

Image courtesy The Group for Women, Norfolk, VA.

5. The image shown below demonstrates which type of pathologic state?

a. cystic mass

b. solid mass

c. complex mass

d. calcified structure

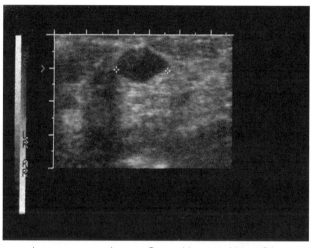

Image courtesy Acuson Corp., Mountain View, CA.

6. Which statement best describes the image shown below?

a. cystic mass with posterior through transmission

b. solid mass with smooth borders

c. mixed echogenically solid mass with irregular borders

d. isoechoic solid mass with irregular borders

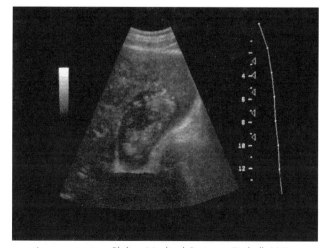

Image courtesy Philips Medical Systems, Bothell, WA.

7. Which statement best describes the image shown below?
   a. cystic mass with posterior through transmission
   b. solid mass with smooth borders
   c. primarily solid complex mass
   d. isoechoic solid mass with irregular borders

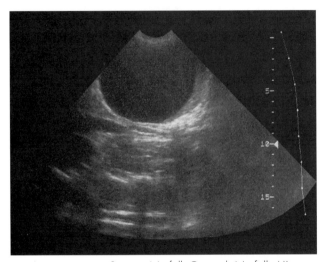

Image courtesy Sentara Norfolk General, Norfolk, VA.

8. Which statement best describes the image shown below?
   a. cystic mass with posterior through transmission
   b. solid mass with smooth borders
   c. primarily solid complex mass
   d. calcific mass with posterior shadowing

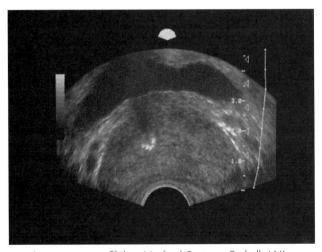

Image courtesy Philips Medical Systems, Bothell, WA.

9. Which statement best describes the image shown below?
   a. cystic mass with posterior through transmission
   b. solid mass
   c. primarily solid complex mass
   d. calcific mass with posterior shadowing

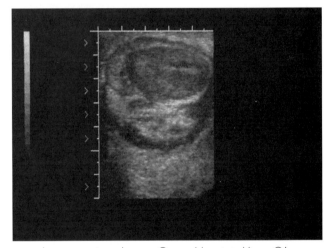

Image courtesy Acuson Corp., Mountain View, CA.

10. Which of the following statements best describes the typical appearance of a liver containing metastatic tumors?
    a. homogeneous and hyperechoic
    b. homogeneous and hypoechoic
    c. heterogeneous with areas of hypoechogenicity
    d. multiple intrahepatic masses with irregular borders and variable echogenicity
    e. both c and d may be appropriate

11. A true cyst
    a. has smooth walls
    b. has no internal echoes
    c. may contain anterior echoes
    d. has posterior through transmission
    e. has all of the above

12. Since it is recommended that sonographers not state a diagnosis when reporting the findings of pathology during an ultrasound examination, it is necessary only for sonographers to be able to recognize textural appearances. It is not important for them to be familiar with the pathologic processes associated with the area of interest.

    a. true

    b. false

13. Which of the following statements is correct?

    a. solid masses may have variable echogenicity

    b. all cystic masses have smooth borders

    c. complex masses are never found in conjunction with adjacent vasculature

    d. posterior through transmission occurs because very little sound passes through a mass

14. Ultrasound is able to definitively identify all pathologic processes within the abdomen.

    a. true

    b. false

Match the following:

15. decreased echogenicity _____

16. posterior through transmission _____

17. posterior shadowing _____

18. mixed echogenicity _____

19. septation _____

    a. complex mass

    b. increased echogenicity posterior to a mass

    c. thin membranous component within a cystic mass

    d. hypoechoic

    e. anechoic area posterior to a calcific mass with clean borders

20. All posterior shadowing arises from pathologic conditions.

    a. true

    b. false

21. After reviewing the following images of the gallbladder, write your technical observation:

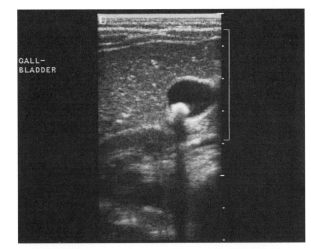

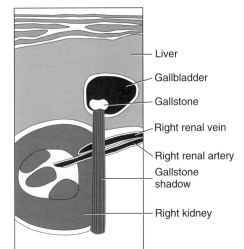

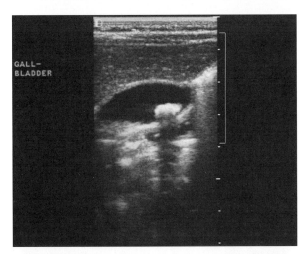

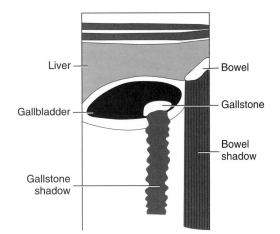

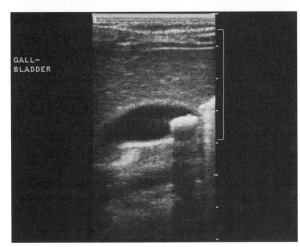

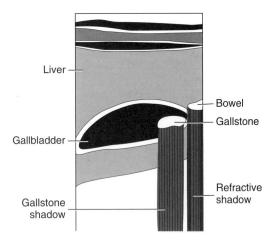

22. The following images are of the liver in a patient with known pancreatic carcinoma. Describe the liver in sonographic terms.

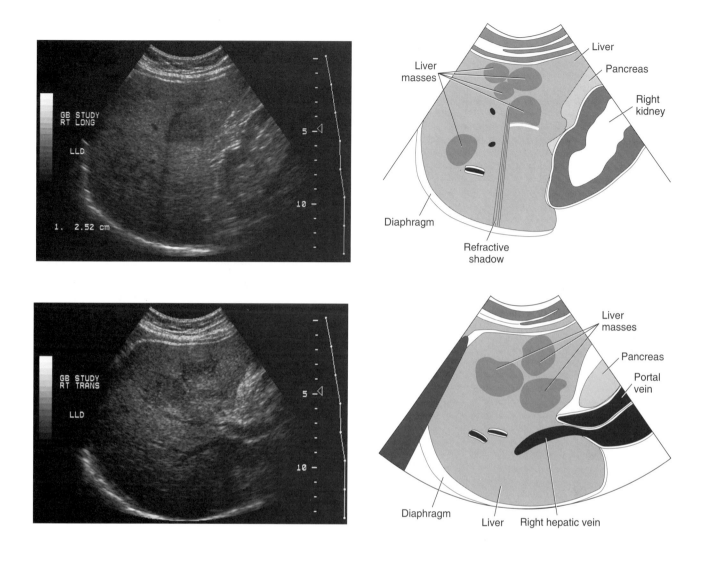

23. After reviewing the next images, write your technical observations. A 16-year-old female presents with a palpable left adnexal mass. Last menstrual period 2 weeks ago. Periods normal.

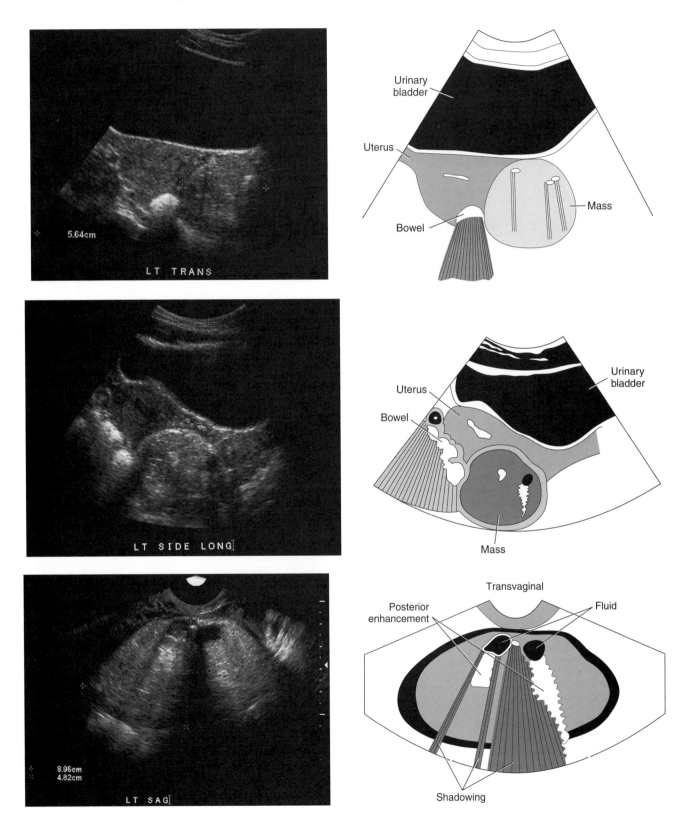

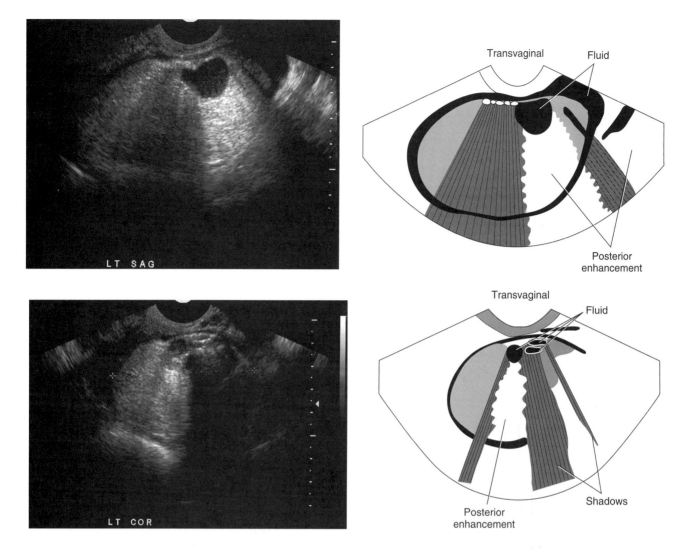

24. This image demonstrates a mass (indicated by the calipers) within the breast of a 50-year-old female. Describe the mass in sonographic terms.

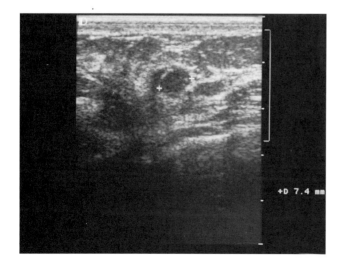

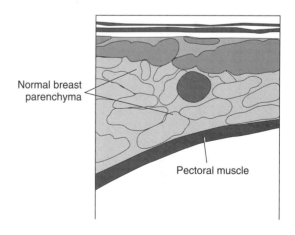

Identify the structures indicated in the following illustrations. These figures duplicate those found in *Sonography: Introduction to Normal Structure and Function.* Refer to the textbook if you need help.

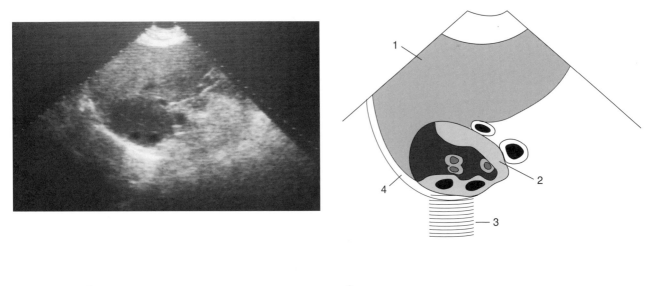

1 _____   3 _____

2 _____   4 _____

Figure 26-1 Right lower quadrant image.

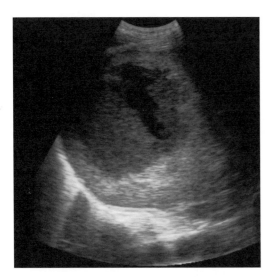 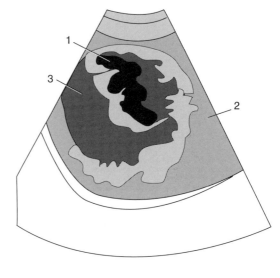

1 _____   3 _____

2 _____

Figure 26-2 Intrahepatic mass.

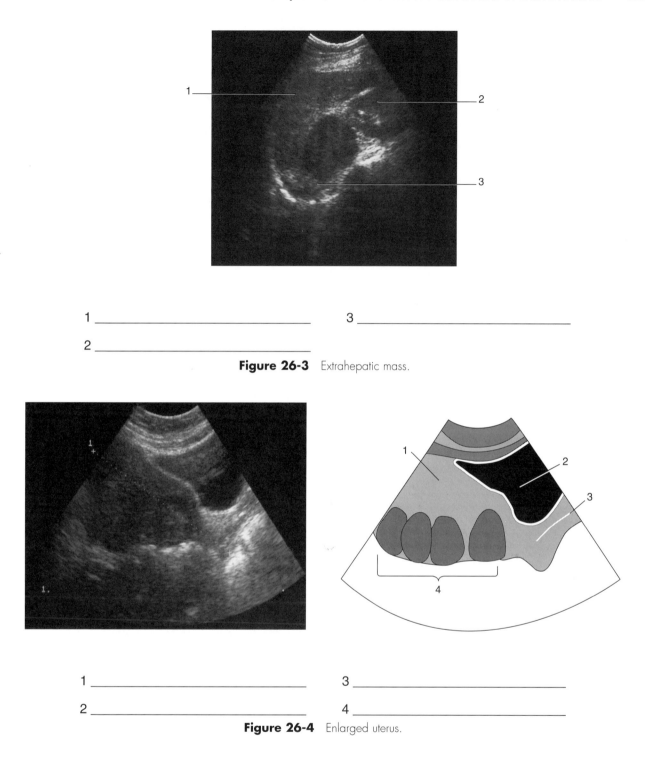

1 _____   3 _____

2 _____

Figure 26-3 Extrahepatic mass.

1 _____   3 _____

2 _____   4 _____

Figure 26-4 Enlarged uterus.

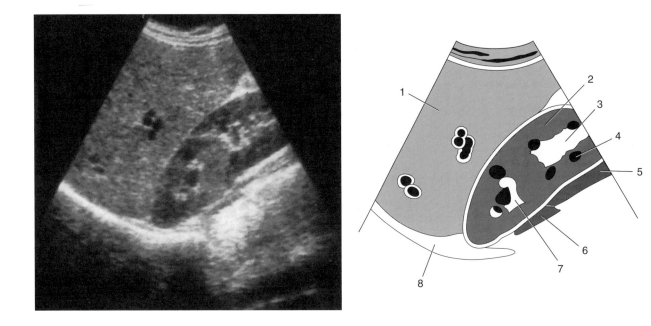

1 _____	5 _____
2 _____	6 _____
3 _____	7 _____
4 _____	8 _____

Figure 26-5 Normal liver and right kidney.

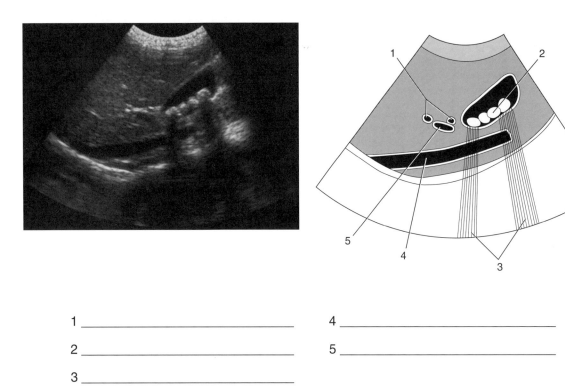

1 _____	4 _____
2 _____	5 _____
3 _____	

Figure 26-6 Gallbladder.

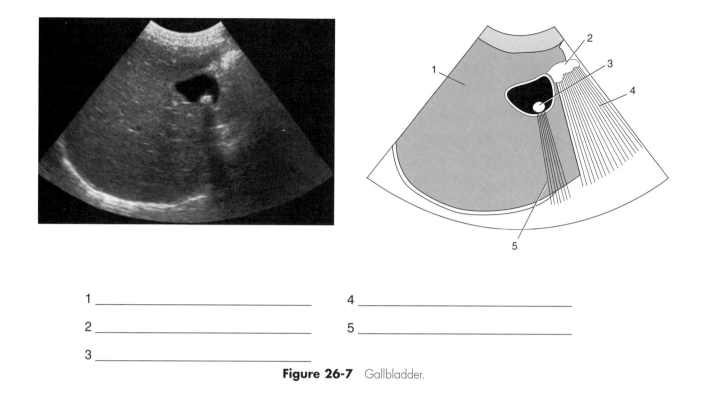

1 _____   4 _____

2 _____   5 _____

3 _____

Figure 26-7 Gallbladder.

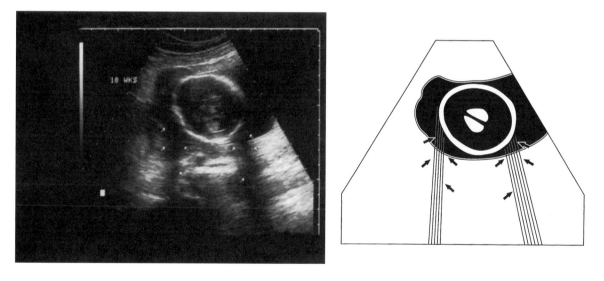

1 _____

Figure 26-8 Fetal skull. (Half-tone image courtesy The Group for Women, Norfolk, VA.)

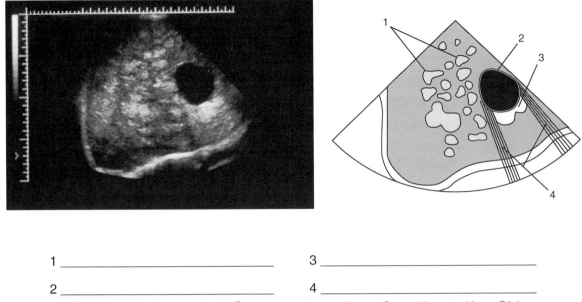

1 _____ 3 _____

2 _____ 4 _____

Figure 26-9 Liver masses. (Half-tone image courtesy Acuson Corp., Mountain View, CA.)

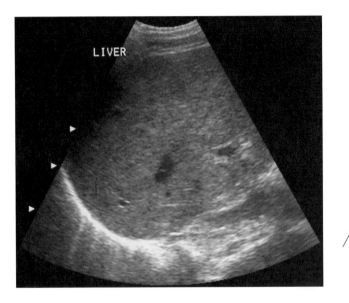

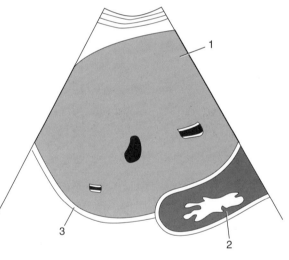

1 _____ 3 _____

2 _____

Figure 26-10

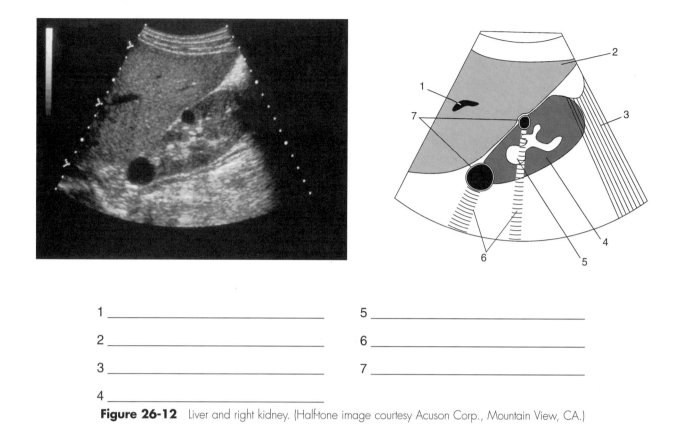

1 _____	5 _____
2 _____	6 _____
3 _____	7 _____
4 _____	

Figure 26-12 Liver and right kidney. (Half-tone image courtesy Acuson Corp., Mountain View, CA.)

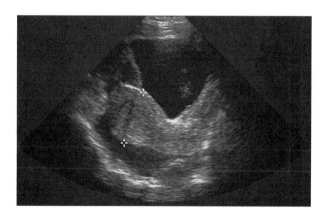
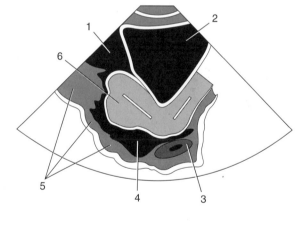

1 _____	4 _____
2 _____	5 _____
3 _____	6 _____

Figure 26-13 Pelvic image.

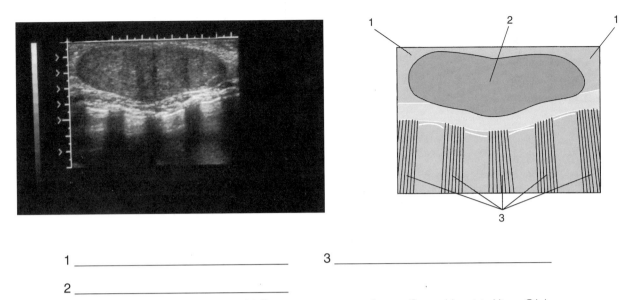

1 _____   3 _____

2 _____

Figure 26-15 Breast mass. (Half-tone image courtesy Acuson Corp., Mountain View, CA.)

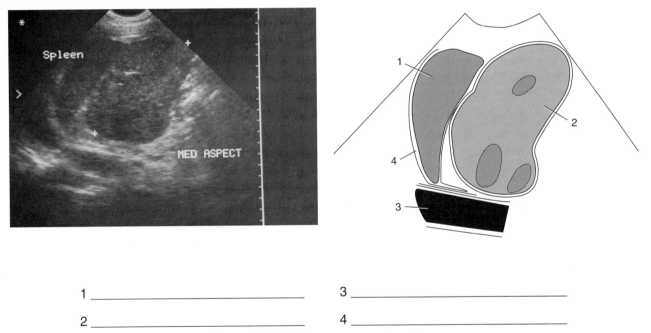

1 _____   3 _____

2 _____   4 _____

Figure 26-16 Mass isosonic to the spleen.

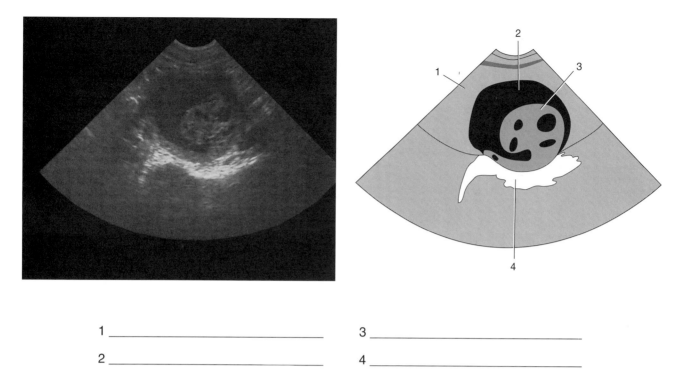

1 _____   3 _____

2 _____   4 _____

Figure 26-17 Complex masses. (Half-tone image courtesy Norfolk General Hospital, Norfolk, VA.)

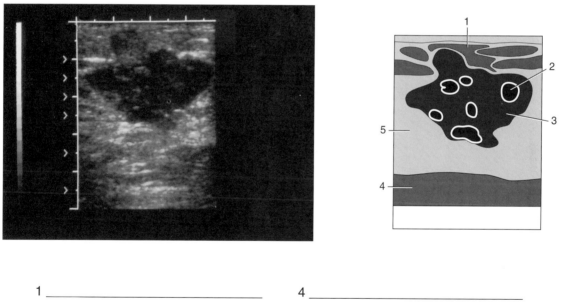

1 _____   4 _____

2 _____   5 _____

3 _____

Figure 26-18 Breast mass. (Half-tone image courtesy Acuson Corp., Mountain View, CA.)

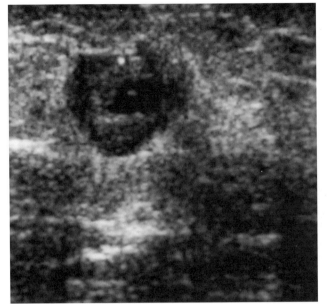

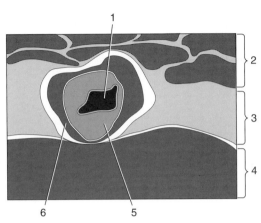

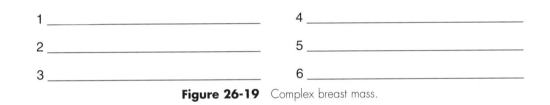

1 _____   4 _____

2 _____   5 _____

3 _____   6 _____

Figure 26-19 Complex breast mass.

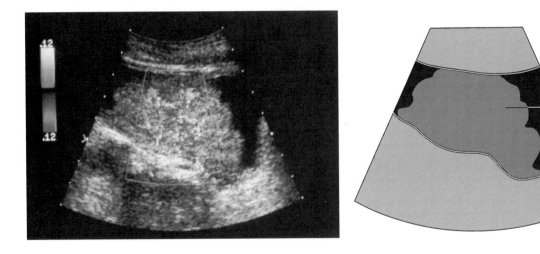

1 _____

2 _____

Figure 26-21 Bladder mass. (Half-tone image courtesy Acuson Corp., Mountain View, CA.)

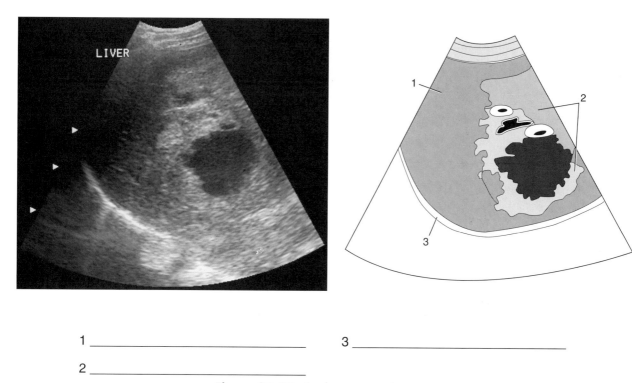

1 _____   3 _____

2 _____

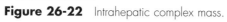

Figure 26-22 Intrahepatic complex mass.

CHAPTER 27

Three-Dimensional Ultrasound

REVIEW QUESTIONS

1. Applications for three-dimensional (3D) ultrasound do NOT include which of the following?
   a. abdominal
   b. endovaginal
   c. small parts
   d. musculoskeletal
   e. none of the above
   f. all of the above

2. A volume data set is the acquisition of patient
   a. algorithms
   b. anatomy
   c. physiology
   d. measurements

3. In order to display the volume data set on a flat screen, the following format must be used
   a. multiplanar
   b. maximum mode
   c. 3D rendering
   d. minimum mode

4. The two primary methods of acquiring volumes are (select two answers)
   a. manual acquisition
   b. maximum mode
   c. automatic acquisition
   d. minimum mode

5. The most accurate volume data set can be acquired from
   a. manual acquisition
   b. maximum mode
   c. automatic acquisition
   d. minimum mode

6. The most important step in acquiring 3D ultrasound images is
   a. volume acquisition
   b. reconstruction
   c. rendering
   d. how to move the transducer

7. Which 3D rendering mode is probably most familiar?
   a. reconstruction mode
   b. surface mode
   c. maximum mode
   d. minimum mode

8. Four-dimensional (4D) ultrasound can be used in which of the following procedures? (Select two answers.)
   a. endovaginal
   b. fetal viability
   c. endorectal
   d. needle biopsy

9. Low-frequency transducers work best in a 3D examination of the breast.
   a. true
   b. false

10. 3D acquisition can occur with color Doppler.

    a. true

    b. false

11. 3D acquisition cannot occur with power Doppler.

    a. true

    b. false

12. 3D imaging can create imaging planes that were not possible to achieve during a normal examination, and thus result in improved visualization of structures.

    a. true

    b. false

Identify the structures indicated in the following illustrations. These figures duplicate those found in *Sonography: Introduction to Normal Structure and Function.* Refer to the textbook if you need help.

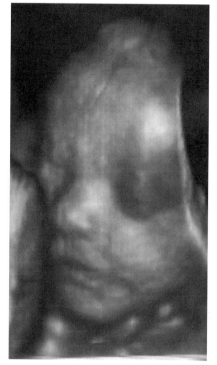

Figure 27-1 _____ mode image.

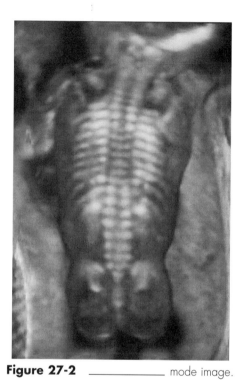

Figure 27-2 _____ mode image.

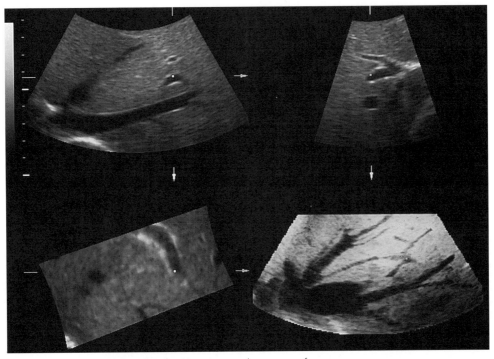

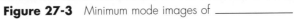

Figure 27-3 Minimum mode images of _____ .

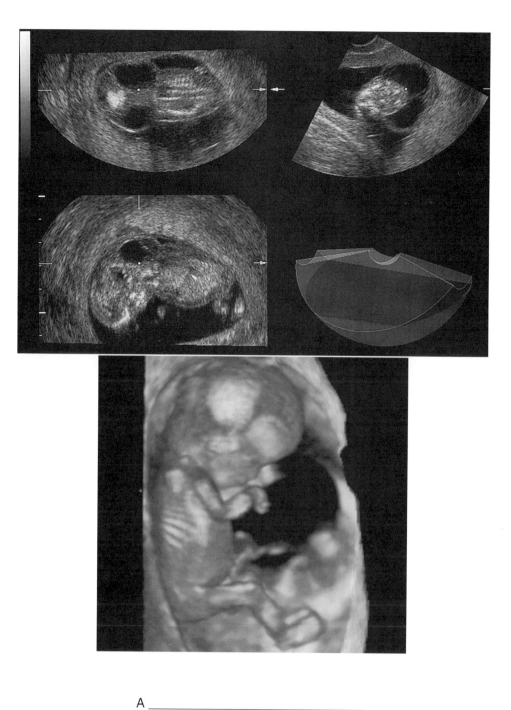

A _____

Figure 27-4

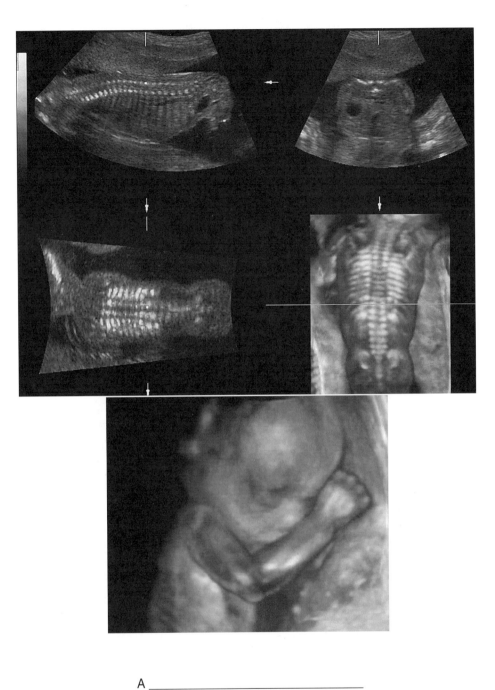

A

Figure 27-5

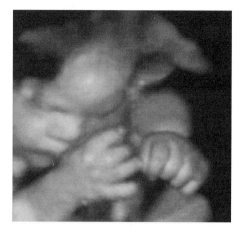

A _____

Figure 27-6

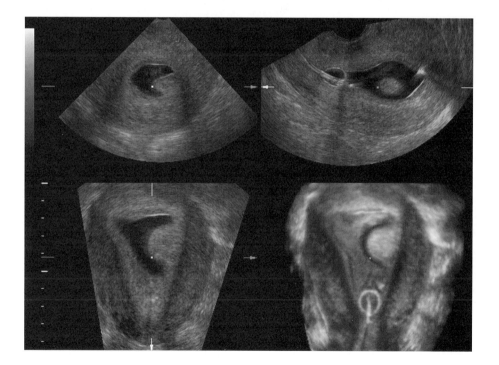

A _____

Figure 27-7

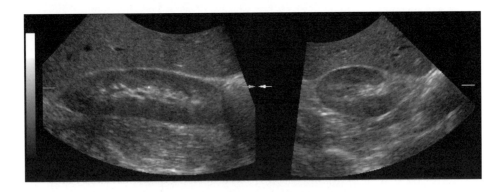

A _____

Figure 27-8

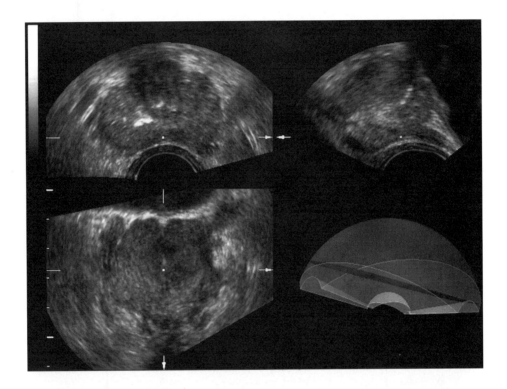

A _____

Figure 27-9

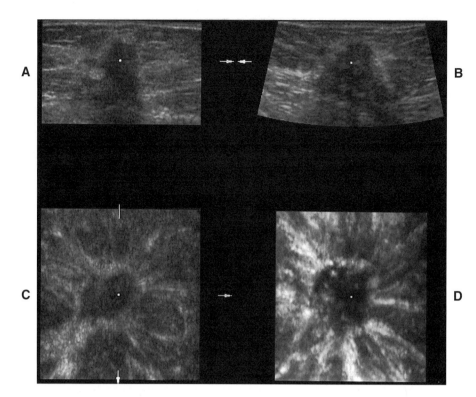

A _____

B _____

C _____

D _____

Figure 27-10

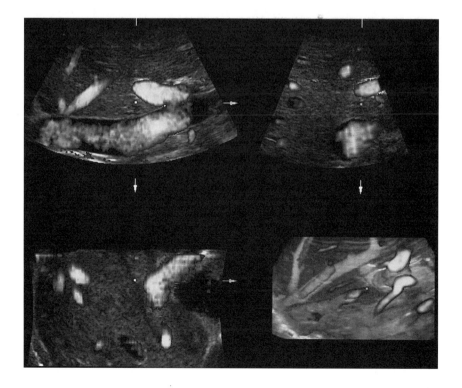

A _____

Figure 27-11

CHAPTER 28

Interventional and Intraoperative Ultrasound

REVIEW QUESTIONS

1. Percutaneous means
   a. the act of pouring over or through, especially the passage of a fluid through the vessels of a specific organ
   b. to sample
   c. performed through the skin
   d. to suture

2. Ultrasound-guided biopsies assist needle placement for
   a. fluid sampling
   b. small organ or stone extraction
   c. amniocentesis
   d. tissue sampling

3. An option for sterile transducer sheaths during interventional ultrasound is
   a. an alcohol bath
   b. sterile gel
   c. a rubber glove
   d. a water path

4. Ultrasound-guided aspirations assist needle placement for
   a. fluid sampling
   b. small organ or stone extraction
   c. amniocentesis
   d. tissue sampling

5. During intraoperative ultrasound procedures, sterile gel is
   a. not used
   b. used as a scanning couplant
   c. used as a couplant between the transducer and probe cover
   d. used in place of sterile sheaths

6. During intraoperative ultrasound procedures, the transducer is
   a. placed on a sterile water path
   b. in direct contact with the skin surface
   c. in direct contact with organs and vessels
   d. laparoscopic only

7. Nephrostomy is an ultrasound-guided
   a. villi sampling
   b. percutaneous tube placement
   c. percutaneous biopsy
   d. percutaneous stone extraction

8. A percutaneous cholangiogram is an ultrasound-guided
   a. bile aspiration
   b. evaluation of the gallbladder
   c. gallbladder biopsy
   d. evaluation of the biliary ducts

9. Endoluminal ultrasound

    a. is utilized for percutaneous tube placement

    b. is used to evaluate vessels and grafts during surgery

    c. is not currently practiced

    d. is limited to neurosurgical procedures

10. Chorionic villi sampling is

    a. a percutaneous biopsy

    b. collected during amniocentesis

    c. limited to intraoperative surgical procedures

    d. collected during a nephrostomy procedure

Identify the structures indicated in the following illustrations. These figures duplicate those found in *Sonography: Introduction to Normal Structure and Function.* Refer to the textbook if you need help.

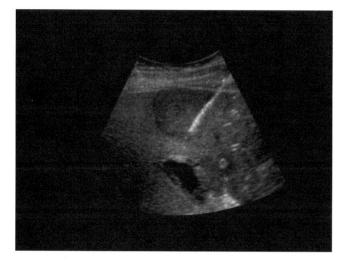
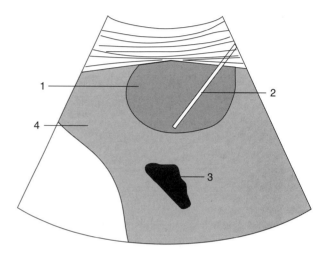

1 _____

2 _____

3 _____

4 _____

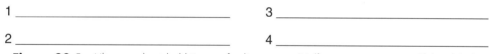

Figure 28-1 Ultrasound-guided biopsy of a liver mass. (Half-tone image courtesy Philips Medical Systems, Bothell, WA.)

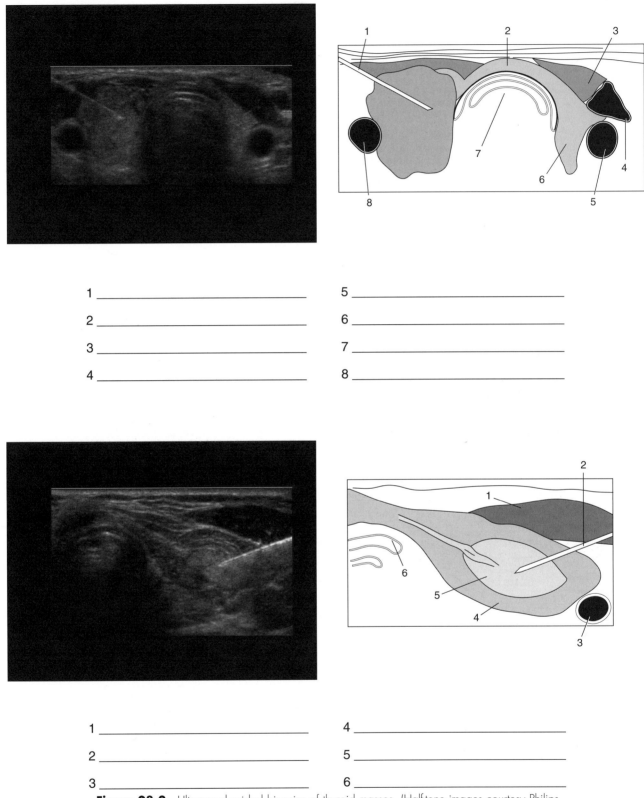

1 _____   5 _____

2 _____   6 _____

3 _____   7 _____

4 _____   8 _____

1 _____   4 _____

2 _____   5 _____

3 _____   6 _____

Figure 28-2 Ultrasound-guided biopsies of thyroid masses. (Half-tone images courtesy Philips Medical Systems, Bothell, WA.)

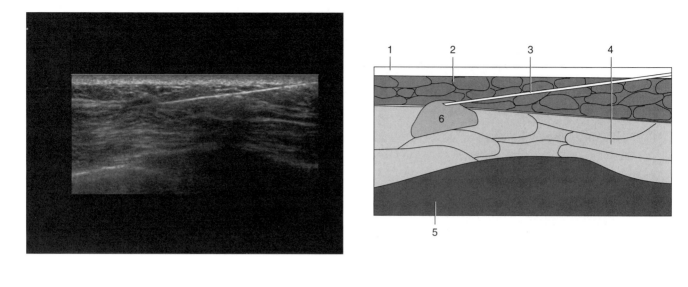

1 _____ 4 _____

2 _____ 5 _____

3 _____ 6 _____

Figure 28-3 Ultrasound-guided breast mass biopsy. (Half-tone image courtesy Philips Medical Systems, Bothell, WA.)

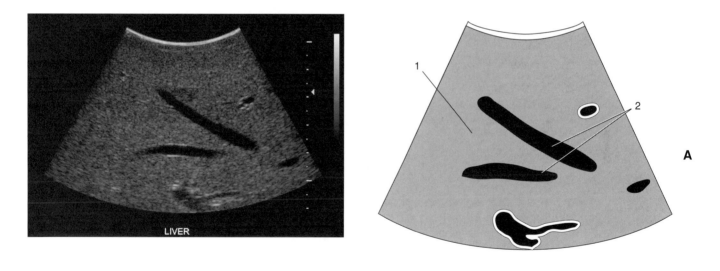

1 _____ 2 _____

Figure 28-5 Intra-abdominal intraoperative ultrasound images. **A,** Transverse section of the liver. (Half-tone image courtesy Philips Medical Systems, Bothell, WA.)

continued

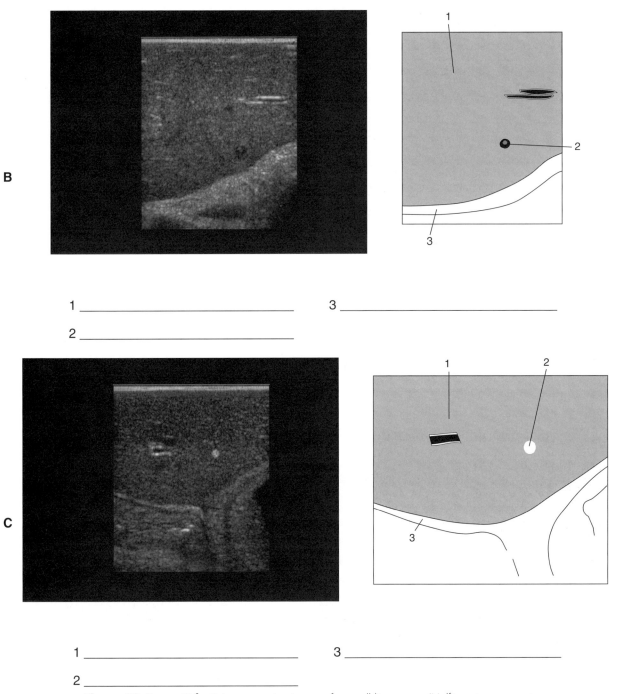

B

1 _____   3 _____

2 _____

C

1 _____   3 _____

2 _____

Figure 28-5, cont'd   B, Intraoperative image of a small liver mass. (Half-tone image courtesy Philips Medical Systems, Bothell, WA.) C, Intraoperative image of a small liver hemangioma. (Half-tone image courtesy Philips Medical Systems, Bothell, WA.)

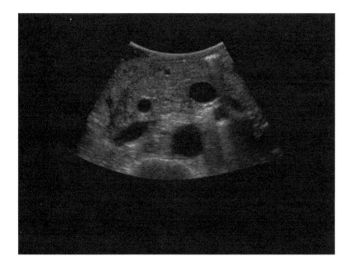
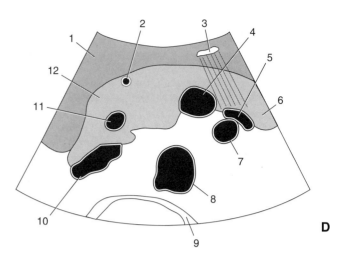

D

1 _____ 7 _____

2 _____ 8 _____

3 _____ 9 _____

4 _____ 10 _____

5 _____ 11 _____

6 _____ 12 _____

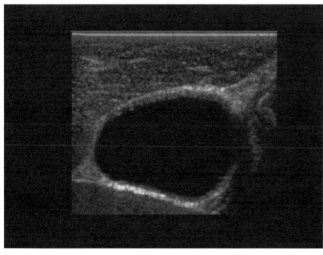
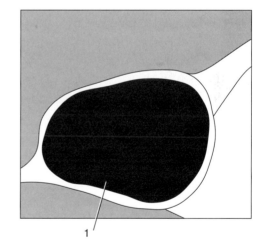

E

1 _____

Figure 28-5, cont'd D, Intraoperative, transverse, midline section of the abdomen. (Half-tone image courtesy Philips Medical Systems, Bothell, WA.) E, Intraoperative view of the gallbladder. (Half-tone image courtesy Philips Medical Systems, Bothell, WA.)

continued

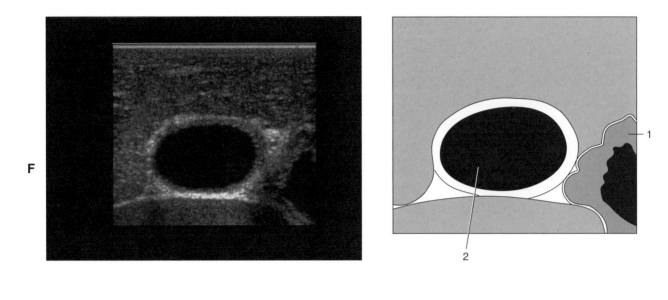

F

1 _____   2 _____

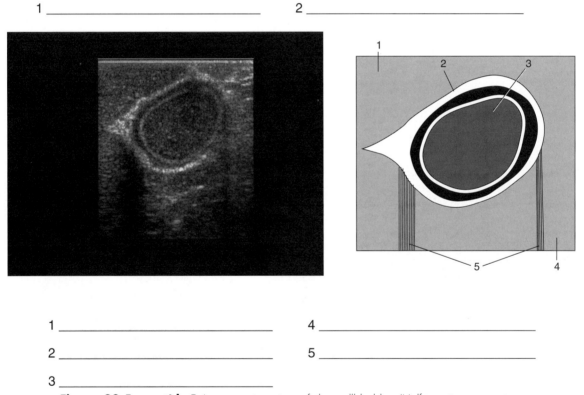

G

1 _____   4 _____

2 _____   5 _____

3 _____

Figure 28-5, cont'd F, Intraoperative view of the gallbladder. (Half-tone image courtesy Philips Medical Systems, Bothell, WA.) G, Intraoperative image of a gallbladder with sludge. (Half-tone image courtesy Philips Medical Systems, Bothell, WA.)

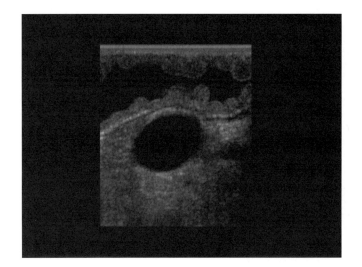

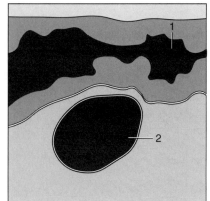

H

1 _____   2 _____

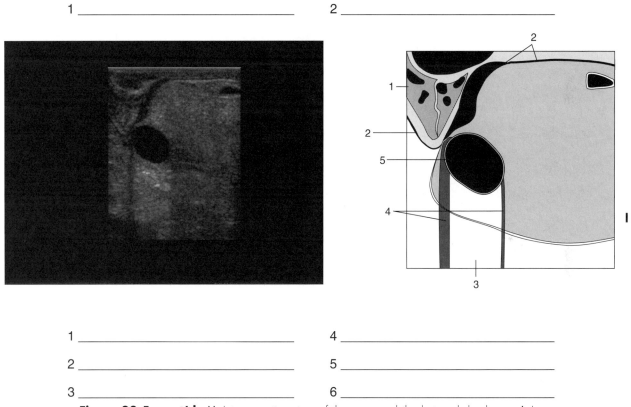

I

1 _____   4 _____

2 _____   5 _____

3 _____   6 _____

Figure 28-5, cont'd H, Intraoperative view of the common bile duct and duodenum. I, Intraoperative image of the common bile duct. (Half-tone images courtesy Philips Medical Systems, Bothell, WA.)

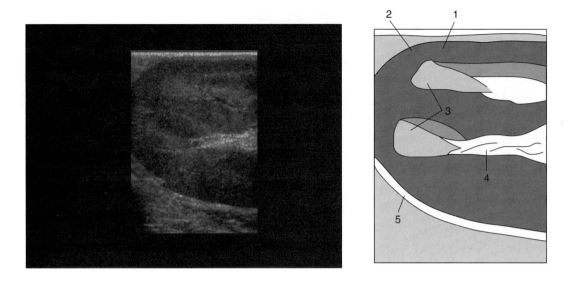

1 _____   4 _____

2 _____   5 _____

3 _____

Figure 28-6 Intraoperative transverse section of the kidney. (Half-tone image courtesy Philips Medical Systems, Bothell, WA.)

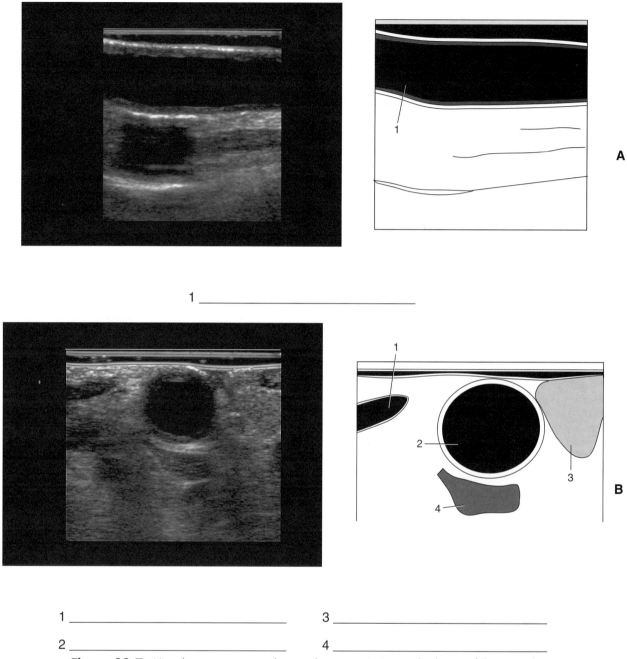

1 _____

1 _____   3 _____

2 _____   4 _____

Figure 28-7 Vascular intraoperative ultrasound images. **A,** Longitudinal view of the internal carotid artery. (Half-tone image courtesy Philips Medical Systems, Bothell, WA.) **B,** Intraoperative transverse view of the internal common carotid artery. (Half-tone image courtesy Philips Medical Systems, Bothell, WA.)

continued

E

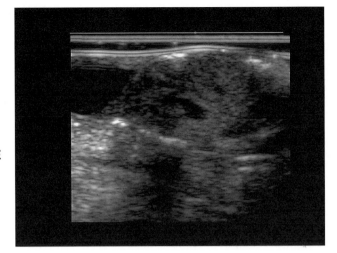
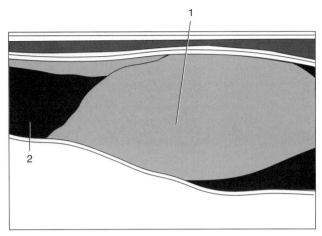

1 _____ 2 _____

F

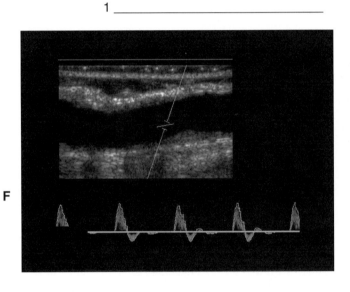
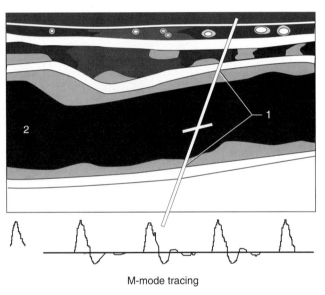

M-mode tracing

1 _____ 2 _____

Figure 28-7, cont'd E, Intraoperative image of the internal carotid artery with plaque. (Half-tone image courtesy Philips Medical Systems, Bothell, WA.) **F**, Intraoperative image of an arterial graft with Doppler tracing. (Half-tone image courtesy Philips Medical Systems, Bothell, WA.)

Answers

INTRODUCTION

1. c	**4.** a	**7.** d	**10.** f
2. b	**5.** b	**8.** c	
3. c	**6.** d	**9.** d	

CHAPTER 1

1. b	**11.** a	**21.** a	**31.** a
2. a	**12.** d	**22.** b	**32.** d
3. a	**13.** c	**23.** c	**33.** b
4. d	**14.** b	**24.** c	**34.** d
5. c	**15.** c	**25.** a	**35.** b
6. b	**16.** c	**26.** b	**36.** c
7. b	**17.** a	**27.** d	**37.** c
8. b	**18.** a	**28.** d	
9. c	**19.** b	**29.** c	
10. a	**20.** d	**30.** c	

CHAPTER 2

1. c	**11.** a	**21.** a	**31.** b
2. c	**12.** c	**22.** b	**32.** d
3. a	**13.** d	**23.** c	**33.** a
4. c	**14.** c	**24.** b	**34.** d
5. b	**15.** c	**25.** c	**35.** b
6. d	**16.** a	**26.** c	**36.** d
7. a	**17.** a	**27.** b	**37.** c
8. b	**18.** b	**28.** c	
9. c	**19.** d	**29.** c	
10. b	**20.** d	**30.** c	

CHAPTER 3

1. d	**5.** a	**9.** c	**13.** d
2. b	**6.** d	**10.** b	**14.** c
3. d	**7.** d	**11.** a	**15.** a
4. b	**8.** a	**12.** b	**16.** b

17. c	**21.** c	**25.** a	**29.** c
18. c	**22.** d	**26.** b	
19. c	**23.** c	**27.** d	
20. b	**24.** b	**28.** d	

CHAPTER 4

1. b. The pancreas is a retroperitoneal organ.

2. a. The gallbladder is an intraperitoneal organ.

3. c. The left renal vein lies transversely as it runs from the kidney to the inferior vena cava.

4. c. The portal vein lies in a transverse oblique position.

5. d. Medial—the anatomic areas appreciated on a sagittal section are anterior, posterior, superior, inferior.

6. c. Anterior—the anatomic areas appreciated on a coronal section are lateral, medial, superior, inferior.

7. a. Superior—the anatomic areas appreciated on a transverse section are anterior, posterior, right lateral, left lateral from either an anterior or posterior approach, or lateral, medial, anterior, posterior from either a right lateral or left lateral approach.

8. d. The location of the transducer and sound wave approach.

9. b. Sonographic appearance—the size, shape, and adjacent relationships of structures are the same on an ultrasound image section and the cadaver section.

10. b. Annular array is a type of ultrasound transducer.

11. a. Inferior

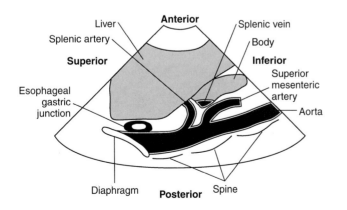

12. b. Lateral

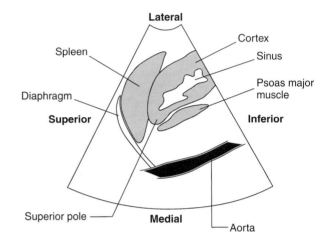

13. b. Posterior

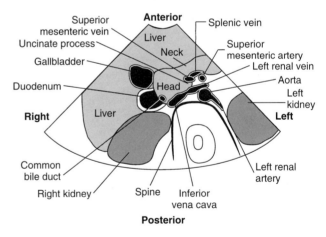

14. c. Right lateral.

15. c. pancreas neck and the uncinate process.

16. b. Kidneys, adrenal glands, pancreas, inferior vena cava, spleen, ascending colon, descending colon.

17. c. Ovaries, uterus, majority of the intestines.

18. a. Extends from the diaphragm to the pelvis and covers the width of the abdomen.

19. b. is a diverticulum of the greater sac located posterior to the stomach.

20. d. mesentery

21. d. Muscular bands that arise from the lumbar vertebrae and insert into the diaphragm.

22. b. posterior

23. c. lateral, posterior

24. c. less than echogenic

25. b. normal lymph nodes, normal fallopian tubes, normal ureters.

CHAPTER 5

1. b
2. d
3. a
4. d
5. a
6. b
7. c
8. a
9. c

10. b
11. a
12. c
13. a
14. d
15. b
16. b
17. d
18. a

19. d
20. a
21. fusiform
    saccular
    dissecting
22. tunica intima
    tunica media
    tunica adventitia

CHAPTER 6

1. a
2. c
3. a
4. c
5. b
6. a
7. a
8. b

9. a
10. b
11. a
12. d
13. c
14. b
15. a
16. c

17. a
18. d
19. c
20. a
21. duplex Doppler sonography
    color flow Doppler
    impedance flow plethysmography

CHAPTER 7

1. d
2. b
3. a
4. a

5. a
6. c
7. a
8. b

9. b
10. a
11. d
12. b

13. c
14. a

CHAPTER 8

1. c. The celiac artery arises from the anterior wall of the abdominal aorta.

2. d. portal vein

3. a. The infrarenal abdominal aorta supplies blood flow to the high-resistance vascular beds of the lumbar arteries and the peripheral arterial system of the lower limbs.

4. c. Low-resistance vascular waveforms are characterized by high forward diastolic flow components.

5. a. The postprandial SMA signal is characterized by constant forward diastolic flow consistent with the metabolically imposed change from high-resistance (fasting) to low-resistance vascular beds.

6. c. The signals suggest elevated renal vascular resistance consistent with intrinsic medical renal disease

7. b. The portal vein and its branches are intra-abdominal vessels

8. c. The portal vein is formed by the confluence of the splenic and superior mesenteric veins.

9. d. The portal triad is comprised of the main portal vein, hepatic artery, and common bile duct.

10. b. The first two phases represent reflections of right atrial and ventricular diastole. The third phase is characterized by systolic flow reversal and results from contraction of the right atrium.

11. a. The flow patterns in the portal venous system are a reflection of changes in respirophasicity and intraabdominal pressure. This results in a continuous, mildly disordered flow pattern with low peak and mean velocities.

12. c. Hematocrit does not appear to have a direct effect on blood flow patterns in the portal vein.

13. d. The left renal artery lies inferior to the left renal vein.

14. a. between the anterior aortic wall and the superior mesenteric artery

15. c

16. a

17. d

CHAPTER 9

1. a
2. c
3. b
4. c
5. d
6. a
7. c
8. b
9. d
10. b
11. d
12. c
13. c
14. a
15. b
16. d

17. a,d
18. c
19. d
20. b
21. c
22. c
23. a
24. b
25. d
26. a
27. c
28. a
29. c
30. a
31. d
32. a

33. a. The gallbladder, divides the anterior right lobe from the medial left lobe.
b. The ligamentum teres, divides the medial left from the lateral left lobe.
c. The inferior vena cava, separates the right from the caudate lobe.
d. The ligamentum venosum, divides the caudate from the lateral left lobe.

34. porta hepatis

35. F

36. F, C

37. C

38. F

39. P

40. P

41. E

CHAPTER 10

1. c. The gallbladder lies in the gallbladder fossa located on the posterior and inferior portion of the right lobe of the liver.

2. b. The porta hepatis is a fissure on the visceral surface of the liver where the portal vein and the hepatic artery enter and the hepatic ducts leave.

3. a. The proximal portion of the biliary duct is the common hepatic duct.

4. d. The right and left hepatic ducts are intrahepatic.

5. a. The distal portion of the biliary duct is the common bile duct.

6. b. The portal triad consists of the portal vein, hepatic artery, and common bile duct.

7. c. Normal biliary duct diameter is 1 mm to 7 mm.

8. b. 3 mm or less is normal for gallbladder wall thickness.

9. d. The fundus of the gallbladder is usually just anterior to the superior pole of the right kidney.

10. b. The sonographic appearance of the bile-filled biliary system is anechoic with echogenic walls.

11. c	20. a
12. b	21. c
13. a	22. b
14. d	23. b
15. a	
16. d	
17. d	
18. a	
19. b	

CHAPTER 11

1. Head (bordered by the inferior vena cava and superior mesenteric vein); Neck (bordered by the superior mesenteric vein); Body (bordered by the superior mesenteric artery and splenic vein; Tail (bordered by the splenic vein).

2. Head (pancreaticoduodenal arteries, pancreatic arcade, gastroduodenal artery); Body and Tail (splenic artery branches, specifically, dorsal pancreatic, pancreatica magna, caudal pancreatic arteries).

3. Trypsin (protein); Amylase (carbohydrates); Lipase (fats).

4. Insulin (changes glucose to glycogen); Glucagon (changes glycogen back to glucose); Somatostatin (inhibits alpha and beta cells).

5. The gastroduodenal artery and common bile duct appear as two small, anechoic areas in the head of the pancreas. The gastroduodenal artery is more anterior than the common bile duct. Both vessels appear circular on transverse images, elongated on sagittal images.

6. The pancreas appears more echodense than the liver, but is less homogeneous.

7. Longitudinal. Transverse images show the long axis of the pancreas.

8. The body of the pancreas.

9. The uncinate process.

10. The common bile duct and duct of Wirsung (main pancreatic duct) usually enter the ampulla of the duodenum together. The accessory duct (duct of Santorini) enters the duodenum approximately 2 cm superior to the main duct and common bile duct.

11. digestive/hormonal

12. epigastrium and left hypochondrium

13. amylase: digests carbohydrates
    lipase: acts on fats
    trypsin, chymotrypsin, carboxypeptidase: help break down proteins
    nucleases: work on nucleic acids
    sodium bicarbonate: neutralizes hydrochloric acid

14. duct of Wirsung/ ampulla of Vater

15. islets of Langerhans

16. duct of Santorini

17. (1) head /C-loop
    (2) neck/anterior
    (3) body/anterior
    (4) tail/hilum

18. splenic

19. a posteromedial projection of pancreatic tissue that extends from the head

20. total length: ranges between 12 and 13 cm approximately 2.5 cm thick, 3 to 5 cm wide because a portion of the gland may be enlarged but still fall within normal limits

21. common bile duct and gastroduodenal artery

22. pancreaticoduodenal/ splenic

23. echodense/ homogeneous

24. transverse
    long

CHAPTER 12

1. The urinary system maintains the body's chemical equilibrium through the excretion of urine, a waste product. Other functions include detoxifying the blood, regulating blood pressure, and maintaining the proper balance of pH, minerals, iron, and salt levels in the blood.

2. The kidneys are anterior to the diaphragm and the psoas, quadratus lumborum, and transversus muscles.

3. The right kidney is posterior to the right lobe of the liver, right adrenal gland, second part of the duodenum, hepatic flexure of the colon, and the jejunum or ileum of the small intestine.

4. The left kidney is posterior to the tail of the pancreas, the left adrenal gland, the spleen and splenic vein, the jejunum, the stomach, and the splenic flexure of the colon.

5. The ureters are retroperitoneal structures that extend inferiorly along the psoas muscle to the urinary bladder. The duodenum, terminal ileum, and right colic, ileocolic, and gonadal (testicular or ovarian) vessels are anterior to the right ureter. The colon and the left colic and left gonadal vessels are anterior to the left ureter. The abdominal portions of both ureters pass anterior to the psoas muscle and bifurcation of the common iliac arteries. The pelvic portions of the ureters pass posterior to the ductus deferens in the male and uterine artery in the female.

6. The urinary bladder is retroperitoneal and lies posterior to the symphysis pubis. The male urinary bladder is anterior to the seminal vesicles and rectum, and superior to the prostate gland. The female urinary bladder is anterior to the vagina, posterior cul-de-sac, and rectum.

7. Normal sizes of urinary system structures are:
   Adult kidney: 9-12 cm in length, 4-6 cm in width, 2.5-4 cm in depth
   Ureters: 28-34 cm in length, 6mm in width
   Distended urinary bladder wall: 3-6 mm
   Female urethra: 4 cm in length
   Male urethra: 20 cm in length

8. The formation of urine begins when blood enters the kidney through the renal artery, which branches into interlobar arteries; these in turn branch into afferent arterioles, which carry blood into the glomerulus of the nephron, the functional unit of the kidney. The glomerulus filters the blood. Waste is excreted in the form of urine, and useful substances are reabsorbed into the bloodstream.

9. The parts of the urinary system and their sonographic appearance are as follows:
   The **true capsule** acts as a protective covering that surrounds the renal cortex. Its sonographic appearance is echogenic.
   The **parenchymal cortex** contains the renal corpuscle, and the proximal and distal convoluted tubules of the nephron; thus, filtration occurs in the cortex. Its sonographic appearance is homogeneous with medium- to low-level echoes that are less than or equal to the echogenicity of the normal liver or spleen. The contour of the normal cortex should appear smooth.
   The **parenchymal medulla** contains the loop of Henle of the nephron, thus reabsorption occurs there. The medulla consists of 8-18 medullary pyramids that appear sonographically as triangular, round, or blunted hypoechoic areas to the more urine-filled anechoic areas.
   The **arcuate vessels** may be seen sonographically as echogenic dots at the corticomedullary junction.

The **renal sinus** is the central portion of the kidney that contains the minor and major calyces, renal pelvis, renal artery and vein, fat, nerves, and lymphatics. The overall sonographic appearance of the sinus is echogenic because it is surrounded by fat. The renal pelvis and calyces are not seen if collapsed; otherwise they appear anechoic surrounded by the echogenic fat. The renal artery and vein have echogenic walls and anechoic lumina. Unless enlarged, lymph nodes are not seen. Nerves are not yet appreciated sonographically.

The **ureters** are tubular structures that carry urine from each kidney to the urinary bladder. Normal ureters are not generally seen with sonography. However, "ureteral jets"—the effect of the ureter ejecting urine into the bladder—can be seen during real time examination. The **urinary bladder** is a temporary storage site for urine until it is excreted from the body through the **urethra.** The bladder lumen is not seen sonographically if collapsed; otherwise it appears anechoic. The distended bladder wall appears as a smooth, thin, echogenic line. The urethra, when seen, appears echogenic.

10. Ultrasound is used to evaluate the urinary system for the following reasons:
    renal size
    detection and composition of renal masses and cysts
    urinary system obstruction
    renal abscess
    renal hematoma
    enlarged ureters
    urinary bladder masses
    Doppler evaluation of renal blood flow abnormalities
    sonography-guided biopsies of renal parenchyma or masses
    sonography-guided fluid aspirations
    renal transplant

11. Urinary system normal variants recognized by ultrasound are:
    dromedary hump: localized bulge(s) on the lateral border of the kidney that has the same sonographic appearance as normal renal cortex.
    hypertrophied column of Bertin: an enlarged portion of the renal cortex that varies in size and may indent the renal sinus. It has the same sonographic appearance as normal renal cortex.
    double collecting system: occurs when the renal sinus is divided. Each sinus has a renal pelvis. A bifid (double) ureter may also be present. The sonographic appearance is the same as normal renal cortex and sinus.

    horseshoe kidney: occurs when the kidneys are connected, usually at the lower poles. It has the same sonographic appearance as normal renal cortex.
    renal ectopia: occurs when one or both kidneys are found outside the normal renal fossa. Locations include the lower abdominal and pelvic region. Other ectopic locations (e.g., thoracic) are rare.

12. Physicians associated with the urinary system include **urologists,** who specialize in the surgical diseases of the urinary system in women and genitourinary tract in men. The **nephrologist** specializes in medical diseases of the kidney and the **radiologist** specializes in the diagnostic interpretation of imaging modalities that assess renal disease.

13. Diagnostic tests commonly used to evaluate the urinary system include the radiologic examination **IVP (intravenous pyelogram),** in which a contrast medium (dye) is injected into a vein and x-ray films are taken at specific time intervals to observe kidney function and urinary system anatomy. The test is performed by a radiologic technologist and a radiologist. The examination is interpreted by a radiologist. **CT or CAT scan (computerized axial tomography)** is a radiologic examination in which cross-sectional x-ray images are obtained of the kidneys and other urinary system structures to assess anatomy. A contrast medium may be administered to differentiate between pathology and normal anatomy. This test is performed by a radiologic technologist and a radiologist. The examination is interpreted by the radiologist.

14. The normal laboratory value for **BUN (blood urea nitrogen)** is 26 mg/dl, which represents normal renal function. The normal value for **Cr (creatinine)** is 1.1 mg/dl, which represents normal renal function. Elevations of these values may indicate renal disease.

15. Hormones that affect the kidneys include **aldosterone,** which increases salt and water reabsorption by the kidneys; **renin,** which helps the kidneys maintain blood pressure; and **antidiuretic hormone (ADH),** which also increases water reabsorption.

16. d

17. two kidneys (right and left)
    two ureters (one for each kidney)
    urinary bladder
    urethra

18. b

19. a

20. d

21. true capsule: tough, fibrous, protective covering that surrounds each kidney; appears highly echogenic surrounding the cortex of the kidney.

cortex: the area immediately inside the fibrous capsule that does the work of the kidney. Filtration takes place in the cortex. It appears as mid-gray or medium- to low-level homogeneous echoes (less than or equal to the normal liver or spleen).

arcuate vessels: small arteries and veins that help transport blood to and from the renal parenchyma located at the corticomedullary junction. They appear on sonogram as hyperechoic dots.

medullae: area between cortex and sinus. Medullary pyramids appear hypoechoic to anechoic.

sinus: the central portion of the kidney (includes the minor and major calyces, the renal pelvis, renal artery and vein, fat nerves, and lymphatics). The sinus appears echodense and highly reflective because of the fat it contains. The renal pelvis, if seen, will appear anechoic.

22. the area where the renal artery enters the kidney and the renal vein and ureter exit.

23. the urinary bladder holds urine received from the kidneys and transported through the ureters, which insert posteriorly on either side of it. If collapsed, it is not visible. If distended, its lumen should normally be anechoic as it is filled with urine. In transverse cuts it is somewhat squared with rounded sides. The wall appears as a smooth, hyperechoic, thin line. The urinary bladder lies posterior to the symphysis pubis. In the male it is anterior to seminal vesicles and rectum, and superior to the prostate gland. In the female it is anterior to the vagina, posterior cul-de-sac, and rectum.

24. urine being ejected into the bladder from the ureters. They appear as hyperechoic "bursts" in real-time that quickly disappear. They enter the bladder posteriorly, on either side from the corresponding ureter.

25. b

CHAPTER 13

1. d	**9.** c	**17.** a	**25.** a
2. b	**10.** b	**18.** b	**26.** a
3. a	**11.** d	**19.** b	**27.** a
4. b	**12.** b	**20.** d	**28.** b
5. d	**13.** d	**21.** c	**29.** d
6. b	**14.** c	**22.** c	**30.** b
7. d	**15.** a	**23.** d	
8. b	**16.** d	**24.** a	

CHAPTER 14

1. c	13. d	25. b	37. d
2. f	14. b	26. d	38. a
3. a	15. a	27. d	39. c
4. a	16. c	28. c	40. d
5. b	17. b	29. a	41. a
6. c	18. a	30. e	42. b
7. b	19. a	31. c	43. b
8. d	20. c	32. b	44. c
9. a	21. b	33. d	45. c
10. c	22. d	34. d	46. d
11. b	23. c	35. b	
12. a	24. a	36. d	

CHAPTER 15

1. a. 46XY is the normal male karyotype whereas 46XX indicates a normal female.

2. b. Normal seminal vesicles measure approximately 5 cm in length and *less than* 1 cm in diameter. Seminal vesicles measuring greater than 1 cm in diameter are abnormal and should be further investigated for pathology such as obstruction or tumor invasion.

3. a. The ductus epididymis is located within the scrotum, but is not found within the testis.

4. e. The left testicular vein drains into the left renal vein, while the right testicular vein drains into the inferior vena cava. This is important because in the presence of a left varicocele (dilatation of the scrotal veins), the left kidney should be scanned to rule out an obstruction of the left renal vein.

5. c. The ejaculatory ducts are not located within the spermatic cord. Each spermatic cord contains the ductus deferens, testicular arteries, venous pampiniform plexus, lymphatics, autonomic nerves, and fibers from the cremaster muscles.

6. a. The peripheral zone accounts for approximately 70% of the normal prostate gland.

7. b. The penis contains two corpora cavernosa and a single corpus spongiosum.

8. c. The body of the epididymis is not seen in the examination of a normal scrotum. The head of the epididymis is normally visualized, but if the body and tail can be visualized, this usually indicates pathology.

9. b. Normal seminal vesicles appear less echogenic (hypoechoic) than the normal prostate.

10. a. The peripheral zone occupies the posterior and lateral portions of the prostate gland and should have a homogeneous echotexture. The other zones cannot be individually distinguished on transrectal ultrasound.

11. a. The shape of the prostate is semilunar superiorly near the base, and more rounded inferiorly at the apex.

12. b. The cavernosal arteries are located with the corpus cavernosum of the penis.

13. b. Penile sonography is used most frequently for the detection of vasculogenic impotence.

14. c. The mediastinum testis is much more echogenic than the head of the epididymis, testis, or seminal vesicles.

15. b. The lumen of the deep arteries is echolucent, and is best demonstrated in the transverse view of the penis. Although the walls of the deep artery are echogenic, the lumen itself is echolucent.

CHAPTER 16

1. c		**8.** d		**15.** d		**22.** a
2. c		**9.** b		**16.** c		**23.** b
3. a		**10.** a		**17.** b		**24.** a
4. c		**11.** a		**18.** a		**25.** b
5. a		**12.** b		**19.** d		
6. d		**13.** b		**20.** d		
7. b		**14.** d		**21.** c		

CHAPTER 17

1. c		**8.** e		**15.** c		**22.** e
2. d		**9.** e		**16.** a		**23.** e
3. d		**10.** c		**17.** a		**24.** b
4. b		**11.** d		**18.** c and d		**25.** d
5. c		**12.** c		**19.** c		
6. c		**13.** d		**20.** a		
7. d		**14.** b		**21.** b		

CHAPTER 18

1. d

2. c

3. c

4. c

5. e

6. b

7. b. The umbilical cord consist of two umbilical arteries and one umbilical vein.

8. b. Maternal marginal veins are anechoic tubular structures normally seen on the uterine surface of the placenta.

9. c, Placenta previa occurs when a portion of the placenta covers the internal os of the cervix.

10. d. BPD can be obtained through any plane of section intersecting the thalami and third ventricle.

11. c. Cisterna magna appears as an anechoic, subarachnoid space.

12. c. The foramen ovale is the atrial septal opening.

13. b. The thalami are centrally located in the brain and appear homogeneous and mid gray.

14. a. The fetal colon typically appears hypoechoic to adjacent structures.

15. a. Sonographic identification of the fetal urinary bladder is necessary to establish renal function.

16. b. Adrenal glands appear hypoechoic to the liver, spleen, and renal cortex.

17. e. Bone density, attenuates sound waves.

18. c. Muscles usually appear hypoechoic to adjacent structures.

19. c. HC is obtained through a *single* plane of section, perpendicular to the *thalami, third ventricle, cavum septum pellucidum, and tentorium.*

20. a. AC is obtained through a *single* plane of section where the *right* and *left portal veins* are continuous with one another.

CHAPTER 19

1. Fetal biophysical variables observed and scored to predict perinatal outcome include:
    Fetal Heart Rate, Fetal Body Movements, Fetal Tone, Fetal Breathing Movements, Amniotic Fluid Volume, and Placental Grading

2. c. Neurological dysfunctions are associated with abnormal fetal aortic flow velocity waveforms.

3. d

4. a

5. e

6. b. AFP (alpha-fetoprotein) is the component of amniotic fluid that increases beyond normal limits when certain defects are present.

7. Biophysical Profile, Doppler, Amniocentesis, Chorionic Villus Sampling, Fetal Blood Sampling, and Fetal Intravascular Transfusion are ultrasound studies utilized for high-risk pregnancies.

8. The amniotic fluid index (AFI) is the sum of the anteroposterior measurement of the deepest amniotic fluid pocket in each of four quadrants evenly dividing the gravid uterus. The sum should equal at least 8 cm to be considered normal.

9. Abnormal biochemical screening, previous child with a chromosomal disorder, neural tube defect, or malformation syndrome, intrauterine growth retardation, maternal diabetes, postdates, multiple pregnancy, and advanced maternal age are considered high-risk pregnancies with indications for specific prenatal ultrasound evaluations or ultrasound-guided procedures.

10. a. Scores lower than 8 on a Biophysical Profile are usually followed up with additional testing or induced labor.

11. e. A twin gestation is dichorionic-diamniotic when division of the zygote occurs prior to the 4th day post fertilization.

12. c. Conjoined or "Siamese" twins are the result of division of the embryonic disk more than 13 days post fertilization.

13. a. The 6th through 10th gestational weeks. At this point, sonographic identification of the number of gestational sacs is an accurate method for predicting chorionicity.

14. e. Twin fetuses of opposite gender are always dichorionic and diamniotic.

15. b. The interfetal membrane is identifiable in a diamniotic twin gestation.

CHAPTER 20

1. b	8. b	15. c	22. a
2. d	9. b	16. a	23. d
3. c	10. d	17. c	24. a
4. c	11. c	18. b	25. d
5. b	12. d	19. b	26. c
6. b	13. b	20. a	27. c
7. b	14. d	21. a	28. d

CHAPTER 21

1. c	6. d	11. b	16. a
2. b	7. c	12. b	17. a
3. a	8. b	13. a	18. a
4. e	9. d	14. a	19. b
5. d	10. d	15. b	20. a

CHAPTER 22

1. a	6. d	11. b	16. b
2. c	7. a	12. a	17. b
3. d	8. d	13. a	18. d
4. c	9. a	14. c	19. c
5. b	10. b	15. a	20. c

CHAPTER 23

1. Generally, the heart provides the driving force that propels blood through the vessels for the distribution of nutrients, gases, minerals, vitamins, hormones, and blood cells to the tissues, and for collection of waste products for excretion.

2. The heart is located in the lower anterior chest posterior to the sternum and anterior to the thoracic vertebrae and esophagus. It rests upon the diaphragm in the middle mediastinum, bounded laterally by the right and left lungs; two thirds of the heart lie to the left of the midsagittal plane and one third lies to the right.

3. Blood enters the right atrium from the superior and inferior venae cavae, passes through the tricuspid valve and into the right ventricle. From the right ventricle, blood flows through the pulmonary valve into the main pulmonary artery, and into the right and left pulmonary artery branches to the lungs. Oxygenated blood returning from the lungs enters the left atrium from the four pulmonary veins. From the left atrium, blood flows through the mitral valve, into the left ventricle, and out through the aorta to the head and body.

4. The pulmonary circulation is the flow of blood from the right heart to the lungs for oxygenation.

5. The systemic circulation is the delivery of oxygenated blood to the head and body from the left heart.

6. The heart muscle has a soft, homogeneous, even-textured echogenicity. The color appears medium to, in some cases, a dark gray. The valves and chordae appear slightly more echogenic than the medium gray heart muscle. The valves appear as thin, flexible linear structures that are freely mobile. The pericardium is the most echogenic structure, with a smooth, white, linear appearance. The cavities, being filled with blood, are black. The left ventricle is shaped somewhat like a bullet (ellipsoid) and the right ventricle more like a triangle. The right atrium should receive the inferior and superior venae cavae. The left atrium should receive four pulmonary veins.

7. The sinoatrial node (SA node) sets the pace of the heart. When the SA node fires, impulses travel through a pathway called internodal tracts to both atria. They immediately contract. As the impulses travel to the atria, they also travel to the atrioventricular node (AV node). At this point, there is a short delay in activation and transmission. After this delay, the AV node fires, sending impulses along the bundle of His. From the bundle, impulses move through the Purkinje fibers into the myocardium. The cardiac conduction system enables the heart to produce a synchronous, coordinated, effective heartbeat.

8. The heart is perfused by two coronary arteries: the right and left coronary arteries. A major branch of the right coronary artery is the posterior descending coronary artery. The left coronary artery divides almost immediately, upon exiting the aorta, into the left circumflex and the left anterior descending coronary artery.

   The heart is drained by the cardiac veins. Generally, they course with the coronary arteries. Most drain into the coronary sinus and empty into the right atrium. The remainder drain directly into the right atrium.

9. Cardiologist

10. Chest x-ray studies are performed by a radiologic technologist and interpreted by a radiologist. EKGs (or ECGs) are performed by a technician and interpreted by a cardiologist.

11. The oxygen content in the right side of the heart is normally lower than in the left side. Pressures on the right side (pulmonary circulation) are lower than those on the left side (systemic circulation).

12. Parasternal Left
    Apical
    Subxiphoid
    Suprasternal Notch
    Parasternal Right
    Supraclavicular Fossa

13. Aortic valve level
    Mitral valve level
    Papillary muscle level

14. True

15. Left Ventricle
    Mitral valve inserted more superiorly on the septum (two-leaflet valve)
    Two papillary muscles
    Thicker myocardium
    No moderator band
    Smooth-walled

Right Ventricle
    Tricuspid valve inserted more inferiorly on the septum (three-leaflet valve)
    Three or more papillary muscles
    Thinner myocardium (as opposed to the left ventricle)
    Has a moderator band
    Heavily trabeculated wall

16. Anterolateral papillary muscle: 3-4 o'clock
    Posteromedial papillary muscle: 8 o'clock

17. Sinoatrial

18. P-wave: atrial contraction
    QRS: ventricular contraction
    T-wave: ventricular resting state (recovery of electrical charge)

19. b

20. Endocardium

21. Epicardium
    Visceral pericardium
    Parietal pericardium

22. Space between the visceral and parietal pericardium. It contains pericardial fluid.

23. a

24. An echocardiographic study performed while the patient is stressed (increased heart rate) used mainly to check for wall motion abnormalities.

25. An echocardiographic study performed by placing the transducer in the patient's esophagus and stomach to get images of the heart.

26. Left anterior descending (LAD)
    Left circumflex (LCS)

27. Increases the heart rate

28. b

29. b

CHAPTER 24

1. b

2. e

3. b

4. d

5. d

6. a

7. b

8. a

9. d

10. d

11. b

12. d

13. b

14. a

15.

16. a

17. b

18. c

19. d

20. d

21. d

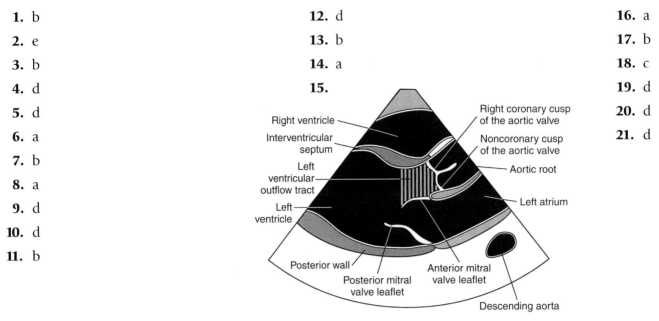

Right ventricle

Interventricular septum

Left ventricular outflow tract

Left ventricle

Posterior wall

Posterior mitral valve leaflet

Right coronary cusp of the aortic valve

Noncoronary cusp of the aortic valve

Aortic root

Left atrium

Anterior mitral valve leaflet

Descending aorta

CHAPTER 25

1. b

2. c

3. b

4. c

5. c

6. a

7. a

8. c

9. b

10. b

11. b

12. a

13. c. Indirect physiologic testing assesses the functional significance of flow-reducing disease downstream from the site of the lesion.

14. b

15. b. They pass through the upper six cervical vertebrae.

16. c

17. c. Flow in the low-resistance internal carotid artery demonstrates constant forward flow throughout the cardiac cycle.

18. a. A pressure-flow gradient develops as the result of dilatation of the bulb compared to the distal common carotid and internal carotid arteries. This results in separation of the flow stream, into central forward flow and reverse flow near the posterolateral wall of the bulb.

19. c. constant for the speed of sound in soft tissue. Such factors as the hematocrit, or viscosity, etc., would need to be known in order to calculate the speed of sound in various fluids.

20. d. The remaining vessel should be the superficial femoral artery.

21. b. It lies on the tibia

22. b. In the normal peripheral artery at rest, there should be a significant pressure gradient between the aortic pressure and the distal tibial arteries. This results in an ankle-to-brachial ratio greater than 1.0.

23. a. Loss of the reverse diastolic flow component is associated with exercise or flow-reducing disease, not age.

24. d. The average peak systolic velocity of 90 cm/sec in the aorta decreases normally to an average of 60 cm/sec in the popliteal artery.

25. c . Pulsatile flow is associated with systemic fluid overload, tricuspid insufficiency, etc.

26. d. Common iliac veins are duplicated infrequently.

27. c. The venous wall is only one tenth as thick as the wall of an artery and has very little elastin.

CHAPTER 26

1. b

2. a

3. b

4. c

5. c

6. c

7. a

8. d

9. b

10. e

11. e

12. b

13. a

14. b

15. d

16. b

17. e

18. a

19. c

20. b

21. "Multiple echogenic foci within the gallbladder (GB) that shadow and demonstrate movement. GB wall is slightly thickened. Common hepatic duct is within normal limits." *Pathology: Cholelithiasis (gallstones) with cholecystitis (inflammation of the GB).*

22. "The liver appears heterogeneous. Multiple, solid, intrahepatic masses are visualized. Three anterior masses appear hypoechoic with slightly irregular borders. They range from the largest, measuring 3.5 cm long axis, 3 cm anteroposteriorly, to the smallest, measuring 1.5 cm long axis, 1 cm anteroposteriorly. Single isosonic mass located in the superoposterior portion of the lobe. Borders appear uniform. Long axis measures 4.8 cm. Anteroposterior measure 4 cm. The vasculature is somewhat obscure and not readily defined." *Pathology: Metastatic disease to the liver from the pancreatic primary. Vasculature is obliterated by compression of the vessel from diffuse tumor infiltrate.*

23. "The uterus appears homogeneous. The body is being displaced anteriorly by a complex mass in the left adnexa that extends into the cul-de-sac. Mass is primarily solid, with scattered areas of fluid and calcifications. It measures 8.9 × 4.8 × 5.6 cm. No free fluid is seen." *The benign cystic teratoma contains tissues from all three fetal layers including the endoderm, mesoderm, and ectoderm. This explains why these masses can be composed of any type of tissue, including skin, hair, fat, teeth, bone, and fluid. Cystic teratomas are the most common tumor seen in patients younger than 20 years of age. In females, they are usually associated with the ovaries.*

24. "Hypoechoic solid mass. Appears irregular in contour. Measure 10.8 × 10.4 mm." *This type of mass is bothersome for a malignant tumor because of the irregular contour, solid consistency, and the age of the patient. Benign masses tend to have smooth, regular borders with a homogenous pattern or contain fluid.*

CHAPTER 27

1. e

2. b

3. a

4. a, c

5. c

6. a

7. b

8. b, d

9. b

10. a

11. b

12. a

CHAPTER 28

1. c, performed through the skin

2. d, tissue sampling

3. a, an alcohol bath

4. a, fluid sampling

5. c, used as a couplant between the transducer and probe cover.

6. c, in direct contact with organs and vessels.

7. b, percutaneous tube placement.

8. d, evaluation of the biliary ducts.

9. b, is utilized to evaluate vessels and grafts during surgery.

10. a, a percutaneous biopsy.